EmbryoGenetics

EmbryoGenetics

Editors

Carlos Simón
Carmen Rubio

MDPI • Basel • Beijing • Wuhan • Barcelona • Belgrade • Manchester • Tokyo • Cluj • Tianjin

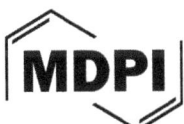

Editors
Carlos Simón
Valencia University
Spain

Carmen Rubio
Director of Embryo Genetics Research
Spain

Editorial Office
MDPI
St. Alban-Anlage 66
4052 Basel, Switzerland

This is a reprint of articles from the Special Issue published online in the open access journal *Genes* (ISSN 2073-4425) (available at: https://www.mdpi.com/journal/genes/special_issues/EmbryoGenetics).

For citation purposes, cite each article independently as indicated on the article page online and as indicated below:

LastName, A.A.; LastName, B.B.; LastName, C.C. Article Title. *Journal Name* **Year**, *Volume Number*, Page Range.

ISBN 978-3-0365-1152-8 (Hbk)
ISBN 978-3-0365-1153-5 (PDF)

© 2021 by the authors. Articles in this book are Open Access and distributed under the Creative Commons Attribution (CC BY) license, which allows users to download, copy and build upon published articles, as long as the author and publisher are properly credited, which ensures maximum dissemination and a wider impact of our publications.

The book as a whole is distributed by MDPI under the terms and conditions of the Creative Commons license CC BY-NC-ND.

Contents

About the Editors vii

Carmen Rubio and Carlos Simón
Embryo Genetics
Reprinted from: *Genes* **2021**, *12*, 118, doi:10.3390/genes12010118 1

Blanca Simon, David Bolumar, Alicia Amadoz, Jorge Jimenez-Almazán, Diana Valbuena, Felipe Vilella and Inmaculada Moreno
Identification and Characterization of Extracellular Vesicles and Its DNA Cargo Secreted During Murine Embryo Development
Reprinted from: *Genes* **2020**, *11*, 203, doi:10.3390/genes11020203 5

Anna Idelevich and Felipe Vilella
Mother and Embryo Cross-Communication
Reprinted from: *Genes* **2020**, *11*, 376, doi:10.3390/genes11040376 23

Manuel Viotti
Preimplantation Genetic Testing for Chromosomal Abnormalities: Aneuploidy, Mosaicism, and Structural Rearrangements
Reprinted from: *Genes* **2020**, *11*, 602, doi:10.3390/genes11060602 37

Nathan R. Treff, Jennifer Eccles, Diego Marin, Edward Messick, Louis Lello, Jessalyn Gerber, Jia Xu and Laurent C.A.M. Tellier
Preimplantation Genetic Testing for Polygenic Disease Relative Risk Reduction: Evaluation of Genomic Index Performance in 11,883 Adult Sibling Pairs
Reprinted from: *Genes* **2020**, *11*, 648, doi:10.3390/genes11060648 73

Pere Mir Pardo, José Antonio Martínez-Conejero, Julio Martín, Carlos Simón and Ana Cervero
Combined Preimplantation Genetic Testing for Autosomal Dominant Polycystic Kidney Disease: Consequences for Embryos Available for Transfer
Reprinted from: *Genes* **2020**, *11*, 692, doi:10.3390/genes11060692 83

Carmen M. García-Pascual, Luis Navarro-Sánchez, Roser Navarro, Lucía Martínez, Jorge Jiménez, Lorena Rodrigo, Carlos Simón and Carmen Rubio
Optimized NGS Approach for Detection of Aneuploidies and Mosaicism in PGT-A and Imbalances in PGT-SR
Reprinted from: *Genes* **2020**, *11*, 724, doi:10.3390/genes11070724 93

Martine De Rycke and Veerle Berckmoes
Preimplantation Genetic Testing for Monogenic Disorders
Reprinted from: *Genes* **2020**, *11*, 871, doi:10.3390/genes11080871 105

Pradeep Reddy, Felipe Vilella, Juan Carlos Izpisua Belmonte and Carlos Simón
Use of Customizable Nucleases for Gene Editing and Other Novel Applications
Reprinted from: *Genes* **2020**, *11*, 976, doi:10.3390/genes11090976 121

Lorena Rodrigo, Mónica Clemente-Císcar, Inmaculada Campos-Galindo, Vanessa Peinado, Carlos Simón and Carmen Rubio
Characteristics of the IVF Cycle that Contribute to the Incidence of Mosaicism
Reprinted from: *Genes* **2020**, *11*, 1151, doi:10.3390/genes11101151 141

Sandra Garcia-Herrero, Blanca Simon and Javier Garcia-Planells
The Reproductive Journey in the Genomic Era: From Preconception to Childhood
Reprinted from: *Genes* **2020**, *11*, 1521, doi:10.3390/genes11121521 . . . . **155**

About the Editors

Carlos Simón, M.D.; Ph. D.Board Certified and Full Professor of Ob/Gyn at the University of Valencia, Spain; Senior Lecturer PT, BIDMC Harvard University, Boston, MA, USA, Adjunct Professor, Department of Ob/Gyn, Baylor College of Medicine, USA and Head of the Scientific Advisory Board of Igenomix. His main interest is in the understanding of the human embryonic implantation process during the preconception period, considering the embryo, the maternal endometrium, and the cross-communication between them as key elements, using different scientific perspectives. He is author of 493 publications in international peer-review journals, adding up to an accumulated impact factor of 2,393.24. His papers have received a total of 37,363 citations, with an average of 74 per paper. His Google Scholar is 109. Complete list of publications can be found at: https://www.ncbi.nlm.nih.gov/myncbi/simon_c. He is editor of 19 books, and supervisor of 40 PhD Thesis.Pubmed Publication List: https://www.ncbi.nlm.nih.gov/myncbi/simon_cGoogle Scholar: https://scholar.google.es/citations?user=nA_MhRMAAAAJ&hl=es Personal Website: www.carlos-simon.com.

Carmen Rubio, PhD.Senior Research Director in Embryo Genetics at Igenomix, and Igenomix Foundation in Spain. Teaching experience in several Masters in the field of Biotechnology of Reproduction. Trained in science in the University of Valencia, Spain, Dr Carmen Rubio specialized in cytogenetic studies in human reproduction, partly in the University of Barcelona. She completed her PhD in the field of Reproductive Genetics and post-doctoral research included research into male and female meiosis at the laboratory of Drs. Patricia Hunt and Terry Hassold (Washington State University, USA). She has published more than 100 papers in the main peer-reviewed specialist journals in the field, book chapters, as well as numerous lectures at conferences worldwide. After becoming interested in chromosomal aneuploidies in human embryos, she started with cytogenetics analysis of sperm and embryos, moving later to molecular analysis. Currently, she is focused on non-invasive approaches for embryo aneuploidy testing, based on the analysis of the cell-free DNA secreted by preimplantation embryos to the spent culture medium.

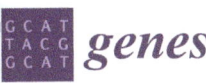

Editorial

Embryo Genetics

Carmen Rubio [1],* and Carlos Simón [2,3,4],*

1. EmbryoGenetics Department, Igenomix, 46980 Valencia, Spain
2. Professor of Obstetrics & Gynecology, Valencia University, 46010 Valencia, Spain
3. Senior Lecturer PT, BIDMC Harvard University, Boston, MA 02215, USA
4. Adjunct Clinical Professor, Department of Ob/Gyn, Baylor College of Medicine, Houston, TX 77030, USA

* Correspondence: carmen.rubio@igenomix.com (C.R.); carlos.simon@igenomix.com (C.S.)

Abstract: Advances in embryo and reproductive genetics have influenced clinical approaches to overcome infertility. Since the 1990s, many attempts have been made to decipher the genetic causes of infertility and to understand the role of chromosome aneuploidies in embryo potential. At the embryo stage, preimplantation genetic testing for chromosomal abnormalities and genetic disorders has offered many couples the opportunity to have healthy offspring. Recently, the application of new technologies has resulted in more comprehensive and accurate diagnoses of chromosomal abnormalities and genetic conditions to improve clinical outcome. In this Special Issue, we include a collection of reviews and original articles covering many aspects of embryo diagnosis, genome editing, and maternal–embryo cross-communication during the implantation process.

Keywords: embryo genetics; infertility; aneuploidies; monogenic disease; polygenic disease; blastocyst; endometrium; implantation

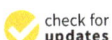

Infertility affects 15% of couples of reproductive age seeking to become parents, which accounted for 48 million infertile couples worldwide in 2010 [1]. The majority of these couples seek specialist medical care. In vitro fertilization (IVF) is the cornerstone of infertility treatment. European statistics indicate that approximately 500,000 IVF cycles are performed annually, resulting in the birth of 100,000 infants, or nearly 5% of all babies born in countries such as Denmark.

Having a baby is just the first challenge to overcome in the reproductive journey; the next and most important is to give birth to a healthy baby free of preventable genetic conditions. Genetic disorders affect 1% of live births and are responsible for 20% of pediatric hospitalizations and 20% of infant mortality. Many such disorders are caused by recessive or X-linked genetic mutations carried by 85% of the human population. Because assisted reproduction has provided us with technologies such as IVF that provide access to human embryos, certain genetic diseases were initially screened by selecting sex. The first live births following preimplantation genetic testing (PGT) to identify sex for X-linked disorders were reported by Alan Handyside in 1990 [2]. This ground-breaking work identified male embryos and selectively transferred unaffected normal or carrier females to avoid genetic diseases, paving the way to extend the concept to PGT for monogenic diseases (PGT-M), including Mendelian single-gene defects (autosomal dominant/recessive and X-linked dominant/recessive), severe childhood lethality or early-onset disease, cancer predisposition, and Human Leukocyte Antigen (HLA) typing for histocompatible cord blood stem cell transplantation.

Later, we moved on to identifying and selecting euploid embryos by analyzing all 23 pairs of chromosomes in 4–8 cells from the trophectoderm, known as PGT for aneuploidy (PGT-A). PGT-A currently leverages next-generation sequencing (NGS) technologies to uncover meiotic- and mitotic-origin aneuploidies affecting whole chromosomes, as well as duplications/deletions of small chromosome regions. A further step forward was the use of structural chromosome rearrangements (PGT-SR) to identify Robertsonian

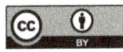

and reciprocal translocations, inversions, and balanced vs. unbalanced rearrangements. Another advancement came with PGT for polygenic risk scoring (PGT-P). This technique has taken us from learning how to read simple words to beginning to understand poetry (i.e., evolving from PGT-M/A/SR to PGT-P for multifactorial, polygenic risk prediction). Common multifactorial diseases, such as diabetes, coronary heart disease, and cancer, are caused by a combination of environmental, lifestyle, and genetic factors; risk scores are now being generated to predict the likelihood of such complex, later-life diseases in embryos. Moreover, we are moving from embryo selection to intervention because the human genetic code is not only readable and writable, but also hackable. Indeed, gene editing is now possible using tools such as (CRISPR)/CRISPR-associated (Cas9), which is applicable to all species, including human embryos.

This Special Issue traverses the field of embryo genetics in ten papers: four reviews and six original articles addressing specific aspects of developments in technology, clinical application, and basic research.

The first review introduces the reproductive journey in the genomic era, from preconception to childhood, leveraging NGS as a genomic precision diagnostic tool to understand the mechanisms underlying genetic conditions, which account for 20–30% of all infant deaths and more than 50% of clinical miscarriages [3]. Genome-wide technologies are applied at different stages of the reproductive health lifecycle from preconception carrier screening and preimplantation genetic testing, to prenatal and postnatal testing.

Six articles cover preimplantation genetic testing at the chromosome and gene levels. A review for genetic disorders covers the evolution of this technology as an established alternative to invasive prenatal diagnosis, as well as future innovations [4]. The development of new algorithms and the declining costs of sequencing are propelling PGT to a sequencing-based, all-in-one solution for PGT-M, PGT-SR, and PGT-A. Along this line, this Special Issue includes an original manuscript for combined PGT-M and PGT-A in autosomal dominant polycystic kidney disease (ADPKD). ADPKD can manifest extrarenally and as seminal cysts that have been associated with male infertility in some cases [5]. The results of this study indicate that AMA couples who are also ADPKD patients have an increased risk of generating aneuploid embryos, but ADPKD-linked male infertility does not promote an increased aneuploidy rate. In a third article, the possibility of testing embryos not only for monogenic diseases, but also for polygenic conditions (PGT-P) is presented, with a strategy of disease relative risk reduction to evaluate the potential clinical utility of embryo selection with PGT-P [6]. The results demonstrate the potential for simultaneous relative risk reduction for all diseases tested in parallel, which include diabetes, cancer, and heart disease, and indicate applicability beyond patients with a known family history of disease.

Of the three articles related to embryo chromosomal abnormalities, the first is a review of state-of-the-art methods for PGT-A, mosaicism, and PGT-SR that reinforces the idea that there is a high incidence of chromosomal abnormalities in early human embryos, resulting in low success rates with assisted reproductive technologies [7]. Chromosomal anomalies are also responsible for a large proportion of miscarriages and congenital disorders. The review covers efforts from 2000–2020 to improve technology to accurately identify embryos containing chromosomal abnormalities. The second article describes an optimized NGS approach for PGT-A and PGT-SR with special emphasis on mosaicism and the development of tailored algorithms and diagnostic tools to identify different levels of mosaicism objectively in order to avoid subjectivity in the diagnosis [8]. The third article addresses different extrinsic factors related to the IVF cycle that could affect the incidence of overall aneuploidy, whole uniform aneuploidy, mosaicism, and segmental aneuploidy. Female and male parental age, ovarian response, embryo vitrification, and sperm concentration were considered in a multivariate analysis [9].

Finally, the development of novel genome editing tools has unlocked new opportunities for gene editing at the embryo level. We incorporate a review of new developments in genome editing techniques to modify specific regions of the genome [10]. Among genome editing tools, the CRISPR/Cas system has proven to be the most popular for both basic research and clinical purposes and was the topic for the Nobel Laureate in Chemistry 2020.

To end this Special Issue, we highlight that other players beyond the embryo are crucial in the reproductive journey. The endometrium is particularly important, with implantation failure resulting from suboptimal endometrial receptivity. As pregnancy progresses, the uterus continues to communicate closely with the embryo/fetus. Recent progress in the availability of high-throughput techniques, including transcriptomics, proteomics, and metabolomics, has allowed the simultaneous examination of multiple molecular changes, enhancing our knowledge in this area. This review covers known mechanisms of mother–embryo cross-communication identified from animal and human studies [11]. Coverage of this topic concludes with an original research article describing the identification and characterization of extracellular vesicles and their DNA cargo that is secreted during embryo development in a murine model [12]. The authors conclude that murine blastocysts secrete extracellular vesicles containing genome-wide sequences of DNA to the medium, reinforcing the relevance of studying these vesicles and their cargo at the preimplantation stage, where secreted DNA may aid in the assessment of the embryo before implantation.

We can conclude that, in the coming years, genetics will dramatically change and improve the field of reproduction and infertility treatments by means of precision medicine.

Funding: This research received no external funding.

Conflicts of Interest: The authors declare no conflict of interest.

References

1. Mascarenhas, M.; Flaxman, S.; Boerma, T.; Vanderpoel, S.; Stevens, G. National, Regional, and Global Trends in Infertility Prevalence Since 1990: A Systematic Analysis of 277 Health Surveys. *PLoS Med.* **2012**, *9*. [CrossRef] [PubMed]
2. Handyside, A.H.; Kontogianni, E.H.; Hardy, K.; Winston, R.M. Pregnancies from biopsied human preimplantation embryos sexed by Y-specific DNA amplification. *Nature* **1990**, *344*, 768–770. [CrossRef] [PubMed]
3. García-Herrero, S.; Simón, B.; García-Planells, J. The reproductive journey in the genomic era: From preconception to childhood. *Genes* **2020**. submitted.
4. De Rycke, M.; Berckmoes, V. Preimplantation Genetic Testing for Monogenic Disorders. *Genes* **2020**, *11*, 871. [CrossRef] [PubMed]
5. Mir Pardo, P.; Martínez-Conejero, J.; Martín, J.; Simón, C.; Cervero, A. Combined Preimplantation Genetic Testing for Autosomal Dominant Polycystic Kidney Disease: Consequences for Embryos Available for Transfer. *Genes* **2020**, *11*, 692. [CrossRef] [PubMed]
6. Treff, N.; Eccles, J.; Marin, D.; Messick, E.; Lello, L.; Gerber, J.; Xu, J.; Tellier, L. Preimplantation Genetic Testing for Polygenic Disease Relative Risk Reduction: Evaluation of Genomic Index Performance in 11,883 Adult Sibling Pairs. *Genes* **2020**, *11*, 648. [CrossRef] [PubMed]
7. Viotti, M. Preimplantation Genetic Testing for Chromosomal Abnormalities: Aneuploidy, Mosaicism, and Structural Rearrangements. *Genes* **2020**, *11*, 602. [CrossRef] [PubMed]
8. García-Pascual, C.; Navarro-Sánchez, L.; Navarro, R.; Martínez, L.; Jiménez, J.; Rodrigo, L.; Simón, C.; Rubio, C. Optimized NGS Approach for Detection of Aneuploidies and Mosaicism in PGT-A and Imbalances in PGT-SR. *Genes* **2020**, *11*, 724. [CrossRef] [PubMed]
9. Rodrigo, L.; Clemente-Císcar, M.; Campos-Galindo, I.; Peinado, V.; Simón, C.; Rubio, C. Characteristics of the IVF Cycle that Contribute to the Incidence of Mosaicism. *Genes* **2020**, *11*, 1151. [CrossRef] [PubMed]
10. Simon, B.; Bolumar, D.; Amadoz, A.; Jimenez-Almazán, J.; Valbuena, D.; Vilella, F.; Moreno, I. Identification and Characterization of Extracellular Vesicles and Its DNA Cargo Secreted During Murine Embryo Development. *Genes* **2020**, *11*, 203. [CrossRef] [PubMed]
11. Reddy, P.; Vilella, F.; Izpisua Belmonte, J.; Simón, C. Use of Customizable Nucleases for Gene Editing and Other Novel Applications. *Genes* **2020**, *11*, 976. [CrossRef] [PubMed]
12. Idelevich, A.; Vilella, F. Mother and Embryo Cross-Communication. *Genes* **2020**, *11*, 376. [CrossRef] [PubMed]

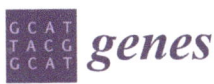

Article

Identification and Characterization of Extracellular Vesicles and Its DNA Cargo Secreted During Murine Embryo Development

Blanca Simon [1,2,†], David Bolumar [1,2,†], Alicia Amadoz [3], Jorge Jimenez-Almazán [3], Diana Valbuena [3], Felipe Vilella [1,*] and Inmaculada Moreno [1,3,*]

1. Igenomix Foundation-INCLIVA Biomedical Research Institute, Ronda de Narcís Monturiol, 11B, 46980 Paterna, Spain; blansi@alumni.uv.es (B.S.); david.bolumar@igenomix.com (D.B.)
2. Department of Pediatrics, Obstetrics and Gynecology, School of Medicine, University of Valencia, Av. de Blasco Ibáñez, 15, 46010 Valencia, Spain
3. Igenomix, R&D, Parque Tecnológico de Paterna, Ronda de Narcís Monturiol, 11B, 46980 Paterna, Spain; alicia.amadoz@igenomix.com (A.A.); jorge.jimenez@igenomix.com (J.J.-A.); diana.valbuena@igenomix.com (D.V.)
* Correspondence: felipe.vilella@igenomix.com (F.V.); Inmaculada.moreno@igenomix.com (I.M.); Tel.: +34-963905310 (F.V. & I.M.)
† These authors contributed equally to this study.

Received: 7 January 2020; Accepted: 12 February 2020; Published: 17 February 2020

Abstract: Extracellular vesicles (EVs) are known to transport DNA, but their implications in embryonic implantation are unknown. The aim of this study was to investigate EVs production and secretion by preimplantation embryos and assess their DNA cargo. Murine oocytes and embryos were obtained from six- to eight-week-old females, cultured until E4.5 and analyzed using transmission electron microscopy to examine EVs production. EVs were isolated from E4.5-day conditioned media and quantified by nanoparticle tracking analysis, characterized by immunogold, and their DNA cargo sequenced. Multivesicular bodies were observed in murine oocytes and preimplantation embryos together with the secretion of EVs to the blastocoel cavity and blastocyst spent medium. Embryo-derived EVs showed variable electron-densities and sizes (20–500 nm) and total concentrations of $1.74 \times 10^7 \pm 2.60 \times 10^6$ particles/mL. Embryo secreted EVs were positive for CD63 and ARF6. DNA cargo sequencing demonstrated no differences in DNA between apoptotic bodies or smaller EVs, although they showed significant gene enrichment compared to control medium. The analysis of sequences uniquely mapping the murine genome revealed that DNA contained in EVs showed higher representation of embryo genome than vesicle-free DNA. Murine blastocysts secrete EVs containing genome-wide sequences of DNA to the medium, reinforcing the relevance of studying these vesicles and their cargo in the preimplantation moment, where secreted DNA may help the assessment of the embryo previous to implantation.

Keywords: extracellular vesicles; exosomes; microvesicles; apoptotic bodies; DNA; preimplantation embryos; murine blastocysts

---

1. Introduction

Embryo-endometrial communication is mediated by different mechanisms including extracellular vesicles (EVs) with a plethora of molecules released to this interface. EVs constitute a novel bidirectional form of cross-talk during embryo implantation, as they are secreted by both the endometrium [1,2], and the embryo [3,4] contributing to new functional perspectives as their cargo is composed by virtually all sorts of biomolecules. In fact, EVs have been described to participate in several reproductive processes, such as gametogenesis, fertilization, embryo development and implantation, and fetal development throughout term (for review see [5]).

EVs are secreted by cells of different human tissues and organs and can be isolated in a variety of biological fluids including blood [6], urine [7], saliva [8], breast milk [9], amniotic fluid [10], ascitic fluid [11], cerebrospinal fluid [12], bile [13], semen [14], and endometrial fluid [2].

Three major types of EVs have been described based on their biogenetic pathway, composition, and physical characteristics such as size or density, namely, apoptotic bodies (ABs), microvesicles (MVs), and exosomes (EXOs) [15,16]. ABs result from the outward budding of the plasma membrane in the context of programmed cell death and their diameter ranges from 50–5000 nm [17,18]. MVs are produced directly by outward budding of the plasma membrane. They are in the size range from 100–1000 nm and are associated to the GTP-binding protein ARF6, which is used for their identification [19]. EXOs originate from the endosomal pathway as late endosomes that evolve into multivesicular bodies and migrate from the perinuclear region to the cell surface by fusion [20,21]. Their sizes range between 30–150 nm and are identified by classical molecular markers such as tetraspanins (CD63, CD9, CD81), flotillin-1, or heat shock 70-kDa proteins, although recent reports considered that other EVs might share these markers [22]. Their cargo portrays their functionality in regulating communication by means of proteins, cytokines, lipids, RNA, or DNA [23].

The embryo also secretes EVs that participate in both the dialogue with the maternal endometrium [24], and in self-paracrine regulation [4]. EVs are secreted by a trophectoderm cell line in the pig model [25], and in the human model [26] stimulating the proliferation of endothelial cells in vitro, thus becoming potential regulators of maternal endometrial angiogenesis. Regarding the nucleic acid cargo of embryo derived EVs, several papers have described the RNA cargo of trophoblast-derived EVs, mainly focusing on miRNA [25], linking miRNA signature with successful pregnancy [27], nevertheless, the DNA cargo of embryo derived EVs has received little attention. The aim of the present study is to identify and characterize embryo derived EVs secreted during murine embryo development, and to analyze their DNA cargo comparatively among the different EVs subpopulations.

2. Materials and Methods

2.1. Mouse Embryo Isolation and Culture

Female B6C3H1/Crl mice of 8-weeks of age (Charles River Laboratories International, Wilmington, MA, USA) were stimulated using 10 IU of Foligon/PMSG (MSD Animal Health, Madrid, Spain) followed by administration of 10 IU of Ovitrelle/hCG (Merck Serono, Darmstadt, Germany) 48 h later. Female mice were mated with males overnight and sacrificed by cervical dislocation 24 h after vaginal plug was observed. At embryonic day 1.5 (E1.5), embryos were extracted by flushing the oviduct with PBS using a 30G syringe needle. Non-fertilized metaphase II (MII) oocytes were also collected. Mouse embryos were washed and cultured in oxygenated G2-Plus media (Vitrolife, Västra Frölunda, Sweden) at 37 °C and 5% CO_2 in groups of 40 embryos per well (Nunc 4-well plates, ThermoFisher Scientific, Whaltham, MA, USA) until day E4.5, reaching the stage of hatching/hatched blastocysts. MII oocytes, embryos at different developmental stages (E2.5, E3.5, and E4.5) and spent culture media from them were collected and preserved accordingly to the objective of the investigation.

The total number of females used was 80. Embryos from 10 animals were used for identification and phenotypic characterization of EVs using electron microscopy and immunogold. Ten animals were used in triplicates (n = 30) for quantification by nanoparticle tracking analysis and 10 in quadruplicates (n = 40) for sequencing experiments. An average of 32 embryos were obtained per female, 50% of them achieved hatching/hatched blastocyst stage by day E4.5. All animal experimentation was conducted at the animal facility located in the School of Pharmacy at the University of Valencia under the protocol code 2015/VSC/PEA/00048, approved by the Ethics Committee of Animal Welfare on 12 March 2015.

2.2. Isolation and Purification of EVs Secreted by Murine Embryos

Conditioned media from embryo culture was collected at day E4.5 and centrifuged at low speed (300× g, 10 min) to remove larger debris. The resulting supernatant was centrifuged at 2,000× g for 10 min to recover ABs as previously described [28]. It was subsequently ultracentrifuged at 185,000× g for 70 min in a P50A3 Hitachi rotor (Hitachi, Tokio, Japan) to collect non-apoptotic EVs (naEVs) that includes MVs and EXOs in the same fraction. All centrifugations were conducted at 4 °C.

2.3. Transmission Electron Microscopy and Immunogold

Oocytes and embryos at different developmental stages (E2.5, E3.5, and E4.5) and pellets containing EVs from spent culture media were fixed overnight in Karnovsky's solution (2.5% glutaraldehyde/2% formaldehyde in phosphate buffer 0.1 M, pH 7.4), washed in PBS and encapsulated in 2% agar in distilled water. Samples were then washed 5 times in PBS for 5 min and stained in a 2% osmium tetroxide 0.2 M PBS solution for 2 h. Then, dehydrated following the next sequence: three washes of 5 min in distilled water at 4 °C, 5-min wash in 30° ethanol, 10-min wash in 50° ethanol, 10-min wash in 70° ethanol twice, 45-min wash in 2:1 90° ethanol + LR-white twice, 45-min wash in 2:1 100° ethanol + LR-White, and O/N wash in 1:2 100° ethanol + LR-white in continuous shaking. Ethanol was let to evaporate, and wash media was changed by 100% LR-White in continuous shaking, for a 30-min incubation. Finally, samples were allowed to polymerize for 1 day at 60 °C, protecting them from the air. Resin-embedded samples were ultrasectioned in 60 nm slices, incubated for 1 h on formvar carbon-coated cooper (regular visualization) and nickel (immunogold visualization) grids, and contrasted with uranyl acetate. Ultrathin cuts were done using a UC6 Leica ultramicrotome (Leica, Wetzlar, Germany) equipped with an Ultra 45° diamond blade (Diatome, Hatfield, PA, USA). Prepared samples were observed using a JEM-1010 transmission electron microscope (Jeol Korea Ltd., Seoul, South Korea) at 80 kV, using a digital camera MegaView III and Olympus Image Analysis Software.

For the immunogold labelling assays, 60 nm sections from previous resin blocks were processed as described by Marcilla and collaborators [29]. Specifically, two different combinations of primary antibodies were used: rabbit α-CD63 (Abcam, ref: ab118307), rabbit α-ARF6 (Abcam, ref: ab77581), and mouse α-DNA (Millipore, Burlington, MA, USA ref: CBL186). All the antibodies were diluted in PBS/0.5% BSA following the manufacturer's datasheets. Then, the grids were washed in PBS/0.5% BSA and incubated with gold-coupled secondary antibodies [goat α-mouse coupled to 10 nm gold particles (BBI solutions, Crumlin, UK, ref: 15736) and goat α-rabbit coupled to 18 nm gold particles (Jackson Immunoresearch, Ely, UK) at 1:20 dilution in PBS/0.5% BSA for 30 min, following datasheets specifications. In parallel, paired grids were incubated only with the secondary antibodies as negative controls. Finally, grids were stained with 2% uranyl acetate and imaged by TEM as previously described.

2.4. Nanoparticle Tracking Analysis

Nanoparticle tracking analysis (NTA) was performed using a NanoSight300 (NS300, Malvern Instruments ltd, Malvern, UK). The naEVs fraction isolated from E4.5 spent media was resuspended in 1 mL of sterile PBS w/o Ca2+/Mg2+ (Biowest, Nuaillé, France, ref. L0615-500). In parallel, an aliquot of fresh embryo culture media was processed as a blank control. Three 60 sec videos were recorded under the static flow conditions for each sample with camera level set at 11. Videos were analyzed with NTA software version 3.2 Dev Build 3.2.16 to determine mean size and estimated concentration of measured particles with corresponding standard error. The NS300 system was calibrated with silica microspheres 100, 167, and 300 nm (Bangs Laboratories, Inc.; Fishers, IN, USA) prior to analysis, as previously demonstrated [30], auto settings were used for blur, minimum track length, and minimum expected particle size.

2.5. DNA Amplification and Sequencing of EVs Derived from Murine Embryos

Sequencing analysis was conducted to assess whether a specific DNA cargo is loaded into EVs secreted by the embryo, namely, ABs and naEVs. Mouse embryos representing the whole murine genome and EVs-depleted supernatant fraction after isolation of EVs (SN) were also sequenced. Because ABs are the result of dying cells, it is expected to have a representation of the total embryo DNA in this fraction. Sequencing of the DNA of ABs was used as an internal control. The negative control was blank medium that had not been in contact with murine embryos (blank). Groups of 10 mice were used to obtain the samples (embryo, ABs, naEVs, SN) in four independent sequencing experiments. DNase treatment of the different EV populations was conducted to evaluate and remove external DNA contamination and its potential bias in the analysis. The samples corresponding to DNase treated and untreated ABs from one of the four replicates were lost due to technical reasons, so only DNA from embryos, treated and untreated naEVs, and SN were included in the analysis for this biological replicate.

Embryos for DNA sequencing corresponding to E4.5 stage, were snap-frozen for initial DNA extraction and kept at −80 °C until processing. At this point, embryos were diluted in nuclease-free water (Ambion, ThermoFisher Scientific, Waltham, MA, USA) at a rate of 1 embryo/µL. DNA from pooled SN from all embryo culture wells and an equal volume of fresh blank media (G2-Plus) was extracted using QIAamp DNA mini kit (Qiagen, Hilden, Germany), eluting in 30 µL of nuclease free-water. For DNase treatment, ABs and naEVs were separated in two equivalent aliquots from pooled spent embryo culture media at the beginning of the isolation process. Once isolated, EVs were resuspended in nuclease-free water and, in the case of DNase treatment, 50 U/mL DNaseI (Sigma-Aldrich, San Luis, MO, USA) in 20 mM Tris-HCl (Thermo Fisher Scientific), 10 mM $MgCl_2$ (Thermo Fisher Scientific), and 1 mM $CaCl_2$ (Sigma-Aldrich, ref. 21115-100ML) were added to a final volume of 5 µL. Samples were then incubated at 37 °C for 30 min for DNase digestion followed by 10 min at 75 °C for DNase inactivation.

Immediately after, DNA amplification was performed using DOPlify whole genome amplification platform (RHS Ltd., Thebarton, Australia) following the manufacturer's instruction. Then, DNA was purified by using AMPure XP (Beckman Coulter, Brea, CA, USA) at a final concentration of 1.8X, in order to recover small-sized DNA fragments, and eluted in a final volume of 20 µL of nuclease-free water. Subsequently, the amplified DNA profiles were analysed by TapeStation 4200 (Agilent, Santa Clara, CA, USA). Finally, samples were sequentially diluted to 0.5 and 0.2 ng/µL to meet libraries kit DNA input requirements by Qubit dsDNA HS Assay (TermoFisher Scientific, Waltham, MA, USA). DNA libraries were built using Nextera XT DNA Library Prep Kit, specifically designed for samples with low DNA input. The experimental procedure was conducted following the protocol provided by the manufacturer, adjusting AMPure XP purification to 1.8X proportion. Then, libraries were pooled and sequenced using a 300 cycles-NextSeq 500/550 v2 High Output cartridge in a NextSeq 550 platform (Illumina, San Diego, CA, USA). To do so, 5 µL of the libraries pool, normalized by the bead method, were diluted in 995 µL of HT1 buffer. Then, 750 µL of the dilution was rediluted in 750 µL of HT1 buffer. The resulting dilution was denaturalized at 98 °C for 4 min, cooled in ice for 5 min and loaded into the sequencing cartridge for sequencing.

2.6. Computational Analysis of Sequencing Results

Raw data pre-processing: Raw data from pair-ended Illumina sequencing was downloaded from Illumina BaseSpace and converted into FASTQ files using bcl2fastq (version 2.16.0.10). Then, each sample was aligned to the mouse reference genome (mm10) using BWA (version 0.7.10) [31]. Reads with mapping quality lower than 10 were filtered out using Samtools (version 1.1) [32] and duplicates were removed with PICARD software (version 1.119). Finally, the coverage of each genome feature was obtained with Bedtools (version 2.17.0) [33] using Ensembl Biomart mm10 annotations. The raw genomic sequences generated in this study are deposited in the SRA database under the accession number PRJNA547453.

Murine-specific DNA sequences: A greater than expected quantity of valid reads were observed in blank media. Using the blank media for a background subtraction with the count per million (CPM) of each gene feature to decrease the background noise is not usually recommended because this data transformation may break the statistical assumptions of later steps. Therefore, the approach used here was to identify and filter murine-specific reads in a common manner for all samples. Then, background noise is considered as a background population (blank) and included in the analysis as another comparison group, whose results could be considered as differences with the background. To identify murine-specific reads, pre-processed data was mapped to the human reference genome (Hg19) using BWA. Then, unmapped reads were filtered using Samtools [32] and read ids were retrieved. Murine-specific reads were retrieved from pre-processed data by read id using PICARD software. Finally, the coverage of each genomic feature was obtained with Bedtools using Ensembl Biomart mm10 annotations.

Differential DNA enrichment of vesicles' cargo: The approach used for the differential DNA enrichment analysis is based on the edgeR methodology [34–36] that uses read counts of genomic features obtained from massively parallel sequencing technologies such as Illumina, 454, or ABI SOLiD applied to different types of experiments such as RNA-seq or ChIP-seq. edgeR can be applied to differential abundance analysis at the gene, exon, transcript, or tag level. In fact, read counts can be summarized by any genomic feature.

Here, differential DNA enriched regions were obtained using the following approach. In order to filter out lowly enriched regions, genomic features with greater than 1 cpm reads mapped in at least 1.5 samples (half of the mean of groups sizes) were kept for the following analyses. Raw counts were normalized using TMM method from edgeR R package [34]. A differential enrichment analysis of genome features was done using a generalized linear model approach for pairwise comparisons between sample types (embryo, ABs, naEVs, SN, blank). Experimental set and treatment were taken as factors in the additive model in order to adjust for differences between groups.

3. Results

3.1. Identification of EVs in Murine Oocytes and Embryos

Ultrastructural visualization of murine oocytes using TEM identified the existence of multivesicular bodies (MVBs) in the cytoplasm. These MVBs showed bilipid membrane vesicles containing smaller vesicular structures of different electron densities and sizes that would give rise to EXOs upon fusion of the MVBs with the oocyte plasma membrane. These structures were identified by their lower electron density, and vesicles of different sizes were observed entering the zona pellucida (Figure 1A). The presence of MVBs was also observed in the blastomeres at different embryo developmental stages (E2.5 and E3.5), migrating from the cytoplasm to the plasma membrane where their content was secreted outwards through the zona pellucida (Figure 1B). Interestingly, large vesicles including complex structures were also observed in the intercellular space (Figure 1C). At the blastocyst stage (day E4.5), the secretion of vesicular structures was observed both into the extracellular medium through the zona pellucida (zp), as well as into the blastocoel (bl) cavity (Figure 1D).

3.2. EVs Isolated from Blastocyst Culture Media

In order to study naEVs-including MVs and EXOs-produced and released by murine blastocysts, spent media at developmental day E4.5 was ultracentrifuged and gathered naEVs where quantified by NTA. The vesicular fraction showed vesicle profiles compatible in size with that of EXOs and MVs. The total concentration of naEVs from spent media was $1.74 \cdot 10^7 \pm 2.60 \cdot 10^6$ particles/mL, with a size profile showing two main populations. A first population extended from approximately 50–170 nm and accounted for $9.87 \times 10^6 \pm 7.55 \times 10^5$ particles/mL (56.72%) while the second extended from 180–310 nm and were represented by $6.75 \times 10^6 \pm 1.57 \times 10^6$ particles/mL (38.83%) to the total (Figure 2A).

Importantly, standard error of measurements showed that only a small amount of these particles remained constant among replicates (Figure 2A).

Finally, morphological analysis of EVs isolated from spent culture media by TEM showed vesicles of variable appearance, electron densities, and sizes ranging from 20 nm–500 nm, suggesting that EVs secreted by the embryo constitute a heterogenous population including different types of EVs (Figure 2B).

3.3. Phenotypic Characterization of Embryo Secreted EVs

Phenotypic characterization of the EVs secreted by murine embryos to the spent medium was performed using immunohistochemistry coupled to gold nanoparticles using specific surface markers for EXOs (CD63) or MVs (ARF6). As a negative control, paired grids of E4.5 blastocyst were incubated with the secondary antibodies only. Positive ARF6 staining was consistent with an active vesicular biogenesis through phospholipase D pathway in embryos, a mechanism described for inward budding of MVBs membrane in EXOs biogenetic pathway [37] and outward budding of cell plasma membrane in MVs formation [38]. Positivity for CD63, a tetraspanin involved in the formation of EXOs, was considered as canonical marker for these types of EVs that originate from the endosomal pathway (Figure 3A).

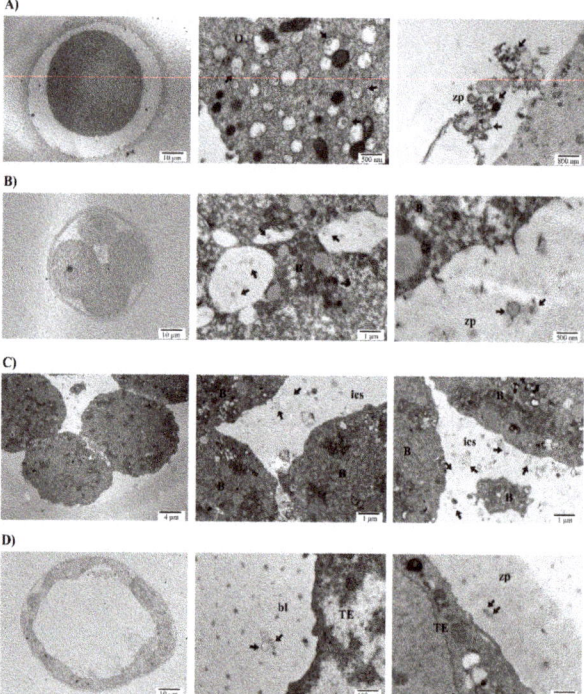

Figure 1. Vesicle production and secretion by murine embryos at different developmental stages shown by TEM. (**A**) Mouse oocyte (left) with magnifications of the production of multivesicular bodies (MVBs) in the cellular cytoplasm (center) and secretion of their content towards the zona pellucida (right). (**B**) E2.5 embryo (left) with magnifications of the cytoplasm containing MVBs (center) and the secretion of extracellular vesicles (EVs) through the zona pellucida (right). (**C**) E3.5 mouse embryo (left) showing MVB secreted to the intercellular space. (**D**) E4.5 blastocyst (left) secreting EVs into the zona pellucida (center) and blastocoel cavity (right). Abbreviations: B, blastomere; bl, blastocoel; O, oocyte; TE, trophectoderm cell; zp, zona pellucida.

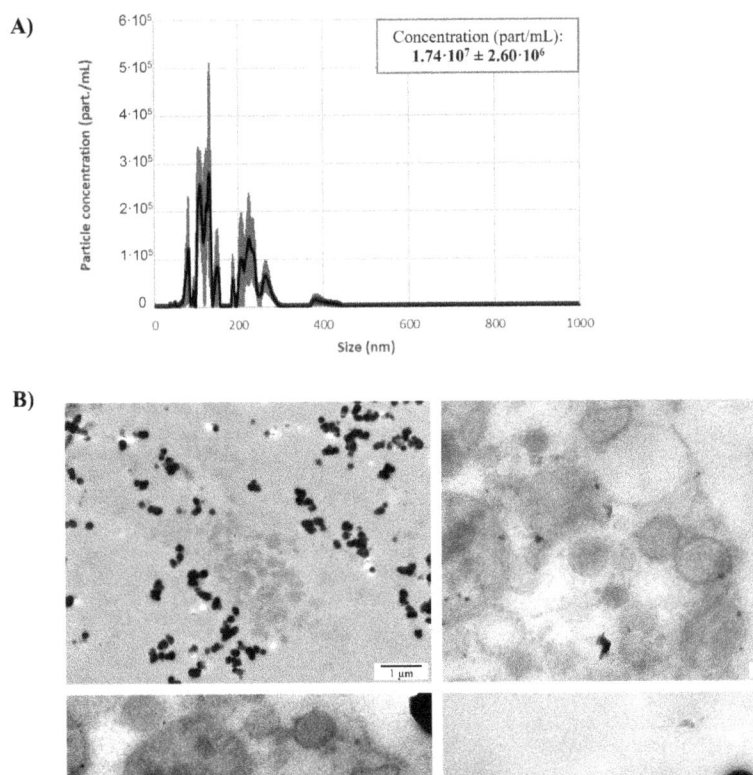

Figure 2. Isolation of naEVs from E4.5 blastocyst spent media. (**A**) Size distribution and quantification using nanoparticle tracking analysis of naEVs isolated from spent blastocyst media. Net particle concentration was calculated after subtracting particles found in the same volume of blank media. Values represent the mean of three independent experiments ±SEM. (**B**) Different images showing morphological characterization of naEVs in spent culture media by TEM. Particles of different aspects, electron densities and sizes ranging from 20–500 nm were observed.

Additionally, immunogold was performed on ultrathin sections to assess the presence of ARF6 and CD63 in naEVs fraction isolated by ultracentrifugation from E4.5 blastocyst spent media. In parallel, to study the potential cargo of DNA in naEVs, DNA targeting antibodies were used. The results revealed positivity for the microvesicular marker ARF6, exosomal marker CD63, and DNA (Figure 3B), thus suggesting the presence of DNA cargo in the EVs secreted by the embryos. Particularly, in our experimental set in which 702 single naEVs were studied, 16.1% of DNA positive EVs were identified.

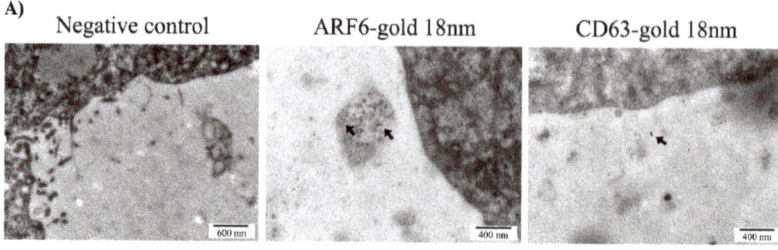

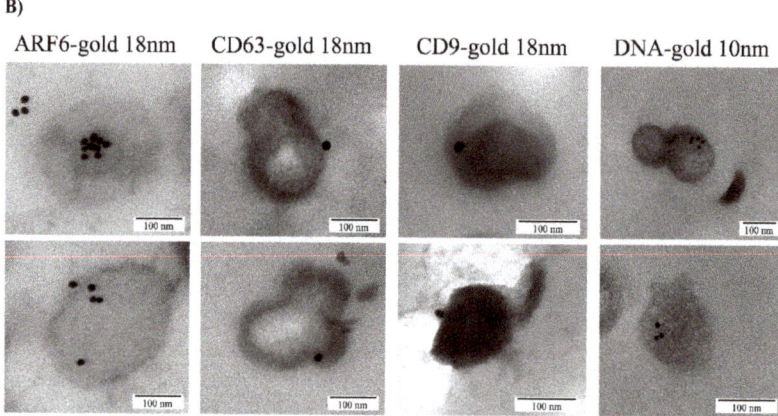

Figure 3. Phenotypic characterization of EVs using immunogold staining. (**A**) Vesicles secreted by the trophoectodermal (TE) cells of murine embryo blastocyst showed positive staining for microvesicles (MVs) and exosomes (EXOs) markers, ARF6 and CD63, respectively. (**B**) Immunogold detection of ARF6, CD63 and DNA in naEVs isolated from spent media of E4.5 blastocysts. ARF6 and CD63 are coupled to 18 nm gold particles; DNA is coupled to 10 nm gold particles. Bars represent 100 μm. Two representative images for each immunogold labeling experiment are included in the figure.

3.4. Characterization of the DNA Cargo of the EVs Secreted by the Embryo

EVs secreted by the embryo, classified as ABs or naEVs, were sequenced and compared. First, DNase treatment was applied to ABs and naEVs fractions and compared to untreated controls to discard the existence of DNA attached to the external membrane of vesicles that could confound with the real cargo. Genomic DNA from the embryos originating the EVs was used as a positive control, SN after the isolation of EVs from the spent media was included as an EVs depleted fraction and oxygenated blank media (G2-plus) as a negative control. Sequencing coverage and mapping statistics are detailed in Table S1. Sequencing of the DNA from different subpopulations revealed no differences among them (Figure 4A). However, DNase treated samples showed a different read count distribution and were differentiated into a separate cluster (Figure 4B, Figure S1), suggesting the existence of external DNA attached to the membrane of vesicles. Paired comparisons of untreated samples showed no statistical differences between the DNA regions observed in ABs and naEVs fractions, neither with the embryo genomic DNA or the EV-depleted SN, but all of them showed significant enrichment in a reduced number of gene sequences compared to the blank media (Figure 4C,D). Eleven of these differential sequences were commonly enriched in all the embryonic fractions against the blank, but no differences among the spent media derived fractions were observed. The complete list of enriched sequences is shown in Table 1 and Tables S2–S5.

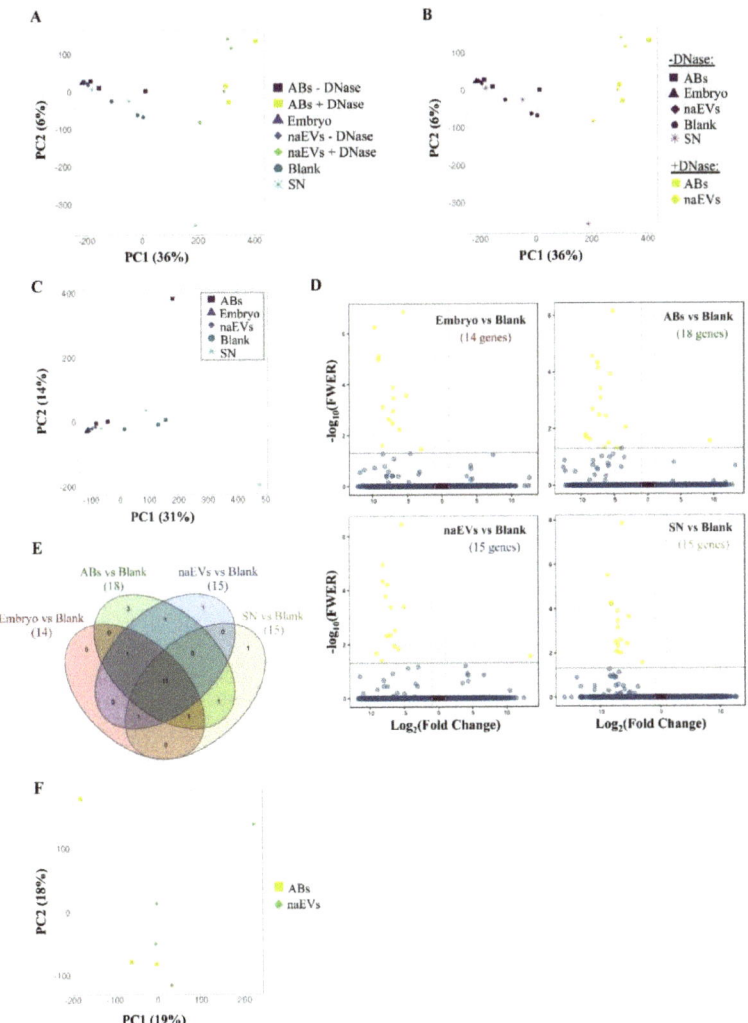

Figure 4. Analysis of the DNA produced and released by the murine embryo to the culture media. (**A**) PCA showing similarity between samples using normalized counts of 27,207 genomic features of the DNase treated and untreated EVs fractions produced by the embryo, the culture media as a negative control (blank), the embryo itself as a positive control, and the SN as an EVs free fraction. (**B**) PCA showing sample distribution by treatment showing separated clusters by treatment. (**C**) PCA of separate analysis using DNase untreated samples, including embryo, Abs, naEVs, SN, and blank control (normalized counts of 26,997 genomic features). PCA shows the similarity between fractions and replicates. (**D**) Volcano plots showing differential enriched genes in the studied fractions (embryo, ABs, naEVs, or SN) compared to the blank control. Negative FC values (left) indicate genes that are enriched in each fraction with respect to the blank medium, while positive values (right) correspond to genes enriched in the blank medium compared to the studied sample. The number of differentially enriched genes is shown in brackets for each comparison. (**E**) Venn diagram showing common and specific enriched genes in pairwise comparisons. (**F**) PCA of DNase treated replicates showed no differences between DNA content in the treated vesicle subpopulations. Abbreviations: AB, apoptotic bodies; naEVs, smaller in size extracellular vesicles (including microvesicles and exosomes); SN, supernatant.

Table 1. Genes enriched in the comparison of the different DNase untreated samples (embryo, ABs, naEVs and SN) against the blank culture medium.

Gene ID	Chr	Embryo vs. Blank		ABs vs. Blank		naEVs vs. Blank		SN vs. Blank	
		log(FC)	FWER	log(FC)	FWER	log(FC)	FWER	log(FC)	FWER
2610005L07Rik	8	7.04	3.50×10^4	7.10	3.79×10^4	6.97	4.26×10^4	7.11	3.48×10^4
Gm10715	9	9.17	1.08×10^5	7.09	8.17×10^4	7.71	1.67×10^4	8.24	6.06×10^5
Gm10717	9	7.71	2.44×10^3	5.89	3.18×10^2	6.50	1.15×10^2	7.13	4.57×10^3
Gm13822	5	7.14	1.35×10^4	7.42	7.34×10^5	7.47	6.25×10^5	7.18	1.27×10^4
Gm17535	9	9.71	5.68×10^7	7.57	4.76×10^5	8.15	1.11×10^5	8.77	3.19×10^6
Gm26624	4	5.22	2.83×10^4	5.62	1.17×10^4	5.09	4.09×10^4	5.37	2.29×10^4
Gm26804	8	7.15	3.47×10^3	7.30	3.35×10^3	7.03	4.63×10^3	6.66	9.83×10^3
Gm7120	13	6.20	5.84×10^3	6.29	3.69×10^3	6.39	3.04×10^3	7.14	7.15×10^4
Pisd-ps1	11	9.14	7.51×10^6	8.38	2.77×10^5	8.17	4.65×10^5	8.12	5.83×10^5
Pisd-ps2	17	8.56	7.81×10^4	8.31	2.08×10^3	7.61	4.78×10^3	7.34	8.52×10^3
Sfi1	11	5.61	1.49×10^7	5.26	7.32×10^7	5.38	3.56×10^7	6.42	1.40×10^8
C230088H06Rik	4	3.10	3.53×10^2	3.38	8.85×10^3			3.18	2.73×10^2
Gm10720	9	7.09	1.11×10^3			5.84	1.44×10^2	6.64	2.54×10^3
Gm14412	2	8.66	2.51×10^2	8.70	2.41×10^2	8.35	3.86×10^2		
C130026I21Rik	1			4.64	4.84×10^2			5.61	3.80×10^3
Gm13251	4			9.41	1.60×10^2	9.08	2.15×10^2		
Cd2bp2	7			−9.38	2.77×10^2				
Fbxw18	9							7.53	2.98×10^3
Gm10306	4					−13.38	2.75×10^2		
Gm13154	4			6.50	4.66×10^2				
Leprot	4			9.29	2.04×10^2				

Abbreviations: ABs, Apoptotic Bodies; Chr, Chromosome; FC, Fold Change; FWER, Family-Wise Error Rate; naEVs, smaller in size extracellular vesicles (including microvesicles and exosomes); SN, supernatant.

DNase treated ABs and naEVs were compared to evaluate their DNA cargo after removal of external DNA. PCA analysis did not cluster separately for both populations and differential enrichment analysis did not evidence any result either (Figure 4F). The absence of differences after DNase treatment may be due to the scarce amount of DNA remaining after treatment, which resulted in poor sequencing outputs (Figure S1, panel C).

Considering these results, the culture media itself was assessed to test whether it could contain contaminating DNA that aligns to the murine genome, masking the results. To evaluate this effect, the reads were aligned to both human and murine genomes. Approximately, 80% of the reads from all the samples, including unused blank media, were able to map both human and murine reference genomes, while only 20% of the reads could be uniquely matched to the murine genome (Figure S2). This fact constituted an important hindrance for the analysis of murine-derived DNA in samples with reduced input and made it impossible to get complete DNA enrichment analyses.

In this context, those DNA sequences that uniquely map the murine genome were analyzed and only those comparisons of murine DNA isolated from embryos or EVs compared to the blank negative controls were considered. PCA analysis of murine-unique sequences showed again a wide dispersion of the different fractions analyzed (Figure 5A) and only DNase treated versus untreated samples clustered separately (Figure 5B and Figure S1, panels D–F). No major differences in DNA regions were found among DNase untreated fractions (Figure 5C). However, a higher amount of gene sequences was found in all the fractions compared to the blank media (Figure 5D) which only showed artefactual mapping to murine DNA (Figure S3). In this case, 169 gene sequences representing all murine chromosomes were found in the different samples studied (embryo, ABs, naEVs, or SN) compared to the blank, while 25 of them were common to all the comparisons. The individual assessment of each fraction compared to the blank rendered a total of 2, 14, 8, and 92 genes enriched in embryo, ABs, naEVs, and SN, respectively. (Figure 5E, Tables S6–S9). Interestingly, the enriched genes found in vesicles were more similar to the DNA found in the embryo, while the SN showed a different pattern of enriched genes compared to embryo, EVs, and blank media (Figure 5E and Table S10).

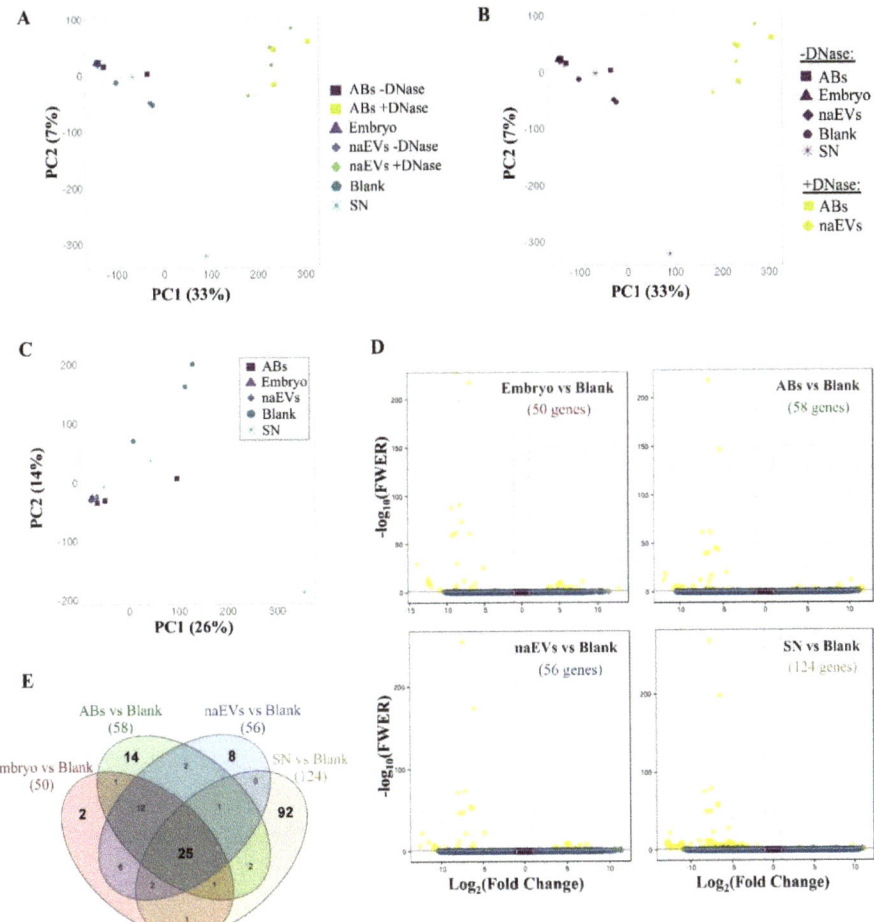

Figure 5. Analysis of murine-specific DNA sequences secreted by the embryo to the culture media. Study of DNA sequences uniquely mapping to Mus musculus reference genome secreted by the murine embryo to the spent media in EVs or as a free form. (**A**) PCA showing similarity between samples using normalized counts of 27,970 genomic features after filtering out human-homologous reads. (**B**) PCA grouping samples by DNase treatment. (**C**) Separate PCA of DNase untreated samples using normalized counts of 27,824 genomic features after filtering out human-homologous reads. (**D**) Volcano plots showing differential enriched genes in the studied fractions (embryo, ABs, naEVs, or SN) compared to the blank control. Negative FC values (left) indicate genes that are enriched in each fraction with respect to the blank medium, while positive values (right) correspond to genes enriched in the blank medium compared to the studied sample. The number of differentially enriched genes is shown in brackets for each comparison. (**E**) Venn diagram showing common and specific enriched genes in pairwise comparisons. Abbreviations: AB, apoptotic bodies; naEVs, smaller in size extracellular vesicles (including microvesicles and exosomes); SN, supernatant.

4. Discussion

The production and secretion of EVs by the embryo have been reported in different species from bovine [39], pig [40], mouse [41], and human [3]. Although different size ranges have been demonstrated among species, all shared phenotypic markers such as CD63 and CD9 [42]. The achievement of blastocyst/hatching stage is key for the release of EVs to the extracellular medium [43]. In humans, the presence of EVs in conditioned media of in vitro cultured human embryos from day three to day five has been previously described as well as their uptake by the maternal side [3]. A similar event occurs in the sheep model, where EVs coming from the conceptus were observed to be internalized by the uterine epithelia, but not in other maternal tissues [24]. Also, of importance is the delivery of EVs between embryo compartments. Particularly, MVs have been observed to be produced by the inner cell mass reaching the trophectoderm, thus promoting its migration and implantation abilities [4]. Our results showed oocytes and embryos in different developmental stages with MVB produced by the blastomeres, as well as secreted vesicles of different sizes (Figure 1A–D). Of note, the existence of large vesicles with complex structures and contents in the intercellular space of the developing embryos was reported, which is in line with Desrochers' group observations (Figure 1C, D). NTA allows a precise measurement and quantification of EVs by their light scattering properties measured directly by a camera. Results showed a polydisperse population with varying sizes (Figure 2A), which were confirmed by deposition, staining, and TEM visualization of the vesicles (Figure 2B). Regarding molecular markers, immunogold staining of ultrathin cuts from EVs produced by the embryos showed the presence of CD63 and CD9 in the EVs, but also of ARF6, a GTP-binding protein involved in MVs synthesis through the phospholipase D pathway [38]. Importantly, gold labelling also revealed the presence of DNA cargo within these EVs (Figure 3). All-in-all, this initial analysis served us to confirm the production of varying in-size/phenotype EVs by the murine embryos to the culture media, and to associate them with EXOs and MVs markers as well as with DNA cargo. However, the quantification of positive vesicles may be impacted by the method used for the isolation of such vesicles. As high recovery methods may result in a great population of vesicles with low purity showing a low percentage of positive vesicles, while methods that yield a very pure population of vesicles may present a higher degree of positivity while missing other vesicular subtypes that may present a different phenotype. In this work, EVs were recovered using high-speed differential ultracentrifugation after intermediate speed apoptotic bodies removal and washes. This is considered an intermediate recovery and intermediate specificity method [44]. Nonetheless, positivity in our experimental set-up is only descriptive as we analyzed immunogold labelling on ultrathin sections, and only a small representation of the total vesicle fraction has been stained and visualized for this purpose.

Different molecules can be analyzed from the spent media with potential different diagnostic usefulness, including RNA [43] and DNA, both nuclear and mitochondrial [45]. DNA content of EVs is currently a developing field of research. Although different studies coincide in that embryo material in the spent medium may be greatly masked by maternal contamination coming from cumulus cells, its putative clinical usefulness has already been proposed for embryo chromosomal non-invasive diagnosis [43,46–50]. DNA secreted by cells can be single or double stranded at the extracellular medium in its free form, but also externally stuck or included in EVs where it is protected from the enzymes present in the medium [51]. Also, it has been reported that different subpopulations of EVs contain different DNA cargo [16], including mtDNA [52]. It was even observed that EVs' DNA can be transported into target cells in either the cytoplasm or nuclei [53] where it serves a function [54]. Nevertheless, there is not much information about the DNA content of EVs produced by preimplantation embryos in culture. A recent study reported the presence of DNA in embryo-derived EVs by flow cytometry, associating higher concentrations of DNA-containing EVs with higher rates of implantation failure after embryo transfer. Nevertheless, this may be explained by the fact that these DNA-containing EVs were mainly apoptotic bodies, thus reflecting poor embryo quality [55]. To our knowledge, there are still no works addressing the potential diagnostic value of embryo derived EVs for the detection of DNA mutations/polymorphisms in the cells of origin, but some works in different biofluids, such as blood, urine, or seminal fluid, have done so, highlighting EVs as potential biomarkers for pathological mutations [56]. In order to go one step further into the analysis of the DNA secreted by the preimplantation embryo, the present study analyzes whether any specific cargo was transported inside the EVs released to the spent media during early embryo development.

Pairwise comparisons of embryo fractions—consisting of full-embryos, ABs, MVs, EXOs and SN—against blank media were performed. Differentially enriched genes were observed in all the fractions analyzed and compared to the blank media (Figure 4), although the number of enriched genes was lower than expected. We hypothesized that the small differences found in the DNA enrichment analysis could be influenced by genetic material present in the blank control. G2-plus is a commercial medium supplemented with human serum albumin, which is a blood derived molecule and so it may drag residual DNA from the original source. The possibility of human–mouse cross-species mapping is not trite since 90% of the mouse and human genomes can be partitioned into corresponding regions of conserved synteny. At the nucleotide level, approximately 40% of the human genome, likely representing most of the orthologous sequences, can be aligned to the mouse genome. Around 80% of the mouse genes have a single identifiable orthologue in the human, while only 1% does not have a known homologue [57]. Our hypothesis was confirmed with 80% of the total reads corresponding to blank media aligning both the human and the murine genomes (Figure S2). The analysis of murine-specific DNA sequences in the blanks evidenced poor DNA size and quality and supported the consideration of these samples as background noise (Figure S3). Under this situation, human-homologous reads were filtered out and pairwise comparisons with murine-specific reads were recalculated (Figure 5). New comparisons provided richer results and even a trend was observed showing a high similarity between EVs and embryo DNA regions, while the SN presented a differential DNA pattern. This would introduce the concept of two differentiated embryo DNA sources: vesicular and cell-free DNA, deserving future analysis. Far from intending to establish any functional conclusion and considering the technical limitations of the data analysis, the results presented herein demonstrate the possibility of detecting specific DNA sequences secreted by the murine embryo over the inherent masking of blank medium and point at a differential DNA profile between EVs and SN, which may be of importance and should be further investigated.

Because DNA potentially stuck to the external surface of EVs may influence the results of the sequencing analysis, paired fractions of ABs and naEVs populations were treated with DNase prior to sequencing. Despite having control for human-homologous sequences effect, no statistically significant genes or DNA regions were obtained when comparing specific subtypes of EVs (ABs and naEVs) after DNase treatment. This may be due to the scarce DNA material left for sequencing after the harsh DNase treatment. Further studies starting from a higher number of vesicles and/or using defined embryo culture media might shed light on this point.

5. Conclusions

Our results demonstrate the existence of EVs produced by the murine oocyte and embryo throughout embryo development. These EVs are secreted to the extracellular space, and can be found in the intercellular space, the blastocoel or even in the spent culture media, after crossing the zona pellucida. The analysis of the different EVs collected from blastocyst spent media showed the presence of DNA representing the full murine genome, with no differences in DNA cargos between the different fractions (ABs and naEVs). Also, vesicle-free DNA was found in the EVs-depleted supernatant of embryo culture. These findings demonstrate that embryo DNA is randomly secreted to the spent culture medium under physiological conditions without the need of aneuploidy or apoptotic events. Furthermore, our results reinforce the relevance of cellular communication between the conceptus and maternal endometrium during implantation and to support the feasibility of non-invasive testing of pre-implantation embryos.

Supplementary Materials: The following are available online at http://www.mdpi.com/2073-4425/11/2/203/s1, Figure S1: DNA sequencing read counts and normalization of the different fractions. Plots showing normalization of samples sequencing reads previous (A, B, C) and after (D, E, F) filtering by specific murine genome. (A and D). All samples populations. (B and E) DNase untreated samples. (C and F) DNase treated EVs. Abbreviations: ABs: Apoptotic bodies; CPM, Counts per million; naEVs: non-apoptotic EVs (including microvesicles and exosomes); SN: supernatant; Figure S2: Mouse-Human cross-mapping. Normalized plot showing the percentages of reads for each sample able to map both to the human and murine reference genomes (purple) and those mapping uniquely to the murine genome (yellow). Abbreviations: ABs: Apoptotic bodies; naEVs: non-apoptotic EVs (including microvesicles and exosomes); SN: supernatant; Figure S3: Quality control of murine specific DNA sequences. (A) Murine genomic sequences detected in blank samples showed poor mapping quality (MAPQ score) compared to embryo-derived samples. Murine genes differentially enriched in the experimental setting showed poor mapping quality (B) and insert insert size (C) in blank samples compared to embryo-derived fractions; Table S1: DNA sequencing reads, and mapping statistics; Table S2: Sequencing analysis data for the enriched genes in the comparison Embryo vs blank control for total gene sequences; Table S3: Sequencing analysis data for the enriched genes in the comparison ABs vs blank control for total gene sequences; Table S4: Sequencing analysis data for the enriched genes in the comparison naEVs vs blank control for total gene sequences; Table S5: Sequencing analysis data for the enriched genes in the comparison SN vs blank control for total gene sequences; Table S6: Sequencing analysis data for the enriched genes in the comparison Embryo vs blank control for gene sequences uniquely binding the Mus musculus reference genome; Table S7: Sequencing analysis data for the enriched genes in the comparison ABs vs blank control for gene sequences uniquely binding the Mus musculus reference genome; Table S8: Sequencing analysis data for the enriched genes in the comparison naEVs vs blank control for gene sequences uniquely binding the Mus musculus reference genome; Table S9: Sequencing analysis data for the enriched genes in the comparison SN vs blank control for gene sequences uniquely binding the Mus musculus reference genome; Table S10: Gene sequences uniquely mapping to the Mus musculus reference genome enriched in the comparisons of the different DNase untreated samples (embryo genomic DNA, ABs, naEVs and SN) vs the blank control. Abbreviations: ABs, Apoptotic Bodies; Chr, Chromosome; FC, FoldChange; FWER, Family-Wise Error Rate; naEVs, non-apoptotic EVs; SN, Supernatant.

Author Contributions: Conceptualization, F.V. and I.M.; methodology, B.S., D.B., and D.V.; software, A.A. and J.J.-A.; validation, D.B., F.V., and I.M.; formal analysis, B.S., D.B., A.A., J.J.-A., D.V., F.V., and I.M.; data curation, A.A. and J.J.-A.; writing—original draft preparation, B.S., D.B., and I.M.; writing—review and editing, B.S., D.B., A.A., J.J.-A., D.V., F.V., and I.M.; funding acquisition, D.B. and F.V. All authors have read and agreed to the published version of the manuscript.

Funding: This research was funded by Igenomix Foundation. D.B. is supported by the grant FPU15/02248 from the Spanish Ministry of Education, Culture and Sports. FV is supported by Instituto de Salud Carlos III through Miguel Servet Program Type II [CPII18/00020] and FIS project [PI18/00957].

Conflicts of Interest: A.A., J.J.-A., D.V. and I.M. are full-time or part-time employed by Igenomix S.L. B.S., D.B. and F.V. declare no competing financial interests.

References

1. Ng, Y.H.; Rome, S.; Jalabert, A.; Forterre, A.; Singh, H.; Hincks, C.L.; Salamonsen, L.A. Endometrial exosomes/microvesicles in the uterine microenvironment: A new paradigm for embryo-endometrial cross talk at implantation. *PLoS ONE* 2013, *8*, e58502. [CrossRef] [PubMed]
2. Vilella, F.; Moreno-Moya, J.M.; Balaguer, N.; Grasso, A.; Herrero, M.; Martínez, S.; Marcilla, A.; Simón, C. Hsa-miR-30d, secreted by the human endometrium, is taken up by the pre-implantation embryo and might modify its transcriptome. *Development* 2015, *142*, 3210–3221. [CrossRef] [PubMed]
3. Giacomini, E.; Vago, R.; Sanchez, A.M.; Podini, P.; Zarovni, N.; Murdica, V.; Rizzo, R.; Bortolotti, D.; Candiani, M.; Viganò, P. Secretome of in vitro cultured human embryos contains extracellular vesicles that are uptaken by the maternal side. *Sci. Rep.* 2017, *7*, 880. [CrossRef] [PubMed]
4. Desrochers, L.M.; Bordeleau, F.C.O.; Reinhart-King, C.A.; Antonyak, M.A.; Cerione, R.A. Microvesicles provide a mechanism for intercellular communication by embryonic stem cells during embryo implantation. *Nat Commun.* 2016, *7*, 1–11. [CrossRef] [PubMed]
5. Simón, C.; Greening, D.W.; Bolumar, D.; Balaguer, N.; Salamonsen, L.A.; Vilella, F. Extracellular Vesicles in Human Reproduction in Health and Disease. *Endocr. Rev.* 2018, *39*, 292–332. [CrossRef] [PubMed]
6. Caby, M.-P.; Lankar, D.; Vincendeau-Scherrer, C.; Raposo, G.; Bonnerot, C. Exosomal-like vesicles are present in human blood plasma. *Int. Immunol.* 2005, *17*, 879–887. [CrossRef] [PubMed]
7. Pisitkun, T.; Shen, R.-F.; Knepper, M.A. Identification and proteomic profiling of exosomes in human urine. *Proc. Natl. Acad. Sci. USA* 2004, *101*, 13368–13373. [CrossRef]
8. Ogawa, Y.; Miura, Y.; Harazono, A.; Kanai-Azuma, M.; Akimoto, Y.; Kawakami, H.; Yamaguchi, T.; Toda, T.; Endo, T.; Tsubuki, M.; et al. Proteomic analysis of two types of exosomes in human whole saliva. *Biol. Pharm. Bull* 2011, *34*, 13–23. [CrossRef]
9. Admyre, C.; Johansson, S.M.; Qazi, K.R.; Filén, J.-J.; Lahesmaa, R.; Norman, M.; Neve, E.P.A.; Scheynius, A.; Gabrielsson, S. Exosomes with immune modulatory features are present in human breast milk. *J. Immunol.* 2007, *179*, 1969–1978. [CrossRef]

10. Asea, A.; Jean-Pierre, C.; Kaur, P.; Rao, P.; Linhares, I.M.; Skupski, D.; Witkin, S.S. Heat shock protein-containing exosomes in mid-trimester amniotic fluids. *J. Reprod. Immunol.* **2008**, *79*, 12–17. [CrossRef]
11. Andre, F.; Schartz, N.E.C.; Movassagh, M.; Flament, C.; Pautier, P.; Morice, P.; Pomel, C.; Lhomme, C.; Escudier, B.; Le Chevalier, T.; et al. Malignant effusions and immunogenic tumour-derived exosomes. *Lancet* **2002**, *360*, 295–305. [CrossRef]
12. Vella, L.J.; Sharples, R.A.; Lawson, V.A.; Masters, C.L.; Cappai, R.; Hill, A.F. Packaging of prions into exosomes is associated with a novel pathway of PrP processing. *J. Pathol.* **2007**, *211*, 582–590. [CrossRef] [PubMed]
13. Masyuk, A.I.; Huang, B.Q.; Ward, C.J.; Gradilone, S.A.; Banales, J.M.; Masyuk, T.V.; Radtke, B.; Splinter, P.L.; LaRusso, N.F. Biliary exosomes influence cholangiocyte regulatory mechanisms and proliferation through interaction with primary cilia. *Am. J. Physiol. Gastrointest. Liver Physiol.* **2010**, *299*, G990–G999. [CrossRef] [PubMed]
14. Ronquist, G.; Brody, I. The prostasome: Its secretion and function in man. *Biochim. Biophys. Acta* **1985**, *822*, 203–218. [CrossRef]
15. Akers, J.C.; Gonda, D.; Kim, R.; Carter, B.S.; Chen, C.C. Biogenesis of extracellular vesicles (EV): Exosomes, microvesicles, retrovirus-like vesicles, and apoptotic bodies. *J. Neurooncol.* **2013**, *113*, 1–11. [CrossRef]
16. Lázaro-Ibáñez, E.; Sanz-Garcia, A.; Visakorpi, T.; Escobedo-Lucea, C.; Siljander, P.; Ayuso-Sacido, Á.; Yliperttula, M. Different gDNA content in the subpopulations of prostate cancer extracellular vesicles: Apoptotic bodies, microvesicles, and exosomes. *Prostate* **2014**, *74*, 1379–1390. [CrossRef]
17. Hochreiter-Hufford, A.; Ravichandran, K.S. Clearing the dead: Apoptotic cell sensing, recognition, engulfment, and digestion. *Cold Spring Harb. Perspect. Biol.* **2013**, *5*, a008748. [CrossRef]
18. Wu, Y.; Tibrewal, N.; Birge, R.B. Phosphatidylserine recognition by phagocytes: A view to a kill. *Trends Cell Biol.* **2006**, *16*, 189–197. [CrossRef]
19. Muralidharan-Chari, V.; Clancy, J.W.; Sedgwick, A.; D'Souza-Schorey, C. Microvesicles: Mediators of extracellular communication during cancer progression. *J. Cell Sci.* **2010**, *123*, 1603–1611. [CrossRef]
20. Greening, D.W.; Gopal, S.K.; Xu, R.; Simpson, R.J.; Chen, W. Exosomes and their roles in immune regulation and cancer. *Semin. Cell Dev. Biol.* **2015**, *40*, 72–81. [CrossRef]
21. Colombo, M.; Raposo, G.; Théry, C. Biogenesis, Secretion, and Intercellular Interactions of Exosomes and Other Extracellular Vesicles. *Annu. Rev. Cell Dev. Biol.* **2014**, *30*, 255–289. [CrossRef] [PubMed]
22. Kowal, J.; Arras, G.; Colombo, M.; Jouve, M.; Morath, J.P.; Primdal-Bengtson, B.; Dingli, F.; Loew, D.; Tkach, M.; Théry, C. Proteomic comparison defines novel markers to characterize heterogeneous populations of extracellular vesicle subtypes. *Proc. Natl. Acad. Sci. USA* **2016**, *113*, e968–e977. [CrossRef] [PubMed]
23. Yáñez-Mó, M.; Siljander, P.R.M.; Andreu, Z.; Zavec, A.B.; Borràs, F.E.; Buzás, E.I.; Buzas, K.; Casal, E.; Cappello, F.; Carvalho, J.; et al. Biological properties of extracellular vesicles and their physiological functions. *J. Extracell. Vesicles* **2015**, *4*, 27066. [CrossRef] [PubMed]
24. Burns, G.W.; Brooks, K.E.; Spencer, T.E. Extracellular Vesicles Originate from the Conceptus and Uterus During Early Pregnancy in Sheep. *Biol. Reprod.* **2016**, *94*, 56. [CrossRef] [PubMed]
25. Bidarimath, M.; Khalaj, K.; Kridli, R.T.; Kan, F.W.K.; Koti, M.; Tayade, C. Extracellular vesicle mediated intercellular communication at the porcine maternal-fetal interface: A new paradigm for conceptus-endometrial cross-talk. *Sci. Rep.* **2017**, *7*, 40476. [CrossRef] [PubMed]
26. Salomon, C.; Yee, S.W.; Mitchell, M.D.; Rice, G.E. The possible role of extravillous trophoblast-derived exosomes on the uterine spiral arterial remodeling under both normal and pathological conditions. *Biomed. Res. Int.* **2014**, *2014*, 693157. [CrossRef]
27. Stefanski, A.L.; Martinez, N.; Peterson, L.K.; Callahan, T.J.; Treacy, E.; Luck, M.; Friend, S.F.; Hermesch, A.; Maltepe, E.; Phang, T.; et al. Murine trophoblast-derived and pregnancy-associated exosome-enriched extracellular vesicle microRNAs: Implications for placenta driven effects on maternal physiology. *PLoS ONE* **2019**, *14*, e0210675. [CrossRef]
28. Szatanek, R.; Baran, J.; Siedlar, M.; Baj-Krzyworzeka, M. Isolation of extracellular vesicles: Determining the correct approach. *Int. J. Mol. Med.* **2015**, *36*, 11–17. [CrossRef]

29. Marcilla, A.; Trelis, M.; Cortés, A.; Sotillo, J.; Cantalapiedra, F.; Minguez, M.T.; Valero, M.L.; Sánchez del Pino, M.M.; Muñoz-Antoli, C.; Toledo, R.; et al. Extracellular vesicles from parasitic helminths contain specific excretory/secretory proteins and are internalized in intestinal host cells. *PLoS ONE* **2012**, *7*, e45974. [CrossRef]
30. Gardiner, C.; Ferreira, Y.J.; Dragovic, R.A.; Redman, C.W.G.; Sargent, I.L. Extracellular vesicle sizing and enumeration by nanoparticle tracking analysis. *J. Extracell. Vesicles* **2013**, *2*. [CrossRef]
31. Li, H.; Durbin, R. Fast and accurate long-read alignment with Burrows-Wheeler transform. *Bioinformatics* **2010**, *26*, 589–595. [CrossRef] [PubMed]
32. Li, H. A statistical framework for SNP calling, mutation discovery, association mapping and population genetical parameter estimation from sequencing data. *Bioinformatics* **2011**, *27*, 2987–2993. [CrossRef] [PubMed]
33. Quinlan, A.R.; Hall, I.M. BEDTools: A flexible suite of utilities for comparing genomic features. *Bioinformatics* **2010**, *26*, 841–842. [CrossRef] [PubMed]
34. McCarthy, D.J.; Chen, Y.; Smyth, G.K. Differential expression analysis of multifactor RNA-Seq experiments with respect to biological variation. *Nucleic. Acids. Res.* **2012**, *40*, 4288–4297. [CrossRef]
35. Nikolayeva, O.; Robinson, M.D. edgeR for differential RNA-seq and ChIP-seq analysis: An application to stem cell biology. *Methods Mol. Biol.* **2014**, *1150*, 45–79. [CrossRef]
36. Robinson, M.D.; McCarthy, D.J.; Smyth, G.K. edgeR: A Bioconductor package for differential expression analysis of digital gene expression data. *Bioinformatics* **2010**, *26*, 139–140. [CrossRef]
37. Ghossoub, R.; Lembo, F.; Rubio, A.; Gaillard, C.B.; Bouchet, J.; Vitale, N.; Slavík, J.; Machala, M.; Zimmermann, P. Syntenin-ALIX Exosome Biogenesis and Budding Into Multivesicular Bodies Are Controlled by ARF6 and PLD2. *Nat. Commun.* **2014**, *5*, 3477. [CrossRef]
38. Muralidharan-Chari, V.; Clancy, J.; Plou, C.; Romao, M.; Chavrier, P.; Raposo, G.; D'Souza-Schorey, C. ARF6-regulated Shedding of Tumor Cell-Derived Plasma Membrane Microvesicles. *Curr. Biol.* **2009**, *19*, 1875–1885. [CrossRef]
39. Mellisho, E.A.; Velásquez, A.E.; Nuñez, M.J.; Cabezas, J.G.; Cueto, J.A.; Fader, C.; Castro, F.O.; Rodríguez-Álvarez, L. Identification and characteristics of extracellular vesicles from bovine blastocysts produced in vitro. *PLoS ONE* **2017**, *12*, e0178306. [CrossRef]
40. Saadeldin, I.M.; Kim, S.J.; Choi, Y.B.; Lee, B.C. Improvement of cloned embryos development by co-culturing with parthenotes: A possible role of exosomes/microvesicles for embryos paracrine communication. *Cell Reprogram.* **2014**, *16*, 223–234. [CrossRef]
41. Kim, J.; Lee, J.; Lee, T.B.; Jun, J.H. Embryotrophic effects of extracellular vesicles derived from outgrowth embryos in pre- and peri-implantation embryonic development in mice. *Mol. Reprod. Dev.* **2019**, *86*, 187–196. [CrossRef] [PubMed]
42. Giacomini, E.; Alleva, E.; Fornelli, G.; Quartucci, A.; Privitera, L.; Vanni, V.S.; Viganò, P. Embryonic extracellular vesicles as informers to the immune cells at the maternal-fetal interface. *Clin. Exp. Immunol.* **2019**, *80*, 1948. [CrossRef] [PubMed]
43. Capalbo, A.; Ubaldi, F.M.; Cimadomo, D.; Noli, L.; Khalaf, Y.; Farcomeni, A.; Ilic, D.; Rienzi, L. MicroRNAs in spent blastocyst culture medium are derived from trophectoderm cells and can be explored for human embryo reproductive competence assessment. *Fertil. Steril.* **2016**, *105*, 225–235. [CrossRef] [PubMed]
44. Théry, C.; Witwer, K.W.; Aikawa, E.; Alcaraz, M.J.; Anderson, J.D.; Andriantsitohaina, R. Minimal information for studies of extracellular vesicles 2018 (MISEV2018): A position statement of the International Society for Extracellular Vesicles and update of the MISEV2014 guidelines. *J. Extracell. Vesicles* **2018**, *23*, 1535750. [CrossRef] [PubMed]
45. Hammond, E.R.; McGillivray, B.C.; Wicker, S.M.; Peek, J.C.; Shelling, A.N.; Stone, P.; Chamley, L.W.; Cree, L.M. Characterizing nuclear and mitochondrial DNA in spent embryo culture media: Genetic contamination identified. *Fertil. Steril.* **2017**, *107*, 220–228. [CrossRef]
46. Shamonki, M.I.; Jin, H.; Haimowitz, Z.; Liu, L. Proof of concept: Preimplantation genetic screening without embryo biopsy through analysis of cell-free DNA in spent embryo culture media. *Fertil. Steril.* **2016**, *106*, 1312–1318. [CrossRef]
47. Xu, J.; Fang, R.; Chen, L.; Chen, D.; Xiao, J.-P.; Yang, W.; Wang, H.; Song, X.; Ma, T.; Bo, S.; et al. Noninvasive chromosome screening of human embryos by genome sequencing of embryo culture medium for in vitro fertilization. *Proc. Natl. Acad. Sci. USA* **2016**, *113*, 11907–11912. [CrossRef]

48. Vera-Rodriguez, M.; Diez-Juan, A.; Jimenez-Almazan, J.; Martinez, S.; Navarro, R.; Peinado, V.; Mercader, A.; Meseguer, M.; Blesa, D.; Moreno, I.; et al. Origin and composition of cell-free DNA in spent medium from human embryo culture during preimplantation development. *Hum. Reprod.* **2018**, *33*, 745–756. [CrossRef]
49. Ho, J.R.; Arrach, N.; Rhodes-Long, K.; Ahmady, A.; Ingles, S.; Chung, K.; Bendikson, K.A.; Paulson, R.J.; McGinnis, L.K. Pushing the limits of detection: Investigation of cell-free DNA for aneuploidy screening in embryos. *Fertil. Steril.* **2018**, *110*, 467–475. [CrossRef]
50. Wu, H.; Ding, C.; Shen, X.; Wang, J.; Li, R.; Cai, B.; Xu, Y.; Zhong, Y.; Zhou, C. Medium-based noninvasive preimplantation genetic diagnosis for human α-thalassemias-SEA. *Medicine (Baltimore)* **2015**, *94*, e669. [CrossRef]
51. Thakur, B.K.; Zhang, H.; Becker, A.; Matei, I.; Huang, Y.; Costa-Silva, B.; Zheng, Y.; Hoshino, A.; Brazier, H.; Xiang, J.; et al. Double-stranded DNA in exosomes: A novel biomarker in cancer detection. *Cell Res.* **2014**, *24*, 766–769. [CrossRef]
52. Guescini, M.; Genedani, S.; Stocchi, V.; Agnati, L.F. Astrocytes and Glioblastoma cells release exosomes carrying mtDNA. *J. Neural. Transm. (Vienna)* **2010**, *117*, 1–4. [CrossRef]
53. Waldenström, A.; Gennebäck, N.; Hellman, U.; Ronquist, G. Cardiomyocyte microvesicles contain DNA/RNA and convey biological messages to target cells. *PLoS ONE* **2012**, *7*, e34653. [CrossRef] [PubMed]
54. Cai, J.; Han, Y.; Ren, H.; Chen, C.; He, D.; Zhou, L.; Eisner, G.M.; Asico, L.D.; Jose, P.A.; Zeng, C. Extracellular vesicle-mediated transfer of donor genomic DNA to recipient cells is a novel mechanism for genetic influence between cells. *J. Mol. Cell Biol.* **2013**, *5*, 227–238. [CrossRef] [PubMed]
55. Pállinger, É.; Bognar, Z.; Bodis, J.; Csabai, T.; Farkas, N.; Godony, K.; Varnagy, A.; Buzas, E.; Szekeres-Bartho, J. A simple and rapid flow cytometry-based assay to identify a competent embryo prior to embryo transfer. *Sci. Rep.* **2017**, *7*, 39927. [CrossRef] [PubMed]
56. Kalluri, R.; LeBleu, V.S. Discovery of Double-Stranded Genomic DNA in Circulating Exosomes. *Cold Spring Harb. Symp. Q. Biol.* **2016**, *81*, 275–280. [CrossRef] [PubMed]
57. Mouse Genome Sequencing Consortium; Waterston, R.H.; Lindblad-Toh, K.; Birney, E.; Rogers, J.; Abril, J.F.; Agarwal, P.; Agarwala, R.; Ainscough, R.; Alexandersson, M.; et al. Initial sequencing and comparative analysis of the mouse genome. *Nature* **2002**, *420*, 520–562. [CrossRef]

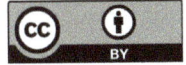

© 2020 by the authors. Licensee MDPI, Basel, Switzerland. This article is an open access article distributed under the terms and conditions of the Creative Commons Attribution (CC BY) license (http://creativecommons.org/licenses/by/4.0/).

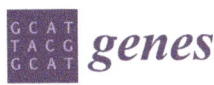

Review

Mother and Embryo Cross-Communication

Anna Idelevich [1] and Felipe Vilella [2,3,*]

1. Igenomix, Boston, MA 02210, USA; anna.idelevich@igenomix.com
2. Igenomix Foundation, Instituto de Investigación Sanitaria Hospital Clínico (INCLIVA), 46010 Valencia, Spain
3. Department of Obstetrics and Gynecology, BIDMC, Harvard University, Boston, MA 02215, USA
* Correspondence: felipe.vilella@igenomix.com; Tel.: +34-963905310

Received: 4 March 2020; Accepted: 30 March 2020; Published: 31 March 2020

Abstract: Endometrial receptivity is a biosensor for embryo quality, as embryos with reduced developmental potential are rejected. However, embryo quality only accounts for an estimated one-third of implantation failures, with suboptimal endometrial receptivity accounting for the remaining two-thirds. As pregnancy progresses, a uterus continues to engage in close communication with an embryo/fetus, exchanging information in the form of endocrine, paracrine, and other cues. Given the long mammalian gestation period, this dialogue is intricate, diverse, and, currently, not fully understood. Recent progress and the availability of high-throughput techniques, including transcriptomics, proteomics, and metabolomics, has allowed the simultaneous examination of multiple molecular changes, enhancing our knowledge in this area. This review covers the known mechanisms of mother–embryo cross-communication gathered from animal and human studies.

Keywords: embryo; uterus; window of implantation

1. Introduction

Infertility is common, with ~12% of women in the United States being unable to conceive [1]. To solve this, patients have turned to in vitro fertilization, with considerable success. According to the European Society of Human Reproduction and Embryology (ESHRE), more than 8 million babies have been born from In vitro fertilisation (IVF) since the world's first IVF-birth in 1978 [2], and currently ~1.6% of all births in the United States now result from this procedure [3]. The success of IVF, however, can vary depending on the cause of infertility. Almost half of infertile cases occur due to endometriosis, but for others, the etiology is unknown [4] and thus a challenge to treat.

Improving the success rate of IVF requires a better understanding of how the embryo interacts with the uterus throughout pregnancy. Embryonic implantation and development are not possible without continuous molecular dialogue. The mother and embryo exchange signals at all times, from embryonic stem-cell differentiation all the way to implantation, decidualization, placentation, and also parturition, resulting in the birth of offspring [5–9].

Pregnancy begins with the union between a haploid (23-chromosome) sperm with a haploid egg, forming a diploid (46-chromosome) single-cell zygote, which continues to undergo mitotic divisions and forms a blastocyst while traveling across the fallopian tube toward the uterus. The blastocyst consists of an inner cell mass and an outer trophectoderm cell layer. During implantation, when the blastocyst adheres to the uterine endometrium, the inner cell mass further differentiates into two cell lineages, the primitive endoderm and the epiblast. The epiblast gives rise to the fetus and the primitive endoderm and trophectoderm give rise to fetal membranes and the placenta, respectively [5,6,10].

Pregnancy relies on blastocyst implantation during a narrow window of uterine receptivity, called the window of implantation; implantation outside this window is associated with spontaneous miscarriages. Uterine sensitivity in mice, is divided into two principal phases: prereceptive (days 1 to 3) and receptive (day 4). The uterine transition to the receptive phase, where blastocysts can implant, requires priming with progesterone hormone (P4) traced on estrogen (E2). Upon closure of this window, the uterus is a hostile milieu, and the blastocyst cannot implant. In humans, the pre-receptive phase occurs after ovulation (7 days, early luteal phase), followed by the receptive (~7–10 days, mid-luteal phase) and nonreceptive (~7–10 to 28–30 days, late-luteal phase) phases until menstruation ensues [5,6,11].

The three main tissue compartments of the uterus—the endometrial epithelium (luminal and glandular) and stroma, and myometrium—support and regulate pregnancy. As the site of blastocyst adhesion, the luminal epithelium is perceived as the crucial site for uterine receptivity and transmits signals to other compartments [12]. Histological aspects of the endometrium when it becomes receptive include: irregular glands with a papillary appearance, migration of vacuoles to a supranuclear position in epithelial cells, edematous uterine stroma, and decidualization [13].

The contact between the receptive endometrium and the competent blastocyst involves a series of stages: apposition, adhesion, and invasion, constituting a successful implantation [13]. During the apposition moment, a multitude of small microvilli protrusions (pinopodes) develop on the apical surface of the luminal epithelium. These microvilli form a single flowerlike shape, which appears only during the window of implantation, and subsequently inter-digitate with the blastocyst. Uterodomes are characterized by the presence of cell-adhesion molecules (i.e., integrins [14,15]). The basal and lateral membranes also undergo transformations, specifically at various junctions [12]. Blastocyst adhesion with the luminal epithelium overlaps with the process of decidualization of the stromal cells. The changes in morphology and function governed by the two main ovarian hormones—E2 and P4—accord with the associated molecular changes, including elevated expression of estrogen receptor 1 (ER1) and the progesterone receptor (PR) as well as a multitude of downstream target genes. These and subsequent events, leading to the progression of pregnancy and completing in the birth of an offspring, involve a complex interplay of endocrine, genetic, and other cues.

Presently, little has been published on the molecular mechanisms that control the dialogue between the early embryo and the mother. Several histological and molecular markers have been identified for endometrial receptivity; however, these await consensus [14,16]. For example, even the presence of uterodomes, characteristic of apposition, is not yet a proven significant biomarker [17,18]. Additionally, preoccupation with one potential biomarker at the expense of exploring others remains a challenge in the field [14,16]. This review summarizes what is known of factors implicated in the communication between the embryo and the mother. We start with presenting several important circulating factors, including hormones, cytokines, chemokines, and extracellular vesicles carrying various signaling components, such as microRNAs, and finish with describing the genetic and epigenetic responses of the uterus and placenta to these circulating factors.

2. Circulating Factors

2.1. Endocrine—Hormones

Hormones have pride of place in the hierarchy of primary determinants for embryo-uterine crosstalk. Ovarian E2 and P4 are crucial for a series of events ranging from uterine receptivity to implantation, decidualization, placentation, and finally birth. E2 and P4 govern the chronological transitions between these events, supporting continuous interactions between the mother and the developing baby [6,11]. Both hormones affect a plethora of growth factors, transcription factors, lipid mediators, cytokines, and cell cycle regulators involved in the course of pregnancy [5].

The role of hormonal signaling has been studied in many model systems. In mice, a "delayed implantation" model is commonly used to assess signaling during pregnancy [19]. This model uses ovariectomy on day 4 before the preimplantation estrogen surge and continued P4 treatment to induce uterine quiescence while maintaining implantation competency, which is resumed upon estrogen repletion. This indicates the importance of these two hormones in controlling uterine receptivity in mice. Specifically, the expression of Sik-SP regulated by E2 is independent of ER but requires the control of estradiol receptor α (ERα) necessary for the coordination of the biphasic responses in the uterus for its growth [20]. However, while P4 is an absolute requirement for implantation in many species, ovarian estrogen rise is not crucial in subhuman primates [6].

In humans, the 28–30-day menstrual cycle begins with menses. The proliferative phase is influenced by rising E2 levels generated from ovarian follicles, which leads to the proliferation of the endometrial epithelium, stroma, and vascular endothelium to regenerate the uterine lining. At midcycle, the gonadotropins: follicle-stimulating hormone (FSH) and luteinizing hormone (LH), induce ovulation on day 14. Subsequently, in the early secretory phase, the endometrium becomes thicker and the corpus luteum forms from the ruptured follicle leading to a P4 upsurge in preparation for implantation. The increase in E2 levels overlaid on P4 define the window of implantation. In the absence of a viable embryo, there is hormone withdrawal and menstruation. The implanting blastocyst secretes chorionic gonadotropin (hCG) to maintain the corpus luteum, and pregnancy ensues [6].

During pregnancy, the expression pattern of ovarian hormones is dynamic and has compartment-specific functions mediated by multiple hormone receptors. Mice lacking Era or both PR isoforms, PR-A and PR-B, are hypoplastic and infertile [21,22]. Just before starts the embryo implantation, PR is expressed in the luminal epithelium. However, at the beginning of embryo implantation, the expression of PR rapidly declines in the luminal epithelium with increased expression in the stroma that persists throughout decidualization [23]. Mice with an epithelial loss of Esr1 show implantation failure and abnormal expression of estrogen related genes. Mice with an epithelial-specific loss of Pgr are unresponsive to P4 treatment and are infertile due to defects in embryo adhesion, stromal cell decidualization, and unrestrained estrogen-induced epithelial cell proliferation [23,24].

Mechanistically, the infertility in these mice is attributed to low expression of leukemia inhibitory factor (LIF), and Indian hedgehog (IHH) [25]. IHH is expressed in epithelial cells and interacts in the stroma with its receptors (Patched and Smoothened), producing the proliferation of the stromal cell. LIF is a cytokine, member of the interleukin-6 family essential for endometrial receptivity and implantation. LIF binds to their LIF receptor (LIFR) that, in partnership with the co-receptor GP130, transduces signals through the signal transducer and activator of transcription 3 (STAT3). Genetic deletion of *GL130* or *STAT3* result in implantation failure [26,27]. Clinically, the role of LIF remains inconclusive. Using a relatively small cohort of hyperstimulated women with diverse etiologies of infertility, administration of LIF did not improve pregnancy outcomes [28].

Overall, steroid hormones affect a plethora of downstream factors crucial for pregnancy progression, acting through bidirectional epithelial-stromal communication. HAND2 is one such ovarian hormone-dependent factor thought to be involved in implantation and decidualization. *Hand2* ablation causes infertility, via a mechanism involving upregulation of fibroblast growth factor-extracellular signal regulated kinase (FGF-ERK) signaling [29]. In contrast, the important homeobox transcription factor *MSX1* is less dependent on E2 and P4 levels [30], but may be vital for fertility. Genetic studies in mice suggest that *MSX1* is necessary for embryo implantation, and subsequent studies in humans revealed that the protein levels of MSX1, were significantly reduced in endometrial biopsies obtained of infertile women [31].

Progesterone resistance—a rapidly expanding topic in clinical research—is linked with reduced endometrial receptivity [16,32]. P4 is anti-inflammatory and induces immune tolerance at implantation. Interference with P4 action using antiprogestins, such as RU-486, causes pregnancy loss and infertility [33]. Furthermore, an early rise in P4 reduces the success rate of embryo transfers, even with frozen embryos known to be competent based on subsequent transfers. There is a 2–3-day temporal window of P4 exposure when receptivity is optimal. Overall, data suggests that abnormal P4 exposure or resistance leads to embryo–uterine asynchrony. P4 is also responsible for timely downregulation of ERs, an effect linked to timely expression of integrin $\alpha\upsilon\beta3$, which plays a role in blastocyst adhesion to the uterus [16,33]. Clinically, endometriosis has also been associated with progesterone resistance, or irresponsiveness to progesterone signaling, guiding the search for suitable biomarkers underlying this effect [34].

2.2. Paracrine—Cytokines, Chemokines

To assess other paracrine factors regulating pregnancy, changes in the level of signaling molecules have been analyzed in maternal blood throughout the course of pregnancy. Using a liquid chip scanning technology, Zhao et al. analyzed 30 circulating factors at 14 time points in pregnant rats [8]. The technology is based on flexible Muti-Analyte Profiling (xMAP), integrating colored microspheres, fluidics, laser technology, and computer programming algorithms. The greatest change in the levels of signaling molecules occurred in the third trimester, with moderate changes in the first trimester, and relatively little changes during the second trimester. During early-pregnancy (days 1–7; first trimester of human pregnancy), the levels of luteinizing hormone (LH) and brain-derived neurotrophic factor (BDNF) were increased and decreased, respectively. In this time frame, sperm–egg binding and fusion occurs, forming the fertilized egg, which moves from the fallopian tube to the uterus and sends stimulatory signals to the endometrium to prepare for blastocyst implantation. Compared with pre-pregnancy levels, the levels of monocyte chemotactic protein 1 (MCP1), interleukin-10 (IL-10), IL-13, and growth-related oncogene (GRO) are elevated at day 5 (equivalent to the second month of human pregnancy). In this window, the so-called "Th2 phenomena" occurs during which maternal T helper 1 (Th1) inhibition and Th2 activation occur, supporting the involvement of the maternal innate and cellular immune response in fetal development and providing mechanisms whereby maternal immune rejection of the fetus is inhibited. However, by day 7 when the fetal heart is fully developed, the reverse occurs. Th2 transforms to Th1 (by the regulation and expression of transcription factors), aiming to activate innate immunity in the embryo.

The shift to mid-pregnancy (days 9–19; second trimester of human pregnancy) results in stabilization of circulating signaling molecules. Growth hormone (GH) and leptin levels increase, promoting muscle growth and fuel anabolism. Th1 and Th2 levels remain stable, indicating adjustment and growth of the fetal immune system and reduction in maternal immune rejection of the fetus, avoiding fetal abortion. Cd4+ regulatory T cells (Tregs) are essential to the maternal immune tolerance, the diminution in number or nonfunctional competence cells are implicated in infertility, miscarriage, preeclampsia and fetal growth restriction [35,36].

During late-pregnancy (days 21–23; third trimester of human pregnancy), IL-2, IL-6, IL-12p70m, IL-18, interferon-g (IFN-g), leptin, and GRO levels increase, while adrenocorticotropic hormone (ACTH) and BDNF levels decrease. At this time, maternal Th1 is rapidly activated, implying immune protection of the mother and fetus in preparation for delivery. Previous studies have also shown that IL-2m, IL-6, and IL18 relate to uterine expansion. Finally, the postpartum period is marked by an increase in vascular endothelial growth factor (VEGF), possibly to repair the wounded tissue, and prolactin (PRL) increases, promoting and maintaining lactation.

Zhao et al. found that over 30 cell types were involved in this intercellular "wireless" communication network and demonstrated common alterations in the level of signaling molecules in maternal serum (such as cytokines, chemokines, and hormones) at various time points throughout pregnancy from pre-implantation to post-delivery in rats. Further investigation of these factors is warranted to evaluate their role in human pregnancy, but separate studies have already identified some paracrine factors in this context. Colony-stimulating factor-1 (*CSF-1*) promotes differentiation of human trophoblast cells into syncytiotrophoblast cells and guide to the production of placental lactogen [37]. Several metalloproteinases have been reported in connection with the invasive ability of the fetal trophoblast, in particular MMP2 and 9 [38,39]. Trophoblastic MMPs are regulated in response to tumor necrosis factor alpha (TNFa), IL-1b, IL-1a, leptin, transforming factor b (TGFb), macrophage colony-stimulating factor (MCSF), and endothelial growth factor (EGF), which are secreted at the fetal–maternal interface from different cells. Endometrial extracellular matrix (ECM) remodeling is essential for successful implantation and placentation and multiple MMPs as well as their substrates are involved in this process. For example, MMP-14 and ADAM10, present in endometrium-derived exosomes, act on IL-8, TGFb, CD44, Notch and its ligand DLL1 promoting their bioactivity [40–43].

For reference, a recent comprehensive review has summarized the roles of MMPs in embryo–maternal crosstalk [44].

2.3. Extracellular Vesicles and Their Cargo—Proteins, Lipids, miRNA

Extracellular vesicles (EVs) were recently shown to play a role in paracrine communication between mother and embryo [9]. EVs comprise a range of membrane enclosed compartments differing in biogenesis, size, and cargo. Their small size facilitates trafficking between local sites. EVs activate surface receptors on target cells, merging with the cell membrane and releasing cargo. EV cargo—proteins, lipids, and genetic material (DNA, RNA, miRNA, and other RNA forms)—reflects the physiological state of the cell of origin and this property has been exploited in the search for biomarkers of various pathologies, including cancer [43,45,46].

Based on their origin and size, EVs are generally subdivided into three classes: apoptotic bodies, microvesicles, and exosomes. Apoptotic bodies are the largest EVs (1–5 µm) and form following cytoplasmic membrane blebbing in cells undergoing programmed cell death, or apoptosis. Molecular markers include: phosphatidylserine (PS) (which serves as the "eat me" signal for phagocytes but is also found in healthy cells), thrombospondin, C3b complement protein, VDAC1 (a protein forming ionic channels in the mitochondrial membrane), and calreticulin (an endoplasmic reticulum protein) [9,47]. Microvesicles are 100–1000 nm, and their molecular markers are ADP-ribosylation factor 6 (ARF6), integrins, selectins, and CD40 ligand. Exosomes are small, virus sized particles (30–150 nm) formed by inward budding of the cytoplasmic membrane. Exosomes were long considered to be nanodust, or dust in electron microscopy, but this perception has changed in recent years, with their role evolving from trash cans to biologically active particles [48,49]. Exosomes play known roles in immunomodulation, their most studied function [46,50], and in angiogenesis, thrombosis [51], and pathologies, such as cancer [47]. The molecular markers of exosomes include: CD63, CD9, CD81, ALIX, TSG101, flotillin-1, HSC70, and syntenin-1 [9]. In general, all EVs have biological and pathological roles and act as messengers in cell-to-cell communication. EVs participate in regulating immune responses, in particular triggering the adaptive immune response and suppressing inflammation [52]. Beyond immunomodulation, EVs contribute to synaptic plasticity, deliver neurotransmitter receptors, play a role in tissue regeneration following injury, and modulate cell phenotype [45].

EVs have only recently become of interest in the growing field of embryo–mother cross communication. Data has accumulated showing key roles of EVs at preconception from gamete maturation to implantation and throughout pregnancy [53]. Ng et al. first showed that EVs contain a specific subset of miRNAs not detectable in the maternal cells, by the human endometrial epithelial cell-line ECC1 [54]. These EVs were later verified to be present in human uterine fluid. Burns et al. demonstrated that the uterine fluid of pregnant sheep contains EVs positive for CD63 and HSP70 (exosomal markers) as well as small RNAs and miRNAs [55]. Greening et al. demonstrated that the proteome of highly purified exosomes from human endometrial epithelial cells is subject to steroid hormonal regulation by estrogen and progesterone and varies with the menstrual cycle [56]. Villela et al. performed a study showing internalization of miR30d by mouse embryos via the trophectoderm that results in indirect overexpression of adhesion related genes—*Itgb3*, *Itga7* and *Cdh* [57]. In this study, treatment of mouse embryos with miR-30d resulted in increased embryo adhesion [57]. In contrast, the same group also showed that miR-30d deficiency results in reduced implantation rates and impaired fetal growth [58]. Heterogeneous nuclear ribonucleoprotein C1 (hnRNPC1) has also been implicated in the mechanism of cell-to-cell communication [59]. These findings support a model in which maternal endometrial miRNAs act as transcriptomic modifiers of the preimplantation embryo. Analysis of human endometrial liquid biopsy (ELB) material in both natural and hormonal replacement therapy (HRT) cycles revealed a panel of differentially expressed miRNAs, including members of the miR-30 family [60]. Recently, embryos were shown to "talk back" via release of progesterone induced protein (PIBF) packaged in EVs that modulate maternal immune response [7,61]. The presence of

EVs in the uterine fluid implies endometrial–embryo cross talk; however, these studies require more thorough exploration.

EV research is rapidly growing, but is still an immature field facing several challenges. Among the notable challenges are a lack of nomenclature for distinct types of EVs based on cellular origin. The terms "microvesicle" and "exosome" have been used mutually in many published manuscripts because of the incomplete understanding of EV biogenesis, inconsistencies and discrepancies in purification protocols, and imprecise characterization [43]. There are many unknowns regarding the biogenesis, route, and function of EVs in reproductive biology. Regardless, EVs are already considered attractive pharmaceutical targets and may be exploited directly as potential therapeutic agents for tissue regeneration and immune response modulation [43]. EVs might additionally be exploited for non-invasive prenatal genetic testing if it is established that embryos transmit EVs carrying genetic material to the mother.

3. Genetic Changes—Receptors, Signaling Molecules

3.1. Uterus

The molecular signature of the uterus at the time of implantation shows elevated expression of several factors, but experts agree that currently, none of these biomarkers have been studied in enough detail to validate their usefulness for assessing endometrial receptivity [14]. Regardless, the emerging evidence about their roles in fertility is worth considering.

Mucin 1 (MUC 1) (a highly glycosylated polymorphic mucin-like protein) secreted by the endometrial luminal epithelium is considered a "barrier to implantation". In humans, MUC1 is expressed in the luteal and pre-implantation phases in a progesterone-dependent manner [62–64]. MUC 1 is more abundant in fertile then infertile women [65]. In baboons, MUC1 was also shown to be progesterone- rather than estrogen-dependent, serving as a marker of the pre-implantation phase [65]. Of interest, a recent study [66] investigating similarities between term pregnancy in eutherian mammals and marsupials found that key biomarkers of implantation, including mucin 1, heparin-binding EGF-like factor (HBEGF), and a range or proinflammatory factors, including IL-6, tumor necrosis factor (TNF), and cyclooxygenase 2 (COX2), are consistent between species, suggesting conserved regulation of embryo implantation. There are transcriptome-wide similarities between the implantation in rabbits and humans and the marsupial adhesion process [66]. Specifically, the marsupial study observed that the biomarker osteopontin was consistent in five human microarray studies in relation to the window of implantation [67].

Osteopontin (OPN) is a glycosylated phosphoprotein expressed in the endometrial epithelium and implicated in adhesion and signaling roles at the embryo–epithelium interface [68,69]. OPN is also a bone associated protein, produced by several bone cell types (osteoblasts and osteoclasts) and extra-osseous tissue (skin, kidney and lung). Due to differences in post-translational modification, OPN's molecule weight ranges from 41 to 75 kDa, and OPN is suggested to have cell type-specific structure and function [70,71]. OPN plays major roles in bone remodeling, inflammation, immune-regulation, and vascularization, as well as in pathologies, including cancer. Several studies have evaluated OPN as a biomarker of tumor progression [70].

Comparative global gene expression studies have demonstrated an increase in OPN in the human endometrium following the LH surge [72], and OPN has been detected in the vicinity of uterodomes and in decidualizing stroma [73]. Moreover, while OPN null mice are fertile, they exhibit reduced pregnancy rates [74]. Mechanistically, OPN interacts with integrins and is classified as a member of the small integrin-binding ligand N-linked glycoprotein (SIBLINGs) family, which includes molecules, such as dentin matrix protein (DMP1), bone sialoprotein (BSP), and others. Binding of OPN to integrins activates their receptors and cytoskeletal proteins, subsequently promoting focal adhesion in the embryo trophectoderm; however, the functional significance of this interaction in endometrial receptivity requires further investigation [75].

Integrins are transmembrane glycoproteins with a and b subunits that mediate several processes, including cell–cell and cell–extracellular matrix (ECM) adhesion. There are integrins expressed constitutively in the luminal epithelium, and others are regulated in a spatial and temporal manner during the menstrual cycle [12,76,77]. Three integrins, A1B1, A4B1, and AVB3, were reported to have unique expression patterns correlating with the window of implantation in women [14,15]. Of these, avb3 is the best characterized. The avb3 integrin emerges on the top of luminal and glandular cell surfaces, coinciding with the aperture of the window of implantation, and its expression continues into pregnancy with expansion of the decidua [33]. The appearance of $\alpha\upsilon\beta3$ integrin on the apical surface of the luminal cells is due to its presence in subnuclear secretory granules [33]. Expression of an intact $\alpha\upsilon\beta3$ heterodimer is regulated by *HOXA10* transcription factor, whose expression together with $\alpha\upsilon\beta3$ is altered in pathologies, including adenomyosis, polycystic ovary syndrome, and endometriosis [14]. However, these observations are opposed by several studies showing no reliable link between integrins and fertility [78,79].

An additional homeobox protein, HOXA11, may have a similar role as HOXA10 in decidualization. Deletion of either protein in mice results in implantation defects [80,81], which are due to uterine (as opposed to embryonic) errors. HOXA10-null mice produce a normal amount of embryos that are capable to implant normally in wild-type surrogate mice; although, wild-type embryos cannot implant in HOXA10-null mice [80,82]. HOXA11−/− mice show a similar phenotype [83]. In the human endometrium, HOXA10 is expressed by stromal and epithelial cells regulated by progesterone in a dependent manner in a menstrual cycle [84]. Precisely how HOXA10 regulates uterine receptivity is unclear, but microarray analysis of murine endometrium transfected with HOXA10 cDNA has identified 40 downstream target genes including clusterin (Clu), phoshoglycerate 3-dehydrogenase (3-Pgdh), and tumor-associated calcium signal transducer 2 (Tacstd2) [85].

3.2. Placenta

The placental interface mediates interaction between the mother and fetus, and changes in placental gene expression have been analyzed to examine how it participates in embryo–mother cross-talk [86]. A recent study conducted single-cell transcriptomics on villous tissue from 2 human term placentas, identifying 87 single-cell transcriptomes. Trophoblast cells at term were concluded to be the most abundant cell type. Single-cell gene expression profiles were segregated into five different clusters (three clusters of cytotrophoblast, decidual cells and extravilous trophoblast), based on combinations of known trophoblast markers (KRT7, KRT8, GCM1, CYP19A1) and diagnostic genes with >10 fold higher expression in uterine vs. immune cells. These transcriptomes were grouped into three large clusters of cytotrophoblast cells. The data were further analyzed with respect to two syncytiotrophoblast transcriptomes, collected from a single placenta by laser microdissection as well as the transcriptomes of primary undifferentiated endometrial stromal fibroblast (ESF), and the transcriptome of in vitro primary differentiated decidual cells. Single-cell data was aligned with tissue-level data to estimate cell origin, and the top 25% (2108) most highly expressed genes were found to comprise 80% of the total aligned placental mRNA.

Based on genetic studies in mice, placenta-derived leptin also has an important role in fertility, and is secreted into maternal and fetal circulation produced by the placental trophoblast. Leptin regulates energy metabolism, feeding, and bone. Released from adipose tissue, leptin travels in the circulation until it reaches leptin receptors in the brain, located in hypothalamic nuclei and other sites [87–89]. Leptin acts on the hypothalamic–pituitary axis to affect steroid hormone release. An absence of leptin (ob/ob mice) is not lethal but results in early onset obesity, extreme insulin resistance, stunted skeletal and brain growth, compromised immune system, and infertility [90]. Interestingly, fertility can be restored in ob/ob mice by exogenous leptin administration, which is characterized by increased LH and FSH. However, fertility is not restored by food restriction in these mice, suggesting that leptin affects the reproductive system independently of metabolism [91,92]. In pregnant mice and humans, the placenta is a major site of leptin expression [90], but it is unclear what role placenta-derived leptin might play in embryonic development [93]. Leptin receptor expression is abundant in placenta. These receptors may pass information about energy metabolism between the mother and the baby [94].

4. Epigenetic and Transcriptomic Changes

Epigenetics is defined as heritable changes in chromosomes without changes in DNA sequence. These changes include histone modification, DNA methylation, and expression of non-coding RNAs. E2 and P4 regulate the expression of their respective receptors, which are important for embryo implantation. Aberrant DNA methylation of the CpG island in the promoter regions of ER or PR has been reported in endometrial carcinoma, suggesting regulation of the uterus by epigenetic mechanisms [95,96]. Factors related to endometrial receptivity, such as *HOXA10* and *MUC1* have also been shown to be controlled by hormone-dependent DNA methylation, which is associated with infertility [97,98], and changes in DNA methylation in the endometrium have been correlated with gene expression during the transition from the pre-receptive to receptive phase in humans [99,100]. Interestingly, comparison of changes in transcriptomes and corresponding DNA methylomes on the same samples revealed association of gene expression and DNA methylation for a number of loci related to endometrial biology [100], suggesting an interplay between hormones and the uterus at the level of the epigenome [101]. In addition, miRNA and circRNA are stably detected in the circulation and EVs. For example, miR-30d is upregulated during the acquiring of receptivity in the endometrium [102], its overexpression induces changes in the transcriptomics and proteomics of the endometrial epithelium [103], and it is involved in the interaction between embryo and uterus, as it is secreted by the uterus and taken up by the embryo [57]. Free hsa-miR-30d and/or exosomes are internalized by embryos through their trophectodermal cells, resulting in overexpression of genes encoding for molecules related to embryonic adhesion (*Itgb3*, *Itga7* and *Cdh5*) [57]. Other miRNA families shown to be important for implantation and that potentially mediate embryo–mother dialog are miR200, Let7, and miR-17-92 clusters [104].

5. Conclusions

For a healthy outcome for the mother and baby, a continuous molecular dialog is crucial. The language is based on endocrine, paracrine, and autocrine factors. Despite gathered knowledge, much remains to be discovered regarding how these factors affect genes in the developing organism and how genetic and epigenetic changes are translated into "readable" information. Estrogen, progesterone, and downstream effectors govern differentiation of the stroma and remodeling of the endometrium, making it receptive for embryo implantation. The embryo also sends various signals to the mother, in the form of EVs carrying miRNA and other material, to which the mother responds. The exact routes of communication are not well understood and further exploration is needed. Better understanding of the physiological mechanisms involved in the mother–baby dialogue during pregnancy should allow identification of reliable biomarkers for endometrial receptivity, aiding the treatment of unexplained infertility and increasing healthy birth rates.

Author Contributions: A.I. and F.V. wrote the paper; all the authors performed the final approval of the manuscript; F.V. contributed to the fundraising. All authors have read and agreed to the published version of the manuscript.

Funding: This work was supported by the Miguel Servet Program Type II of ISCIII [CPII18/00020]; and a FIS project [PI18/00957] to F.V.

Conflicts of Interest: A.I. is a full-time employee of Igenomix S.L.; F.V. declares no competing financial interests.

References

1. Jain, T.; Grainger, D.A.; Ball, G.D.; Gibbons, W.E.; Rebar, R.W.; Robins, J.C.; Leach, R.E. 30 years of data: Impact of the United States in vitro fertilization data registry on advancing fertility care. *Fertil. Steril.* **2019**, *111*, 477–488. [CrossRef] [PubMed]

2. De Geyter, C.; Calhaz-Jorge, C.; Kupka, M.S.; Wyns, C.; Mocanu, E.; Motrenko, T.; Scaravelli, G.; Smeenk, J.; Vidakovic, S.; Goossens, V. European IVF-monitoring Consortium (EIM) for the European Society of Human Reproduction and Embryology (ESHRE) ART in Europe, 2014: Results generated from European registries by ESHRE: The European IVF-monitoring Consortium (EIM) for the European Society of Human Reproduction and Embryology (ESHRE). *Hum. Reprod.* **2018**, *33*, 1586–1601.
3. Levine, A.D.; Boulet, S.L.; Kissin, D.M. Contribution of Assisted Reproductive Technology to Overall Births by Maternal Age in the United States, 2012–2014. *JAMA* **2017**, *317*, 1272–1273. [CrossRef]
4. Miller, J.E.; Ahn, S.H.; Monsanto, S.P.; Khalaj, K.; Koti, M.; Tayade, C. Implications of immune dysfunction on endometriosis associated infertility. *Oncotarget* **2017**, *8*, 7138–7147. [CrossRef] [PubMed]
5. Dey, S.K. How we are born. *J. Clin. Investig.* **2010**, *120*, 952–955. [CrossRef] [PubMed]
6. Cha, J.; Sun, X.; Dey, S.K. Mechanisms of implantation: Strategies for successful pregnancy. *Nat. Med.* **2012**, *18*, 1754–1767. [CrossRef] [PubMed]
7. Szekeres-Bartho, J.; Šućurović, S.; Mulac-Jericevic, B. The Role of Extracellular Vesicles and PIBF in Embryo-Maternal Immune-Interactions. *Front. Immunol.* **2018**, *9*, 2890. [CrossRef]
8. Zhao, M.; Liu, T.; Pang, G. Intercellular wireless communication network between mother and fetus in rat pregnancy-a study on directed and weighted network. *Reprod. Biol. Endocrinol.* **2019**, *17*, 40–45. [CrossRef]
9. Simón, C.; Greening, D.W.; Bolumar, D.; Balaguer, N.; Salamonsen, L.A.; Vilella, F. Extracellular Vesicles in Human Reproduction in Health and Disease. *Endocr. Rev.* **2018**, *39*, 292–332. [CrossRef]
10. Hirota, Y.; Cha, J.; Dey, S.K. Revisiting reproduction: Prematurity and the puzzle of progesterone resistance. *Nat. Med.* **2010**, *16*, 529–531. [CrossRef]
11. Su, R.-W.; Fazleabas, A.T. Implantation and Establishment of Pregnancy in Human and Nonhuman Primates. *Adv. Anat. Embryol. Cell Biol.* **2015**, *216*, 189–213. [PubMed]
12. Murphy, C.R. Uterine receptivity and the plasma membrane transformation. *Cell Res.* **2004**, *14*, 259–267. [CrossRef] [PubMed]
13. Díaz-Gimeno, P.; Ruiz-Alonso, M.; Blesa, D.; Bosch, N.; Martínez-Conejero, J.A.; Alamá, P.; Garrido, N.; Pellicer, A.; Simón, C. The accuracy and reproducibility of the endometrial receptivity array is superior to histology as a diagnostic method for endometrial receptivity. *Fertil. Steril.* **2012**, *99*, 508–517.
14. Lessey, B.A. Assessment of endometrial receptivity. *Fertil. Steril.* **2011**, *96*, 522–529. [CrossRef] [PubMed]
15. Lessey, B.A. Adhesion molecules and implantation. *J. Reprod. Immunol.* **2002**, *55*, 101–112. [CrossRef]
16. Lessey, B.A.; Kim, J.J. Endometrial receptivity in the eutopic endometrium of women with endometriosis: It is affected, and let me show you why. *Fertil. Steril.* **2017**, *108*, 19–27. [CrossRef]
17. Quinn, C.; Ryan, E.; Claessens, E.A.; Greenblatt, E.; Hawrylyshyn, P.; Cruickshank, B.; Hannam, T.; Dunk, C.; Casper, R.F. The presence of pinopodes in the human endometrium does not delineate the implantation window. *Fertil. Steril.* **2007**, *87*, 1015–1021. [CrossRef]
18. Usadi, R.S.; Murray, M.J.; Bagnell, R.C.; Fritz, M.A.; Kowalik, A.I.; Meyer, W.R.; Lessey, B.A. Temporal and morphologic characteristics of pinopod expression across the secretory phase of the endometrial cycle in normally cycling women with proven fertility. *Fertil. Steril.* **2003**, *79*, 970–974. [CrossRef]
19. Yuan, J.; Deng, W.; Cha, J.; Sun, X.; Borg, J.-P.; Dey, S.K. Tridimensional visualization reveals direct communication between the embryo and glands critical for implantation. *Nat. Commun.* **2018**, *9*, 1–13. [CrossRef]
20. Robertshaw, I.; Bian, F.; Das, S.K. Mechanisms of uterine estrogen signaling during early pregnancy in mice: An update. *J. Mol. Endocrinol.* **2016**, *56*, R127–R138. [CrossRef]
21. Lydon, J.P.; DeMayo, F.J.; Funk, C.R.; Mani, S.K.; Hughes, A.R.; Montgomery, C.A.; Shyamala, G.; Conneely, O.M.; O'Malley, B.W. Mice lacking progesterone receptor exhibit pleiotropic reproductive abnormalities. *Genes Dev.* **1995**, *9*, 2266–2278. [CrossRef] [PubMed]
22. Fernandez-Valdivia, R.; Jeong, J.; Mukherjee, A.; Soyal, S.M.; Li, J.; Ying, Y.; Demayo, F.J.; Lydon, J.P. A mouse model to dissect progesterone signaling in the female reproductive tract and mammary gland. *Genesis* **2010**, *48*, 106–113. [CrossRef] [PubMed]
23. Franco, H.L.; Rubel, C.A.; Large, M.J.; Wetendorf, M.; Fernandez-Valdivia, R.; Jeong, J.-W.; Spencer, T.E.; Behringer, R.R.; Lydon, J.P.; Demayo, F.J. Epithelial progesterone receptor exhibits pleiotropic roles in uterine development and function. *FASEB J.* **2012**, *26*, 1218–1227. [CrossRef] [PubMed]
24. Franco, H.L.; Jeong, J.-W.; Tsai, S.Y.; Lydon, J.P.; Demayo, F.J. In vivo analysis of progesterone receptor action in the uterus during embryo implantation. *Semin. Cell Dev. Biol.* **2008**, *19*, 178–186. [CrossRef] [PubMed]

25. Wang, X.; Li, X.; Wang, T.; Wu, S.-P.; Jeong, J.-W.; Kim, T.H.; Young, S.L.; Lessey, B.A.; Lanz, R.B.; Lydon, J.P.; et al. SOX17 regulates uterine epithelial-stromal cross-talk acting via a distal enhancer upstream of Ihh. *Nat. Commun.* **2018**, *9*, 4421–4444. [CrossRef]
26. Song, H.; Lim, H. Evidence for heterodimeric association of leukemia inhibitory factor (LIF) receptor and gp130 in the mouse uterus for LIF signaling during blastocyst implantation. *Reproduction* **2006**, *131*, 341–349. [CrossRef]
27. Sun, X.; Bartos, A.; Whitsett, J.A.; Dey, S.K. Uterine deletion of Gp130 or Stat3 shows implantation failure with increased estrogenic responses. *Mol. Endocrinol.* **2013**, *27*, 1492–1501. [CrossRef]
28. Brinsden, P.R.; Alam, V.; de Moustier, B.; Engrand, P. Recombinant human leukemia inhibitory factor does not improve implantation and pregnancy outcomes after assisted reproductive techniques in women with recurrent unexplained implantation failure. *Fertil. Steril.* **2009**, *91*, 1445–1447. [CrossRef]
29. Mestre-Citrinovitz, A.C.; Kleff, V.; Vallejo, G.; Winterhager, E.; Saragüeta, P. A Suppressive Antagonism Evidences Progesterone and Estrogen Receptor Pathway Interaction with Concomitant Regulation of Hand2, Bmp2 and ERK during Early Decidualization. *PLoS ONE* **2015**, *10*, e0124756. [CrossRef]
30. Daikoku, T.; Cha, J.; Sun, X.; Tranguch, S.; Xie, H.; Fujita, T.; Hirota, Y.; Lydon, J.; DeMayo, F.; Maxson, R.; et al. Conditional deletion of Msx homeobox genes in the uterus inhibits blastocyst implantation by altering uterine receptivity. *Dev. Cell* **2011**, *21*, 1014–1025. [CrossRef]
31. Bolnick, A.D.; Bolnick, J.M.; Kilburn, B.A.; Stewart, T.; Oakes, J.; Rodriguez-Kovacs, J.; Kohan-Ghadr, H.-R.; Dai, J.; Diamond, M.P.; Hirota, Y.; et al. NICHD National Cooperative Reproductive Medicine Network Reduced homeobox protein MSX1 in human endometrial tissue is linked to infertility. *Hum. Reprod.* **2016**, *31*, 2042–2050. [CrossRef] [PubMed]
32. Vercellini, P.; Buggio, L.; Berlanda, N.; Barbara, G.; Somigliana, E.; Bosari, S. Estrogen-progestins and progestins for the management of endometriosis. *Fertil. Steril.* **2016**, *106*, 1552–1571.e2. [CrossRef] [PubMed]
33. Lessey, B.A.; Damjanovich, L.; Coutifaris, C.; Castelbaum, A.; Albelda, S.M.; Buck, C.A. Integrin adhesion molecules in the human endometrium. Correlation with the normal and abnormal menstrual cycle. *J. Clin. Investig.* **1992**, *90*, 188–195. [CrossRef] [PubMed]
34. Rogers, P.A.W.; D'Hooghe, T.M.; Fazleabas, A.; Gargett, C.E.; Giudice, L.C.; Montgomery, G.W.; Rombauts, L.; Salamonsen, L.A.; Zondervan, K.T. Priorities for endometriosis research: Recommendations from an international consensus workshop. *Reprod. Sci.* **2009**, *16*, 335–346. [CrossRef]
35. Robertson, S.A.; Care, A.S.; Moldenhauer, L.M. Regulatory T cells in embryo implantation and the immune response to pregnancy. *J. Clin. Investig.* **2018**, *128*, 4224–4235. [CrossRef]
36. Figueiredo, A.S.; Schumacher, A. The T helper type 17/regulatory T cell paradigm in pregnancy. *Immunology* **2016**, *148*, 13–21. [CrossRef]
37. Strauss, J., III; Lyttle, C.R. *Uterine and Embryonic Factors in Early Pregnancy*; Springer Science & Business Media: New York, NY, USA, 2012.
38. Shimonovitz, S.; Hurwitz, A.; Dushnik, M.; Anteby, E.; Geva-Eldar, T.; Yagel, S. Developmental regulation of the expression of 72 and 92 kd type IV collagenases in human trophoblasts: A possible mechanism for control of trophoblast invasion. *Am. J. Obstet. Gynecol.* **1994**, *171*, 832–838. [CrossRef]
39. Huppertz, B.; Kertschanska, S.; Demir, A.Y.; Frank, H.-G.; Kaufmann, P. Immunohistochemistry of matrix metalloproteinases (MMP), their substrates, and their inhibitors (TIMP) during trophoblast invasion in the human placenta. *Cell Tissue Res.* **1997**, *291*, 133–148. [CrossRef]
40. Cuman, C.; Menkhorst, E.; Winship, A.; Van Sinderen, M.; Osianlis, T.; Rombauts, L.J.; Dimitriadis, E. Fetal–maternal communication: The role of Notch signalling in embryo implantation. *Reproduction* **2014**, *147*, R75–R86. [CrossRef]
41. Arici, A.; Seli, E.; Senturk, L.M.; Gutierrez, L.S.; Oral, E.; Taylor, H.S. Interleukin-8 in the Human Endometrium 1. *J. Clin. Endocrinol. Metab.* **1998**, *83*, 1783–1787. [CrossRef] [PubMed]

42. Tam, E.M.; Moore, T.R.; Butler, G.S.; Overall, C.M. Characterization of the Distinct Collagen Binding, Helicase and Cleavage Mechanisms of Matrix Metalloproteinase 2 and 14 (Gelatinase A and MT1-MMP): The differential roles of the MMP hemopexin c domains and the MMP-2 fibronectin type II modules in collagen triple helicase activities. *J. Biol. Chem.* **2004**, *279*, 43336–43344. [PubMed]
43. El Andaloussi, S.; Mäger, I.; Breakefield, X.O.; Wood, M.J.A. Extracellular vesicles: Biology and emerging therapeutic opportunities. *Nat. Rev. Drug. Discov.* **2013**, *12*, 347–357. [CrossRef] [PubMed]
44. Latifi, Z.; Fattahi, A.; Ranjbaran, A.; Nejabati, H.R.; Imakawa, K. Potential roles of metalloproteinases of endometrium-derived exosomes in embryo-maternal crosstalk during implantation. *J. Cell. Physiol.* **2018**, *233*, 4530–4545. [CrossRef] [PubMed]
45. van Niel, G.; D'Angelo, G.; Raposo, G. Shedding light on the cell biology of extracellular vesicles. *Nat. Rev. Mol. Cell Biol.* **2018**, *19*, 213–228. [CrossRef]
46. Maia, J.; Caja, S.; Strano Moraes, M.C.; Couto, N.; Costa-Silva, B. Exosome-Based Cell-Cell Communication in the Tumor Microenvironment. *Front. Cell Dev. Biol.* **2018**, *6*, 18. [CrossRef]
47. Voloshin, T.; Fremder, E.; Shaked, Y. Small but mighty: Microparticles as mediators of tumor progression. *Cancer Microenviron.* **2014**, *7*, 11–21. [CrossRef]
48. Muller, L. Exosomes: Nanodust? *HNO* **2020**, *68*, 56–59. [CrossRef]
49. Raposo, G.; Nijman, H.W.; Stoorvogel, W.; Liejendekker, R.; Harding, C.V.; Melief, C.J.; Geuze, H.J. B lymphocytes secrete antigen-presenting vesicles. *J. Exp. Med.* **1996**, *183*, 1161–1172. [CrossRef]
50. Kim, H.K.; Song, K.S.; Park, Y.S.; Kang, Y.H.; Lee, Y.J.; Lee, K.R.; Ryu, K.W.; Bae, J.M.; Kim, S. Elevated levels of circulating platelet microparticles, VEGF, IL-6 and RANTES in patients with gastric cancer: Possible role of a metastasis predictor. *Eur. J. Cancer* **2003**, *39*, 184–191. [CrossRef]
51. Janowska-Wieczorek, A.; Majka, M.; Kijowski, J.; Baj-Krzyworzeka, M.; Reca, R.; Turner, A.R.; Ratajczak, J.; Emerson, S.G.; Kowalska, M.A.; Ratajczak, M.Z. Platelet-derived microparticles bind to hematopoietic stem/progenitor cells and enhance their engraftment. *Blood* **2001**, *98*, 3143–3149. [CrossRef]
52. Chaput, N.; Théry, C. Exosomes: Immune properties and potential clinical implementations. *Semin. Immunopathol.* **2011**, *33*, 419–440. [CrossRef] [PubMed]
53. Machtinger, R.; Laurent, L.C.; Baccarelli, A.A. Extracellular vesicles: Roles in gamete maturation, fertilization and embryo implantation. *Hum. Reprod. Update* **2016**, *22*, 182–193. [CrossRef] [PubMed]
54. Ng, Y.H.; Rome, S.; Jalabert, A.; Forterre, A.; Singh, H.; Hincks, C.L.; Salamonsen, L.A. Endometrial exosomes/microvesicles in the uterine microenvironment: A new paradigm for embryo-endometrial cross talk at implantation. *PLoS ONE* **2013**, *8*, e58502. [CrossRef] [PubMed]
55. Burns, G.; Brooks, K.; Wildung, M.; Navakanitworakul, R.; Christenson, L.K.; Spencer, T.E. Extracellular vesicles in luminal fluid of the ovine uterus. *PLoS ONE* **2014**, *9*, e90913. [CrossRef] [PubMed]
56. Greening, D.W.; Nguyen, H.P.T.; Elgass, K.; Simpson, R.J.; Salamonsen, L.A. Human Endometrial Exosomes Contain Hormone-Specific Cargo Modulating Trophoblast Adhesive Capacity: Insights into Endometrial-Embryo Interactions. *Biol. Reprod.* **2016**, *94*, 38. [CrossRef]
57. Vilella, F.; Moreno-Moya, J.M.; Balaguer, N.; Grasso, A.; Herrero, M.; Martinez, S.; Marcilla, A.; Simón, C. Hsa-miR-30d, secreted by the human endometrium, is taken up by the pre-implantation embryo and might modify its transcriptome. *Development* **2015**, *142*, 3210–3221. [CrossRef]
58. Balaguer, N.; Moreno, I.; Herrero, M.; Gónzaléz-Monfort, M.; Vilella, F.; Simón, C. MicroRNA-30d deficiency during preconception affects endometrial receptivity by decreasing implantation rates and impairing fetal growth. *Am. J. Obstet. Gynecol.* **2019**, *221*, 46.e1–46.e16. [CrossRef]
59. Balaguer, N.; Moreno, I.; Herrero, M.; González, M.; Simón, C.; Vilella, F. Heterogeneous nuclear ribonucleoprotein C1 may control miR-30d levels in endometrial exosomes affecting early embryo implantation. *MHR Basic Sci. Reprod. Med.* **2018**, *24*, 411–425. [CrossRef]
60. Grasso, A.; Navarro, R.; Balaguer, N.; Moreno, I.; Alamá, P.; Jimenez, J.; Simón, C.; Vilella, F. Endometrial Liquid Biopsy Provides a miRNA Roadmap of the Secretory Phase of the Human Endometrium. *J. Clin. Endocrinol. Metab.* **2020**, *105*, dgz146. [CrossRef]
61. Pállinger, É.; Bognar, Z.; Bodis, J.; Csabai, T.; Farkas, N.; Godony, K.; Varnagy, A.; Buzas, E.; Szekeres-Bartho, J. A simple and rapid flow cytometry-based assay to identify a competent embryo prior to embryo transfer. *Nat. Publish. Group* **2017**, *7*, 39927–39928. [CrossRef]
62. Aplin, J.D. Embryo implantation: The molecular mechanism remains elusive. *Reprod. Biomed. Online* **2006**, *13*, 833–839. [CrossRef]

63. Hey, N.A.; Graham, R.A.; Seif, M.W.; Aplin, J.D. The polymorphic epithelial mucin MUC1 in human endometrium is regulated with maximal expression in the implantation phase. *J. Clin. Endocrinol. Metab.* **1994**, *78*, 337–342. [PubMed]
64. Wu, F.; Chen, X.; Liu, Y.; Liang, B.; Xu, H.; Li, T.C.; Wang, C.C. Decreased MUC1 in endometrium is an independent receptivity marker in recurrent implantation failure during implantation window. *Reprod. Biol. Endocrinol.* **2018**, *16*, 60–67. [CrossRef] [PubMed]
65. Hild-Petito, S.; Fazleabas, A.T.; Julian, J.; Carson, D.D. Mucin (Muc-1) expression is differentially regulated in uterine luminal and glandular epithelia of the baboon (Papio anubis). *Biol. Reprod.* **1996**, *54*, 939–947. [CrossRef] [PubMed]
66. Griffith, O.W.; Chavan, A.R.; Protopapas, S.; Maziarz, J.; Romero, R.; Wagner, G.P. Embryo implantation evolved from an ancestral inflammatory attachment reaction. *Proc. Natl. Acad. Sci. USA* **2017**, *114*, E6566–E6575. [CrossRef]
67. Aghajanova, L. Leukemia inhibitory factor and human embryo implantation. *Ann. N. Y. Acad. Sci.* **2004**, *1034*, 176–183. [CrossRef]
68. Berneau, S.C.; Ruane, P.T.; Brison, D.R.; Kimber, S.J.; Westwood, M.; Aplin, J.D. Characterisation of Osteopontin in an In Vitro Model of Embryo Implantation. *Cells* **2019**, *8*, 432. [CrossRef]
69. Craciunas, L.; Gallos, I.; Chu, J.; Bourne, T.; Quenby, S.; Brosens, J.J.; Coomarasamy, A. Conventional and modern markers of endometrial receptivity: A systematic review and meta-analysis. *Hum. Reprod. Update* **2019**, *25*, 202–223. [CrossRef]
70. Hao, C.; Cui, Y.; Owen, S.; Li, W.; Cheng, S.; Jiang, W.G. Human osteopontin: Potential clinical applications in cancer (Review). *Int. J. Mol. Med.* **2017**, *39*, 1327–1337. [CrossRef]
71. Christensen, B.; Kazanecki, C.C.; Petersen, T.E.; Rittling, S.R.; Denhardt, D.T.; Sørensen, E.S. Cell type-specific post-translational modifications of mouse osteopontin are associated with different adhesive properties. *J. Biol. Chem.* **2007**, *282*, 19463–19472. [CrossRef]
72. Kao, L.C.; Tulac, S.; Lobo, S.; Imani, B.; Yang, J.P.; Germeyer, A.; Osteen, K.; Taylor, R.N.; Lessey, B.A.; Giudice, L.C. Global gene profiling in human endometrium during the window of implantation. *Endocrinology* **2002**, *143*, 2119–2138. [CrossRef] [PubMed]
73. Quenby, S.; Anim-Somuah, M.; Kalumbi, C.; Farquharson, R.; Aplin, J.D. Different types of recurrent miscarriage are associated with varying patterns of adhesion molecule expression in endometrium. *Reprod. Biomed. Online* **2007**, *14*, 224–234. [CrossRef]
74. Weintraub, A.S.; Lin, X.; Itskovich, V.V.; Aguinaldo, J.G.S.; Chaplin, W.F.; Denhardt, D.T.; Fayad, Z.A. Prenatal detection of embryo resorption in osteopontin-deficient mice using serial noninvasive magnetic resonance microscopy. *Pediatr. Res.* **2004**, *55*, 419–424. [CrossRef] [PubMed]
75. Davidson, L.M.; Coward, K. Molecular mechanisms of membrane interaction at implantation. *Birth Defects Res. C Embryo Today* **2016**, *108*, 19–32. [CrossRef]
76. Singh, H.; Aplin, J.D. Adhesion molecules in endometrial epithelium: Tissue integrity and embryo implantation. *J. Anat.* **2009**, *215*, 3–13. [CrossRef]
77. Bowen, J.A.; Hunt, J.S. The role of integrins in reproduction. *Proc. Soc. Exp. Biol. Med.* **2000**, *223*, 331–343. [CrossRef]
78. Creus, M.; Balasch, J.; Ordi, J.; Fábregues, F.; Casamitjana, R.; Quinto, L.; Coutifaris, C.; Vanrell, J.A. Integrin expression in normal and out-of-phase endometria. *Hum. Reprod.* **1998**, *13*, 3460–3468. [CrossRef]
79. Ordi, J.; Creus, M.; Quintó, L.; Casamitjana, R.; Cardesa, A.; Balasch, J. Within-subject between-cycle variability of histological dating, alpha v beta 3 integrin expression, and pinopod formation in the human endometrium. *J. Clin. Endocrinol. Metab.* **2003**, *88*, 2119–2125. [CrossRef]
80. Benson, G.V.; Lim, H.; Paria, B.C.; Satokata, I.; Dey, S.K.; Maas, R.L. Mechanisms of reduced fertility in Hoxa-10 mutant mice: Uterine homeosis and loss of maternal Hoxa-10 expression. *Development* **1996**, *122*, 2687–2696.
81. Gendron, R.L.; Paradis, H.; Hsieh-Li, H.M.; Lee, D.W.; Potter, S.S.; Markoff, E. Abnormal uterine stromal and glandular function associated with maternal reproductive defects in Hoxa-11 null mice. *Biol. Reprod.* **1997**, *56*, 1097–1105. [CrossRef]
82. Satokata, I.; Benson, G.; Maas, R. Sexually dimorphic sterility phenotypes in Hoxa10-deficient mice. *Nature* **1995**, *374*, 460–463. [CrossRef] [PubMed]

83. Hsieh-Li, H.M.; Witte, D.P.; Weinstein, M.; Branford, W.; Li, H.; Small, K.; Potter, S.S. Hoxa 11 structure, extensive antisense transcription, and function in male and female fertility. *Development* **1995**, *121*, 1373–1385. [PubMed]
84. Taylor, H.S.; Arici, A.; Olive, D.; Igarashi, P. HOXA10 is expressed in response to sex steroids at the time of implantation in the human endometrium. *J. Clin. Investig.* **1998**, *101*, 1379–1384. [CrossRef]
85. Vitiello, D.; Pinard, R.; Taylor, H.S. Gene expression profiling reveals putative HOXA10 downstream targets in the periimplantation mouse uterus. *Reprod. Sci.* **2008**, *15*, 529–535. [CrossRef]
86. Pavličev, M.; Wagner, G.P.; Chavan, A.R.; Owens, K.; Maziarz, J.; Dunn-Fletcher, C.; Kallapur, S.G.; Muglia, L.; Jones, H. Single-cell transcriptomics of the human placenta: Inferring the cell communication network of the maternal-fetal interface. *Genome Res.* **2017**, *27*, 349–361. [CrossRef] [PubMed]
87. Idelevich, A.; Baron, R. Brain to bone: What is the contribution of the brain to skeletal homeostasis? *Bone* **2018**, *115*, 31–42. [CrossRef] [PubMed]
88. Karsenty, G.; Ferron, M. The contribution of bone to whole-organism physiology. *Nature* **2012**, *481*, 314–320. [CrossRef]
89. Nectow, A.R.; Schneeberger, M.; Zhang, H.; Field, B.C.; Renier, N.; Azevedo, E.; Patel, B.; Liang, Y.; Mitra, S.; Tessier-Lavigne, M.; et al. Identification of a Brainstem Circuit Controlling Feeding. *Cell* **2017**, *170*, 429–442.e11. [CrossRef]
90. Herrid, M.; Palanisamy, S.K.A.; Ciller, U.A.; Fan, R.; Moens, P.; Smart, N.A.; McFarlane, J.R. An updated view of leptin on implantation and pregnancy: A review. *Physiol. Res.* **2014**, *63*, 543–557.
91. Chehab, F.F.; Lim, M.E.; Lu, R. Correction of the sterility defect in homozygous obese female mice by treatment with the human recombinant leptin. *Nat. Genet.* **1996**, *12*, 318–320. [CrossRef]
92. Mounzih, K.; Lu, R.; Chehab, F.F. Leptin treatment rescues the sterility of genetically obese ob/ob males. *Endocrinology* **1997**, *138*, 1190–1193. [CrossRef] [PubMed]
93. Thomas, L.; Wallace, J.M.; Aitken, R.P.; Mercer, J.G.; Trayhurn, P.; Hoggard, N. Circulating leptin during ovine pregnancy in relation to maternal nutrition, body composition and pregnancy outcome. *J. Endocrinol.* **2001**, *169*, 465–476. [CrossRef] [PubMed]
94. Hassink, S.G.; de Lancey, E.; Sheslow, D.V.; Smith-Kirwin, S.M.; O'Connor, D.M.; Considine, R.V.; Opentanova, I.; Dostal, K.; Spear, M.L.; Leef, K.; et al. Placental leptin: An important new growth factor in intrauterine and neonatal development? *Pediatrics* **1997**, *100*, E1. [CrossRef] [PubMed]
95. Sasaki, M.; Kotcherguina, L.; Dharia, A.; Fujimoto, S.; Dahiya, R. Cytosine-phosphoguanine methylation of estrogen receptors in endometrial cancer. *Cancer Res.* **2001**, *61*, 3262–3266. [PubMed]
96. Sasaki, M.; Dharia, A.; Oh, B.R.; Tanaka, Y.; Fujimoto, S.; Dahiya, R. Progesterone receptor B gene inactivation and CpG hypermethylation in human uterine endometrial cancer. *Cancer Res.* **2001**, *61*, 97–102. [PubMed]
97. Wu, Y.; Halverson, G.; Basir, Z.; Strawn, E.; Yan, P.; Guo, S.-W. Aberrant methylation at HOXA10 may be responsible for its aberrant expression in the endometrium of patients with endometriosis. *Am. J. Obstet. Gynecol.* **2005**, *193*, 371–380. [CrossRef]
98. Kong, S.; Zhou, C.; Bao, H.; Ni, Z.; Liu, M.; He, B.; Huang, L.; Sun, Y.; Wang, H.; Lu, J. Epigenetic control of embryo-uterine crosstalk at peri-implantation. *Cell. Mol. Life Sci.* **2019**, *76*, 4813–4828. [CrossRef]
99. Kukushkina, V.; Modhukur, V.; Suhorutšenko, M.; Peters, M.; Mägi, R.; Rahmioglu, N.; Velthut-Meikas, A.; Altmäe, S.; Esteban, F.J.; Vilo, J.; et al. DNA methylation changes in endometrium and correlation with gene expression during the transition from pre-receptive to receptive phase. *Nat. Publish. Group* **2017**, *7*, 3916. [CrossRef]
100. Houshdaran, S.; Zelenko, Z.; Irwin, J.C.; Giudice, L.C. Human endometrial DNA methylome is cycle-dependent and is associated with gene expression regulation. *Mol. Endocrinol.* **2014**, *28*, 1118–1135. [CrossRef]
101. Maltepe, E.; Bakardjiev, A.I.; Fisher, S.J. The placenta: Transcriptional, epigenetic, and physiological integration during development. *J. Clin. Investig.* **2010**, *120*, 1016–1025. [CrossRef]
102. Altmäe, S.; Martínez-Conejero, J.A.; Esteban, F.J.; Ruiz-Alonso, M.; Stavreus-Evers, A.; Horcajadas, J.A.; Salumets, A. MicroRNAs miR-30b, miR-30d, and miR-494 Regulate Human Endometrial Receptivity. *Reprod. Sci.* **2012**, *20*, 308–317. [CrossRef] [PubMed]

103. Moreno-Moya, J.M.; Vilella, F.; Martinez, S.; Pellicer, A.; Simón, C. The transcriptomic and proteomic effects of ectopic overexpression of miR-30d in human endometrial epithelial cells. *Mol. Hum. Reprod.* **2014**, *20*, 550–566. [CrossRef] [PubMed]
104. Liu, W.; Niu, Z.; Li, Q.; Pang, R.T.K.; Chiu, P.C.N.; Yeung, W.S.-B. MicroRNA and Embryo Implantation. *Am. J. Reprod. Immunol.* **2015**, *75*, 263–271. [CrossRef] [PubMed]

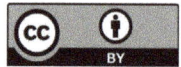

© 2020 by the authors. Licensee MDPI, Basel, Switzerland. This article is an open access article distributed under the terms and conditions of the Creative Commons Attribution (CC BY) license (http://creativecommons.org/licenses/by/4.0/).

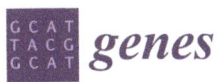

Review

Preimplantation Genetic Testing for Chromosomal Abnormalities: Aneuploidy, Mosaicism, and Structural Rearrangements

Manuel Viotti

Zouves Foundation for Reproductive Medicine and Zouves Fertility Center, 1241 East Hillsdale Blvd, Suite 100, Foster City, CA 94404, USA; manuel@zouvesfoundation.org

Received: 12 May 2020; Accepted: 27 May 2020; Published: 29 May 2020

Abstract: There is a high incidence of chromosomal abnormalities in early human embryos, whether they are generated by natural conception or by assisted reproductive technologies (ART). Cells with chromosomal copy number deviations or chromosome structural rearrangements can compromise the viability of embryos; much of the naturally low human fecundity as well as low success rates of ART can be ascribed to these cytogenetic defects. Chromosomal anomalies are also responsible for a large proportion of miscarriages and congenital disorders. There is therefore tremendous value in methods that identify embryos containing chromosomal abnormalities before intrauterine transfer to a patient being treated for infertility—the goal being the exclusion of affected embryos in order to improve clinical outcomes. This is the rationale behind preimplantation genetic testing for aneuploidy (PGT-A) and structural rearrangements (-SR). Contemporary methods are capable of much more than detecting whole chromosome abnormalities (e.g., monosomy/trisomy). Technical enhancements and increased resolution and sensitivity permit the identification of chromosomal mosaicism (embryos containing a mix of normal and abnormal cells), as well as the detection of sub-chromosomal abnormalities such as segmental deletions and duplications. Earlier approaches to screening for chromosomal abnormalities yielded a binary result of normal versus abnormal, but the new refinements in the system call for new categories, each with specific clinical outcomes and nuances for clinical management. This review intends to give an overview of PGT-A and -SR, emphasizing recent advances and areas of active development.

Keywords: PGT-A; PGT-SR; mosaicism; embryo genetics; chromosomal abnormality

1. Introduction

The modern fertility clinic aspires to achieve a healthy birth using a single embryo transfer (SET). Historically, the transfer of two or more embryos simultaneously was a common ART industry practice, at times resulting in multiple pregnancies and their associated clinical complications [1,2]. A patient's in vitro fertilization (IVF) treatment will frequently produce several embryos available for transfer, and the challenge becomes how best to rank a cohort of embryos in order of highest to lowest likelihood of success. The most rudimentary method to grade embryos is by their appearance, a practice that has been performed since the earliest days of IVF [3]. Although excellent standardization systems for an assessment of embryo morphology have been developed [4], the practice remains subjective, and morphology alone has been shown to be a limited predictor of implantation [5]. When it was understood that early human embryos often harbor chromosomal abnormalities, employing chromosomal profiling to deselect those with copy number and structural anomalies became an attractive prospect. The first application of chromosomal profiling in embryos was to determine their XX/XY status in patients with inherited X-linked conditions, by removing a representative cellular sample from each embryo and analyzing it with molecular methods [6]. This served as proof of concept that autosomal profiling could also become clinically applicable, setting the stage for the development of preimplantation genetic testing (PGT) for aneuploidy (-A) and structural rearrangements (-SR). Over the past two decades, the usage of PGT-A/-SR has experienced tremendous growth, and now accompanies a proportion of ART cycles in many parts of the world [7]. Vocal critics of the technology do exist, and as discussed below, not all clinical data from PGT-A have been positive. However, there are excellent arguments for the appropriate application of PGT-A when the limitations of the technology are understood.

At this point in time, PGT-A is experiencing a massive shift in how it categorizes embryos by their chromosomal profiles (Figure 1). A simple binary grouping of 'normal' or 'abnormal' has become insufficient. Recent data, which will be presented here, argues for a much more refined categorization, and encompasses embryos that are 'euploid', 'aneuploid' (whole chromosome, e.g., monosomy/trisomy), 'mosaic', and 'segmental abnormal'. Additionally, the mosaic and segmental abnormal groups can be refined further according to their characteristics. The goal of such stratification is to obtain an enhanced ranking system to permit selection of the embryo with best likelihood of a positive clinical outcome.

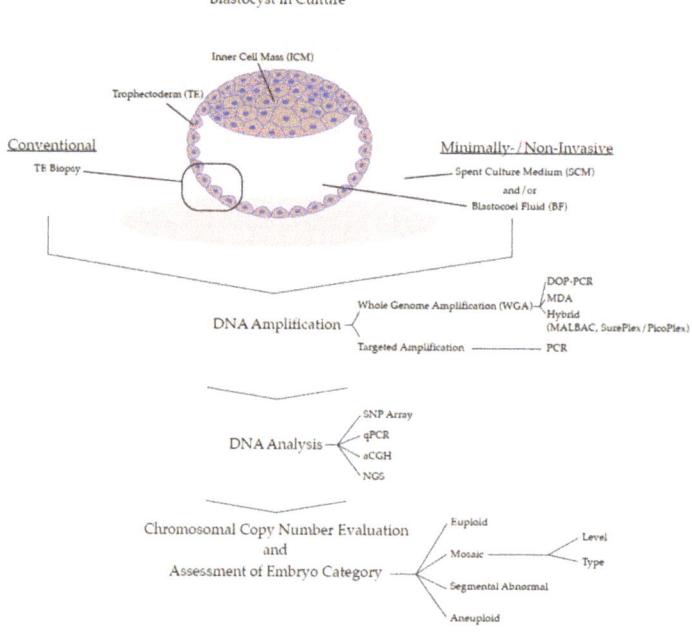

Figure 1. Overview of PGT Methods for 24-Chromosome Analysis.

From a technological standpoint, PGT-A is now coming to a watershed moment in its development and will be shaped by two seemingly opposing forces: simplicity and complexity (Figure 1). On one hand, there is a push to make the process easier, by developing a non-invasive version that would considerably simplify the sample collection step in the laboratory and make it available to a greater number of fertility clinics (but importantly, at the potential expense of data quality). On the other hand, there is demand for more complexity in the data by increasing the resolution of the genome, combining multiple genetic analyses (e.g., copy number and B-allele frequencies, or chromosomal and single gene profiling), or eventually sequencing the entire genome of a candidate embryo. Time will tell which path the technology will take, or whether several parallel versions of PGT-A will co-exist;

what is certain is that the 'genetic revolution' has already transformed embryo selection in IVF and will continue doing so for years to come.

2. Human Reproduction and Chromosomal Abnormalities

The extent to which chromosomal abnormality affects human reproduction is noteworthy. Natural fertility in humans follows an inverse U-curve during maternal reproductive years, and evidence shows that embryonic chromosomal abnormality originating from meiotic errors during oocyte formation is the main cause for the reduced potential toward both ends of the curve [8]. This phenomenon is specific to humans (e.g., chimpanzees' fertility potential remains uniform across maternal reproductive lifespan [9]), and is presumably linked to selective forces balancing risks and evolutionary fitness associated with human childbearing [8]. Even at the peak of a woman's fertility, the incidence of chromosomal abnormality is not negligible—on average affecting ~20% of oocytes [8]. As a result, roughly half of all human preimplantation embryos harbor chromosomal abnormalities [10–12], when in comparison only 1% of early mouse embryos are chromosomally abnormal [13].

Together, these observations suggest that some degree of error-proneness during chromosome segregation in gametogenesis is beneficial to our species. Embryonic chromosomal abnormality should therefore not be regarded as an aberration, but rather an integral and programmed component in the natural process of human reproduction. Further accentuating this point, there is no difference in rates of implantation, miscarriage, and live births between advanced maternal age (AMA) patients and non-AMA patients when chromosomally normal embryos are used for intrauterine transfer [14,15], meaning that the age-related decline in fertility is solely controlled by embryonic abnormality. For the sub-fertility and infertility patient attempting treatment through ART, this peculiarity of human reproduction poses significant problems. The transfer of chromosomally anomalous embryos in the IVF clinic results in failed implantation, miscarriage, or congenital conditions.

3. Overview of Chromosomal Abnormalities in Embryos: Types, Mechanisms, Incidence, and Medical Implications

3.1. Aneuploidy

Aneuploidy is the most common genetic abnormality found in humans, and its high incidence in embryos is the main cause for failed implantation, pregnancy loss, and congenital birth defects [16]. Diploid cells normally contain 46 chromosomes, a state known as euploidy. Aneuploidy is an altered condition involving a deviation in copy number from multiples of 23. Typical examples are monosomy or trisomy, respectively resulting in 45 or 47 chromosomes. Aneuploidy can affect numerous chromosomes in a cell, sometimes referred to as complex aneuploids, or result in nullisomy or polysomy, where none or multiple copies of an individual chromosomes are present.

Aneuploidy in preimplantation embryos is primarily a result of chromosomal/chromatid segregation errors occurring at meiosis (in sperm or egg), uniformly affecting all cells in resulting embryos. Those mechanisms can be broadly grouped into (1) Non-disjunction errors (where homologous chromosomes or sister chromatids fail to separate) and (2) Premature separation (where homologous chromosomes or sister chromatids separate early). A correctly functioning cohesion apparatus between paired entities is therefore vital to preserve euploidy. The vast majority of meiotic errors occur in maternal meiosis (90%–99%) [16,17], of which recent studies estimate ~50%–70% originate at meiosis I, and ~30%–50% at meiosis II [17–20]. Aneuploidy is far less likely to derive from meiotic events in the father, with estimates ranging between 1%–10% [17,21,22]. The dissimilarity in percent aneuploidies originating from female and male gametogenesis is ascribed to several differences which make meiosis in the oocyte more error-prone, including: (1) Oocyte crossover structures during recombination are more frail, (2) Subdued prophase checkpoint control, (3) Decreased efficiency of the spindle assembly checkpoint (SAC), (4) Lower requirements for chromosomal alignment in the spindle equator for onset of anaphase, and (5) Different cell cycle progression [16].

A large percentage of spontaneous abortions in natural and ART pregnancies are ascribed to aneuploidies, as highlighted by a recent study cytogenetically analyzing 2564 samples of fetal tissue from first trimester miscarriages, detecting abnormal karyotypes in 49.5% of cases [23]. Furthermore, about ~4% of stillbirths and ~0.3% of newborns harbor aneuploidies [24]. Because of the strong in utero selection against aneuploidy, its 'true' incidence is determined from studies in fertilized eggs, which is currently impossible for natural conceptions [16]. Overall, about half of ART-generated preimplantation embryos contain uniform aneuploidy when assessed by PGT-A [11,12,25], but there is a distinctive maternal age-related effect. Three studies, each analyzing over 12,000 human blastocysts from ART patients using different genetic testing platforms, came to comparable conclusions: average percent euploid embryos increased from ~60% to ~75% between maternal ages 22 and 28, dipping to ~60% by age 35, followed by a steady decline to ~40% by age 40 until reaching ~10% by age 45 [26–28]. Logically, the incidence of aneuploidy followed the inverse trend, exhibiting its lowest incidence of ~25% at ages 28–29, and a steep rise after age 35, reaching its peak of 90% at age 45 [27]. These observations were recently replicated by a large, single-reference laboratory analysis of over 100,000 blastocyst-stage embryos [11]. Mechanistically, this age-related increase in aneuploidy is thought to be an effect of the prolonged prophase I arrest in oocytes (a state that can last up to 50 years), which results in gradual degradation of the meiotic apparatus [29]. In contrast, the incidence of aneuploidy does not correlate with paternal age [30,31].

Embryonic aneuploidy is also believed to be affected by environmental factors. Some lifestyle conditions of parents, such as obesity, smoking, exposure to radiation, and use of contraceptives have been proposed as candidates to increase meiotic errors [30]. Another source is the hormonal stimulation protocol [32,33]. There is documented variability between IVF clinics in the percentage of aneuploid embryos that are generated [25], suggesting that protocols of oocyte retrieval, intracytoplasmic sperm injection (ICSI), and culture conditions might also contribute to the incidence of meiotic errors.

Aneuploidies analyzed at the blastocyst stage are not evenly distributed over the 23 sets of chromosomes. A review of 5,000 embryos showed that aneuploidies in chromosomes 15, 16, 21, and 22 (relatively small chromosomes) were the most common, while those in chromosomes 1 to 6 (the largest autosomes) were the least common, although by and large the incidence of monosomies and trisomies at this developmental stage were quite similar [30]. A clear exception was chromosome 9, for which trisomies far offset monosomies [30], possibly indicating the presence of genes with essential dosage effects for early development.

All autosomal monosomies and most autosomal trisomies are embryonic lethal, the exceptions being trisomies 13, 18, and 21 which occasionally lead to births resulting in Patau, Edwards, and Down's Syndromes, respectively. The fact that Down's patients can survive well into adulthood suggests that merely having an abnormal chromosomal copy number might not affect viability per se, and rather, it is abnormal transcriptional dosage of genes located in the affected chromosome that compromises development [34]. Incidentally, chromosome 21 is comparatively small and contains relatively few genes, possibly explaining the long-term survival of cells harboring the abnormality. Aneuploidies affecting the sex chromosomes can have a range of clinical implications from undetectable to severe or lethal, depending on the copy number and chromosome affected; 47,XXX and 47,XYY typically result in phenotypically normal females and males, 45,X and 47,XXY lead to Turner and Klinefelter Syndromes, but the X chromosome is absolutely essential as its absence invariably leads to embryonic demise. The absence of one entire set of chromosomes (haploidy) in embryos, or the presence of extra sets (polyploidy), is incompatible with human life. However, it must be noted that these conditions do not fall under the strict definition of aneuploidy (as their chromosomal counts result in multiples of 23).

3.2. Chromosomal Mosaicism

The definition of chromosomal mosaicism is the co-presence of cells with two (or more) different chromosomal constitutions. In the context of PGT-A, the most relevant type is the mix of euploid and aneuploid cells (sometimes referred to as diploid-aneuploid mosaics, hereafter simply referred to as mosaic) because in recent years such embryos have been shown to result in healthy pregnancies when transferred in the clinic [35–40].

Mosaicism originates from mitotic events during post-zygotic development. The best characterized types of mitotic errors resulting in mosaicism are sister chromatid malsegregations [12]: anaphase lagging, mainly resulting in one normal and one monosomic daughter cell (although other patterns of chromosomal inheritance are possible [41]), and non-disjunction, leading to reciprocal trisomic and monosomic daughter cells. Other types of mitotic error resulting in mosaicism are endoreplication, (a diploid cell becomes trisomic by excessive replication of a chromosome), formation of micronuclei (the aberrant establishment of independent nuclear membrane-encapsulated chromosomal material), and centriole/centrosome dysregulation affecting chromatid segregation [42].

The observation that monosomies are commonly found without reciprocal trisomies in mosaic embryos indicates that anaphase lagging might be more frequent than non-disjunction during mitotic errors [43,44]. All these events are mainly attributed to three factors associated with preimplantation embryos: Relaxed control of the cell cycle, aberrations of the centrosome and mitotic spindle, and defects in chromosome cohesion [45]. Cell intrinsic regulation, correction mechanisms, and cell cycle checkpoints are subdued during the first days of post-zygotic development, which is characterized by rapid expansion governed by a strained system of maternal factors before activation of the embryonic genome [45,46]. In this regard, early embryos are comparable to cancers, which experience dysregulated cell cycle control and high rates of aneuploidy [34].

Embryonic mosaicism was first described in 1993 by Delhanty and colleagues performing fluorescent in situ hybridization (FISH) in cleavage-stage embryos, observing different chromosomal counts between cells of a single conceptus [47]. The same phenomenon was also described later in blastocysts by Evsikov and Verlinsky [48]. Modern PGT-A methods can detect mixes of euploid and aneuploid cells with high accuracy, but there is variability between clinics regarding the reported incidence of embryos classified as mosaic with PGT-A at the blastocyst stage. Most recent estimates range between 4%–22% [38,40,49–51]. The reasons for this variation are biological (conditions in laboratories affecting rates of mosaicism) [46,51], as well as technical (lack of standardized system to interpret and report PGT-A results); discussed further below. Estimating rates of mosaicism in preimplantation embryos from natural conceptions is challenging, but observations made in bovine cleavage-stage embryos have revealed that in vitro production engenders a significantly higher incidence of mosaicism than in vivo conception [52]. However, karyotype analysis of neonate umbilical cord blood and placenta showed no difference in rate of mosaicism between samples of natural and IVF conceptions in humans [53].

Contrary to meiotic errors and their age-related accumulation, there appears to be a uniform baseline risk for mitotic errors throughout the maternal reproductive years [54]. Nonetheless, there is a demonstrated reduction in incidence of mosaicism between cleavage and blastocyst stages [54], which further declines through gestation. Mosaicism is detected in ~2.1% of chorionic villus samples (CVS), which tests placental cells [23], and < 0.2% of newborns are estimated to be mosaic, although this is difficult to assess since routine karyotyping of newborns is not performed [49,55]. The attrition of mosaicism through development indicates the presence of selective forces that either cause mosaic embryos to perish, or elicit preferential demise of aneuploid cells in mosaic concepti.

Whether a mitotic error occurs early in development or later influences the percent of cells in the conceptus that contain the abnormality; the closer to the zygote stage, the higher the number of cell divisions that can propagate the aneuploidy. The load of abnormal cells is likely to influence the survival of embryos. Bolton and colleagues have used murine chimera experiments to model mosaicism, showing that embryos with high aneuploid load invariably died [56]. However, embryos with low aneuploid load survived and eliminated abnormal cells by apoptosis in the inner cell mass (ICM, the precursor to the fetus) or attenuated proliferation in the trophectoderm (TE, the precursor to the placenta). This is in accordance with the well-documented fact that aneuploidy generally hinders rates of cell proliferation [34]. A recent study by Mashiko and colleagues used live imaging on an engineered mouse strain with fluorescent nuclei and captured, for the first time, spontaneous mitotic errors and the establishment of mosaicism in developing preimplantation embryos [57]. They observed a correlation between the severity of aneuploidy in the abnormal cell compartment and likelihood to arrest before reaching the blastocyst stage. When transferred, murine blastocysts with visually-confirmed mosaicism resulted in births of healthy pups, suggesting a negative selection against the aneuploid cells through gestation [57]. Extended in vitro culture experiments by Popovic and colleagues with 18 mosaic human blastocysts showed that 58% remained viable in Day 12 outgrowths, of which 80% had resolved the mosaicism and presented euploid profiles, while 20% retained the mosaicism [58]. A mechanism of targeted apoptosis and/or proliferative out-competition of aneuploid cells by euploid cells could explain how a mosaic human embryo might become a healthy baby, as aneuploid cells are effectively diluted out in the course of development. In point of fact, experiments using immunofluorescence have shown significantly different patterns of mitosis and cell death between euploid and mosaic embryos [40], presumably reflecting a process in mosaic embryos of purging aneuploid cells by their directed demise and compensatory proliferation of euploid cells.

An alternative mechanism for the generation of mosaic embryos has been proposed, in which a meiotic error in germ cells could be followed by a mitotic event post-zygotically, 'correcting' the initial aneuploidy. Processes of such intra-cellar correction have been proposed, in which trisomic cells lose the extra chromosome (trisomic rescue) or monosomic cells duplicate the singular chromosome to restore disomy (endoreplication). To date, while one study reported evidence of trisomic rescue pre-zygotically (in oocytes, where a meiosis I error was corrected at meiosis II) [59], such mechanisms have not been convincingly demonstrated in human embryos. These hypothetical events would often result in uniparental disomy (UPD), which in IVF embryos is extremely rare, estimated at 0.06% [60]. Experimental data from extended in vitro culture experiments suggest the contrary, that uniform (non-mosaic) euploid or aneuploid embryos tend to maintain their initial ploidy in both ICM and TE lineages [58]. An embryo with aneuploidy stemming from a meiotic event is therefore bound to retain the chromosomal abnormality and result in failed implantation, miscarriage, or liveborn syndrome.

The medical consequence of mosaicism is a subject of current investigation. Regarding clinical outcomes, recent data indicate that mosaic preimplantation embryos can result in successful pregnancies and healthy births, but at lower rates compared to euploid embryos [35–40]. In gestation, mosaicism is implicated in confined placental mosaicism (CPM), where cells with different ploidy are present specifically in the placenta and fetal cells are normal. The majority of pregnancies diagnosed with CPM continue to term with no complications [61], but some result in intrauterine growth retardation (IUGR), placental insufficiency, and potentially miscarriage [62,63]. The real medical meaning of mosaicism in newborns and adults remains elusive. On one hand, chromosomal mosaicism has been associated with various conditions, including psychiatric disorders, autoimmune disease, and congenital malformations [64]. On the other hand, there is a documented high incidence of mosaicism in various tissues of healthy persons including brain, blood, and skin [65,66].

3.3. Segmental Abnormalities

Segmental abnormalities (sometimes referred to as partial aneuploidies or structural aberrations) affect sub-chromosomal sections, and in the context of PGT-A they typically denote regional losses or gains. The size of a segmental abnormality detectable by modern PGT-A platforms is usually 10–20 Mb and above [67,68], but in some instances the identified segments are as small as 1.8 Mb [69].

Segmental abnormalities originate from faulty corrections of chromosome breakage, so their etiology is altogether different to that of whole chromosome aneuploidies. Double strand breaks (DSBs) occur during DNA synthesis when replicative forks stall and collapse, for reasons such as DNA damage, absence of DNA-synthesis constituents, or strain associated with DNA secondary structure [70,71]. In gametes, there are programmed strand breaks to enable meiotic recombination, which can go awry and result in chromosomal breakage [72]. DSBs can also result from exogenous factors such as oxidative stress or the effect of mutagens. Generally, DSBs elicit a DNA repair mechanism, and failure to execute it typically activates the apoptotic process [73]. Those pathways are often compromised in preimplantation embryos, which are characterized by rapid cell division, compromised repair mechanisms, lax cell cycle checkpoints, and deregulated apoptosis [74]. When a cell 'repairs' a DSB incorrectly, it can result in duplication or deletion of the segment containing the break.

Segmental copy number variants can originate pre- or post-zygotically, respectively affecting all embryonic cells or only a subset. An estimated ~32% of segmental abnormality is meiotic in nature and present throughout the cells of the remaining blastocyst [75], meaning that the majority of instances are of mitotic origin and present in a mosaic pattern [75,76]. Segmental abnormalities can occur in any chromosome, their incidence across the genome largely correlates with chromosomal size, and the frequency of losses and gains is roughly equal [75]. One possible outlier is the high incidence of segmental gains in the q-arm of chromosome (Chr) 9 [74,75]. A study has described loci in the genome of preimplantation embryos with higher likelihood of segmental abnormalities, possibly related to heterochromatic composition of those regions [70].

Approximately ~6%–15% of ART-created blastocysts contain segmental abnormalities when evaluated by current PGT-A methods with the described resolution, either exclusively or in conjunction with whole chromosome aneuploidies [70,74,75]. When only considering instances with no concomitant whole chromosome aneuploidy, the incidence of blastocysts with segmental losses or gains is ~2.4%–7.5% [11,70,74,75]. Incidence of segmental abnormalities in blastocysts do not correlate with medical indication or patient age [70,74,75]. Segmental abnormalities are thought to account for 6% of clinical miscarriages [77] and affect close to 0.05% of newborns [78]. In persisting to term, segmental copy number variants can result in various syndromes and conditions, for example Cri-du-chat (caused by terminal deletion in the p arm of Chr 5), or Charcot–Marie–Tooth disease type 1A (caused by an interstitial duplication in the p arm of Chr 12) [79].

3.4. Structural Rearrangements

Balanced translocations, Robertsonian translocations, insertions, and inversions are abnormalities that change the natural order of chromosomal segments, but leave copy numbers unaltered. Carriers of such anomalies are typically asymptomatic, but recombination and sorting at meiosis can produce chromosomal copy number abnormalities in egg and sperm. This results in fertility problems, increased likelihood of pregnancy loss, and heightened chances of producing offspring with physical and mental disabilities. Therefore, whereas PGT-A is a screening tool for chromosomal abnormalities that arise spontaneously, PGT-SR is a targeted test performed when known chromosomal abnormalities are present in parental genomes. PGT-SR requires a personalized review of parental karyotypes, as the resulting cohort of embryos are tested for instances of recombination producing unbalanced chromosomal configurations in at-risk regions. Occasionally, PGT-SR is also performed when a familial abnormality involves segmental copy number variants, typically with small deletions and duplications that result in relatively mild symptoms in prospective parents. Individualized case evaluation determines whether a given PGT platform has the resolution to detect copy number alterations for a specific segment.

Most PGT-SR is performed with standard PGT-A platforms (as long as the affected regions are above the platform's resolution) as embryos with unbalanced translocations can be identified by displaying segmental losses or gains in the regions involved in the translocation. Nonetheless, this type of PGT-SR cannot distinguish between those embryos in a cohort that are euploid and those that carry the balanced translocation. Although replacing balanced embryos should result in phenotypically normal births, the offspring will, later in life, encounter the same problems as their carrier parents, including reduced fertility, increased miscarriages, and having affected children. A more sophisticated version of PGT-SR can differentiate between euploid and balanced embryos, by analyzing the sequences or genetic markers in/around breakpoint regions [80–83]. Although much more involved than routine PGT-SR, this method can be opted for when patients want to preclude the transfer of balanced embryos, or when the reciprocal translocation affects the X chromosome, considering that the phenotype of balanced carriers is unpredictable due to random inactivation of one X chromosome in female embryos [84].

4. Development of PGT for Chromosomal Abnormalities

4.1. Early Methods of PGT-A

The first clinical instance of chromosomal profiling in human embryos occurred in 1990, but not for aneuploidy [6]. Handyside and colleagues analyzed individual blastomeres of cleavage-stage embryos (Day 3 post fertilization) from a mother that carried a X-linked condition, and amplified a Y-specific repeat sequence using polymerase chain reaction (PCR). In 1992, fluorescent in situ hybridization (FISH) using X- and Y- probes were used in the clinic, again to treat families at risk of transmitting sex-linked disorders [85]. The first direct investigation of embryonic aneuploidy occurred in 1993, using a FISH test for chromosomes with known liveborn syndromes (13, 18, and 21) in addition to the sex chromosomes (X, Y) [47,86,87]. This was the birth moment of PGT-A and PGT-SR. FISH can be adapted to examine several regions within a single chromosome by using multiple probes, for example, by simultaneously using one centromeric and two sub-telomeric probes. This is applicable for patients carrying balanced translocations, identifying the embryos that inherited the translocation in an unbalanced way.

Over the two decades that followed, cleavage-stage PGT-A by FISH grew as an adjunct to the IVF cycle under the recommendations to transfer normal embryos and discard abnormal embryos. Nonetheless, the technology remained limited by the number of chromosomes each test could examine. Although some groups have been successful at implementing this technology clinically to examine up to 12 chromosomes at once [88], this still left half of the chromosomes undiagnosed. This important limitation, as well as the demanding nature of the technique, has led to FISH being largely replaced with other PGT-A platforms. FISH still plays a role in some specific PGT-SR cases, for example, in instances of very distal breakpoints, such that conventional PCR-based methods are inadequate [89]. Furthermore, blastomere collection at the cleavage stage has the potential to decrease embryo viability [90], encouraging development of biopsy isolation techniques at other embryonic timepoints.

Another potential source of genetic material to be evaluated both in its effect on embryo viability and its ability to reflect the chromosomal constitution of the resulting embryo was that of polar bodies (PBs) [91]. Most aneuploidies originate from meiotic errors in the female, such that the PB can contain the reciprocal aneuploidy to that of the associated oocyte (or zygote). For example, in a non-disjunction event, a PB could contain monosomy 21 while the oocyte contains trisomy 21. Nonetheless, many types of aneuploidy in the embryo would not be detected by this method (non-reciprocal aneuploidies, paternal meiotic errors, mitotic events). Furthermore, given that 30%–50% of oocyte-derived chromosomal imbalances originate at the second meiotic division [19,20], there is a necessity to analyze both PBs, considerably increasing the cost of the procedure. In addition, a number of studies investigating PGT-A based on PB analysis have shown high rates of false results [19,92], and negative impact on embryo viability [93]. Irrespective of these caveats, PB analysis persists in countries that legally restrict direct embryo testing [7].

Together, these shortcomings of the original, FISH-based version of the technology (sometimes referred to as PGS 1.0), combined with clinical analyses showing poor performance [94], set the stage for the development of 24-chromosome analysis.

4.2. Development of PGT-A for All Chromosomes

Expansion of the system to investigate all chromosomes (sometimes referred to as PGT-A 2.0) was transformative to the field. A diploid human cell contains approximately 6.6 picograms of DNA, which is too little (even when 5–10 cells are collected in a biopsy) to perform molecular analysis by conventional approaches. The key step was the development of amplification methods that multiplied the DNA in the biopsy. This process has been dubbed whole genome amplification (WGA), and generates sufficient DNA with appropriate genome coverage for full 24 chromosome analysis. Several chemistries have been developed or adapted for this purpose, each with its strengths and weaknesses: Degenerate oligonucleotide primed PCR (DOP-PCR), multiple displacement amplification (MDA), and hybrid methods, including multiple annealing and looping based amplification cycles (MALBAC), and SurePlex/PicoPlex, all comprehensively reviewed and compared before [95,96]. Once the DNA is amplified, it can be used for varying methods of downstream analysis: comparative genome hybridization (CGH) [97,98], arrayed CGH (aCGH) [99,100], single nucleotide polymorphism (SNP) arrays [101], or next generation sequencing (NGS) [67,102]. Ultimately, their goal is one and the same; revealing aneuploidy by identifying regions of the genome that are under- or overrepresented. Another strategy, known as targeted amplification, involves PCR-based replication of strategic regions spread out across the genome. The products can subsequently be quantified by quantitative PCR (qPCR), or by sequencing [103,104]. In comparison to WGA methods of PGT-A, targeted amplification can increase sequencing depth in the targeted regions, but might do so at the expense of breadth of genomic coverage.

At present, the optimal PGT-A solution lies at the intersection between sequence information (coverage breadth and depth) and cost/ease of use. Among all the options, WGA-based NGS has emerged as the most popular method across the PGT-A landscape. The technique has low depth of sequencing, but relatively high breadth of genome coverage, which is suitable for copy number analysis. Decreasing cost of sequencing might make true, 'deep' whole genome sequencing for each embryo a reality in the future.

4.3. Contemporary PGT-A

In recent years, there has been a progressive, worldwide move toward biopsy collection at the blastocyst stage [7], where cells are removed from the TE (the precursor to the placenta). Isolation of a TE biopsy was first described in 1990 by Dokras and colleagues [105]. Since then, different approaches have been described and are continuously being evaluated and refined, for example the use of assisted hatching or laser manipulation [5,106–111]. Two advances in embryology have made the shift to the blastocyst stage possible. One was the development of more physiological culture media, making it possible to consistently grow embryos to the blastocyst stage [112,113]. The other was an improved cryopreservation method of rapid freezing (known as vitrification), which ensures very high survival of blastocysts [114]. Together, they have made it possible to grow embryos until days 5, 6 or 7 post fertilization, at which point TE biopsies are collected and blastocysts are vitrified and stored until PGT-A results are available and transfer is scheduled.

Collecting a blastocyst-stage TE biopsy is advantageous compared to a single blastomere (or two) at the cleavage stage, for several reasons, including: (1) A TE biopsy removes a smaller percentage of the total cells of the embryo, and only detaches cells destined to become placenta as opposed to fetal tissue, (2) Analyzing the content of 5–10 cells provides more DNA, decreasing the chances of failed reactions and technical artifacts due amplification bias or allele drop out (ADO) [115,116], (3) Assessing a group of cells of the TE makes it possible to detect mosaicism within the biopsy, (4) The documented attrition of inviable embryos between cleavage and blastocyst stage [15] translates into fewer unnecessary tests, and (5) The particularly high incidence of mosaicism at the cleavage stage [97], which becomes partly resolved by the blastocyst stage [117], reduces the likelihood of false results.

If performed properly by trained hands, surgically removing 5–10 TE cells is not thought to affect blastocyst viability in an appreciable manner. Perhaps the best evidence comes from an elegant double embryo transfer experiment with blastocyst pairs of similar grade, in which only one blastocyst underwent biopsy collection, showed equal likelihood of implantation [90]. Recently it was reported that even repeat biopsies with two subsequent freeze-thaw cycles did not significantly affect embryo viability [118]. Conceptually those findings are not entirely surprising, considering that monozygotic twinning arises from a split of an embryo at the blastocyst stage, meaning that half of the cells in the blastocyst (TE and ICM) are sufficient to sustain normal fetal development.

The PGT-A technology that is currently most widespread is WGA, followed by NGS [67]. Compared to aCGH, its popular predecessor, WGA-based NGS is thought to provide superior resolution and dynamic range [76,119,120], resulting in improved rates of favorable outcomes in the clinic [38,121–123]. Analysis at the blastocyst-stage involves pooling DNA from 5–10 cells in the TE biopsy. The bioinformatic analysis of resulting data produces a representative average karyotype profile encompassing all 24 chromosomes. A relatively low coverage sequencing (with ≤0.1× depth) suffices for robust chromosomal copy number analysis [102,124], explaining why prevalent NGS-based PGT-A methods are occasionally said to use 'low-pass' or 'shallow' sequencing. Reads are aligned to a human refence genome and grouped together into 'bins' spread out over the chromosomes. The karyotype profiles indicate the copy number for each bin, which can be uniform along a chromosome or variable, indicating segmental abnormalities. Clear nullisomies, monosomies, disomies, trisomies, tetrasomies, and so forth produce data aligning to respective copy numbers 0,1,2,3,4 etc. Profiles with values falling between whole numbers are consistent with intra-blastocyst mosaicism. For example, values aligning at 2.5 for a chromosome are consistent with a 50% mix of cells with disomy and trisomy in the TE biopsy. Currently, many laboratories utilize the 20%–80% span in karyotype profiles to define a region consistent with mosaicism [125]. When values deviate <20% from whole numbers, they are not considered in the mosaic region because they fall inside the normal noise range. Numerous groups have performed detailed mixing experiments of DNA or cells with different karyotypes to model mosaicism, generally finding that WGA-based NGS is excellent at identifying it in whole chromosomes as well as segmental regions [37,39,40,76,126,127].

It must be noted that technical noise, artifacts of imperfect WGA or sequencing reactions, and suboptimal biopsy collection techniques, might also result in profiles that falsely indicate mosaicism [116]. When results appear noisy the confidence of identifying true intra-blastocyst mosaicism is compromised. Currently there are no guidelines for how to deal with such cases. In addition, a TE biopsy containing cells with reciprocal aneuploidies (due to sister chromatid non-disjunction) might yield skewed results, including possibly a disomic looking karyotype and concealing an instance of mosaicism [128]. The probability of such an event is currently unknown but likely to be small, particularly considering that reciprocal aneuploidies are not the predominant pattern of mosaicism in embryos [43,44].

Most modern PGT-A platforms are validated to detect segmental copy number variants of 10–20 Mb or larger, but often have the capability to detect smaller segment variants, some as small as 1.8 Mb [69,76,129]. The resolution is crucial for detection of segmental losses or gains associated with characterized newborn syndromes, of which the majority are in the 1–10 Mb range [130]. Some are even smaller, warranting future efforts to further increase the resolution of routine PGT-A (see Section 7.2).

5. Considerations on the Clinical Use of PGT for Chromosomal Abnormalities

5.1. How Reliable Is PGT-A?

There is broad consensus that contemporary PGT-A methods are superbly robust at evaluating the content of the input material. Consistency in results can be confirmed by re-sequencing WGA material from TE biopsies, or re-amplifying and sequencing aliquots of DNA or cells from lines with known karyotypes. This type of exercise typically indicates near 100% technical accuracy [67,76,100–103]. However, there are potential biological sources of error in PGT-A that must be taken into consideration. A human blastocyst is comprised of 64–128 cells (equaling 6–7 post-fertilization cell divisions) [131], meaning that a 5–10 cell TE biopsy contains 3.9% to 15.6% of all cells in the conceptus. Due to chromosomal mosaicism, a concern is that the TE biopsy is an imperfect representative of the embryo [55]. Thus, even when PGT-A accurately reflects the content of the TE biopsy, the result is meaningless if the TE biopsy is a poor proxy for the associated blastocyst.

Estimating the incidence of false results due to embryo-scale mosaicism has been the goal of several studies–even in the era of FISH and aCGH (comprehensively summarized by Capalbo and Rienzi [132]), broadly showing high concordance rates between TE and ICM. A number of recent publications have conducted serial biopsy experiments in blastocysts donated to research using NGS-based PGT-A. Evaluation of concordance between samples can be computed in two ways: Ploidy concordance (compares overall status of euploidy/mosaicism/aneuploidy) or full karyotype concordance (compares chromosomal profiles to evaluate if they are identical). For example, two biopsies can be aneuploid (ploidy concordant) but contain different aneuploidies (full karyotype discordant).

Huang and colleagues analyzed ICM and four TE biopsies in 44 blastocysts originally categorized as whole chromosome aneuploid (e.g., monosomy/trisomy), observing all were aneuploid in the four biopsies (100% ploidy concordance) [133]. There was perfect karyotype concordance amongst the four biopsies in 39 blastocysts (88.6% full karyotype concordance). In 7 blastocysts with original categorization of segmental abnormality, ploidy concordance was 100% but full karyotype concordance was reduced to 57.4% [133]. A study by Sachdev and colleagues investigated 32 blastocysts and calculated per chromosome concordances between TE biopsy and ICM biopsy, determining rates of 99.5% for euploid results, 97.3% for aneuploid results, but only 35.2% for mosaic results [134]. A study by Lawrenz and colleagues compared PGT-A results from three biopsies for each of the 84 embryos included in the study: one blastomere biopsy, one TE biopsy, and one ICM biopsy [135]. The ploidy concordance between the blastomere and ICM was 69.8% for aneuploidy and 90.3% for euploidy, but concordance was higher between TE and ICM, namely 92.5% for aneuploidy and 93.2% for euploidy. Discordance between TE and ICM largely stemmed from the detection of structural abnormalities in either of the lineages. Of the blastomere-ICM discordances, 84.2% had an aneuploid blastomere but a euploid ICM, and 78.6% of times the matching TE biopsy did reflect the euploidy of the ICM. Thus, the findings of the Lawrenz study showed that a TE biopsy is a superior representative of the ICM (which will become the fetus) to a cleavage-stage biopsy.

Of note, the Huang, Sachdev, and Lawrenz studies did not consider intra-biopsy mosaicism, so ploidy was euploid/aneuploid binary (in which case typically low mosaic profiles become categorized as euploid and high mosaic profiles become categorized as aneuploid). The next set of studies considered mosaicism within individual biopsies. A study by Victor and colleagues compared a TE biopsy to its paired ICM, and observed that in 90 out of 93 blastocysts, a TE biopsy containing whole chromosome aneuploidy corresponded to whole chromosome aneuploidy in the ICM (96.8% ploidy concordance) [136]. In one case the ICM was euploid, and in two cases the ICM was mosaic. However, when considering TE biopsies with exclusively segmental abnormalities, the same study observed ploidy concordance with the ICM in only 2 out of 7 cases [136]. In another study, the same group re-biopsied embryos with an initial mosaic profile in the TE, and observed that the mosaicism was only reflected in 3 out of 8 cases (out of which two contained the reciprocal error) (40).

Popovic and colleagues analyzed two sets of blastocysts [126]. The first set had an original TE biopsy PGT-A result, which when compared to the ICM showed high concordance for whole chromosome aneuploidy (10 out of 10 samples) and segmental abnormality (6 out of 6). However, when the initial TE biopsy was mosaic, concordance with the ICM was seen in only 1 out of 4 samples, as the other 3 had euploid ICMs. For segmental mosaic TE biopsies, the ICM was aneuploid in 1 out of 4 samples, and the other 3 had euploid ICMs. The second set of blastocysts in the study had not been subjected to PGT-A in the clinic, and serial biopsies (1 ICM and 4 TE) were collected for each. Out of 21 blastocysts with a euploid ICM, 14 had perfect ploidy concordance in all biopsies (66.7%), while the remaining 32.3% had ploidy discordance in at least one TE biopsy. When excluding abnormalities of mosaic or segmental nature, the ploidy concordance across all biopsies increased to 95.2% of blastocysts. Out of 10 blastocysts with uniform (non-mosaic) aneuploidy in the ICM, 80%

were aneuploid across all TE biopsies. Finally, out of 3 blastocysts with a mosaic ICM, all three had at least one euploid TE biopsy.

Navratil and colleagues compared a TE biopsy to the entire embryo, observing euploidy concordance in 18 out of 19 blastocysts (94.7%), and whole chromosome aneuploidy concordance in 58 out of 62 blastocysts (93.5%) [137]. Segmental abnormalities showed significantly reduced concordance, as it was only detected in 14 out of 31 blastocysts (45.2%), and mosaic TE biopsies correctly predicted the equivalent mosaicism in the remaining blastocyst in 7 out of 26 instances (26.9%) [137].

Ou and colleagues focused entirely on segmental abnormalities and reported concordance between original TE biopsy and entire embryo in 43 out of 63 cases (68%) [138] When a similar experiment was conducted by Girardi and colleagues with multifocal biopsies, this time collecting four TE biopsies and an ICM biopsy for each blastocyst, it was observed that segmental losses or gains in any single TE biopsy were predictive of the ICM ~50% of times, but only ~32% of embryos contained the same segmental abnormality in all five biopsies [75]. In stark contrast, that same group found there to be discordance of whole chromosome aneuploidy in only 4 out of 390 (~1%) analyzed TE-ICM pairs [75], although it must be noted that the study did not consider intra-biopsy mosaicism.

Another potential source of biological error in PGT-A is the cell-cycle state of the probed cells. The worry revolves around S-phase, when DNA is replicated in a way that is not even across the genome and begins multifocally in tens of thousands of genomic regions called origin of replication. The resulting PGT-A profile of a single cell in S-phase could theoretically produce false positive profiles consistent with segmental abnormalities [139]. All cells in a TE biopsy would need to be synchronized and spontaneously engage the same origin of replication (something that is highly variable among cells [140]) to falsely mimic a uniform segmental gain, which is implausible. Nonetheless, including one or more cells in S-phase in the biopsy could conceptionally result in 'noisy' profiles [141], possibly consistent with mosaic profiles. However, a study by Ramos and colleagues on cell lines and embryos has shown that this effect is negligible with contemporary WGA methods for PGT-A [142].

The emerging theme from this set of combined findings is that a single TE biopsy detecting either uniform euploidy or whole chromosome aneuploidy is an excellent predictor of the state of the remaining embryo (likely reflecting a meiotic error), but segmental abnormalities and intra-biopsy mosaicism (mitotic error) have a vastly reduced predictive power.

5.2. Discussion on the Clinical Merits of PGT-A

After the development of FISH-based PGT-A, a collection of studies describing its use in the clinic propelled the adoption of the technology [143–146]. However, a number of randomized control trials (RCTs) published between 2004 and 2010 produced controversial results regarding its effect on clinical outcomes, and a comprehensive meta-analysis performed by Mastenbroek and colleagues in 2011 ultimately showed no benefit of PGT-A, and even described a detrimental effect [94]. This was true for all patient groups analyzed: good prognosis, advanced maternal age, and repeat implantation failure. The findings were mainly ascribed to four principal limitations of PGT-A at the time: (1) FISH only evaluated a subset of chromosomes, (2) Biopsy of one cell (or two) at the cleavage stage, a preimplantation timepoint with a particularly high incidence of mosaicism [146,147], potentially leading to false results, (3) Harm done to the embryo by removing a considerable portion of its biomass, (4) Technical challenges of producing clear results by FISH on a single cell. While a subsequent RCT by Rubio and colleagues showed a positive effect in AMA patients [148], the findings of the Mastenbroek meta-analysis in 2011 largely discredited FISH-based PGT-A [94]. However, almost concurrently to its publication, new technologies permitting 24-chromosome analysis in blastocysts were validated and launched for clinical use [98].

Since the advent of 24-chromosome PGT-A, an extensive body of evidence, encompassing numerous observational studies and RCTs, describes the benefits of the technology on clinical outcomes. Some of the most prominent are highlighted here.

The first RCT in the era of 24-chromosome analysis was published in 2012 by Yang and colleagues, where aCGH-based PGT-A and morphology assessment were used in one arm of the study (group A, n = 425 blastocysts), compared to morphology assessment alone in the other arm (group B, n = 389 blastocysts) [149]. Participants were all good-prognosis patients under 35 years old, and received fresh single embryo transfer (SET) at day 6. Group A had a better implantation rate than group B (70.9% and 45.8%, respectively; p = 0.017), as well as higher ongoing pregnancy rate (69.1% vs. 41.7%, respectively; p = 0.009).

That same year (2012), Scott and colleagues published a 'non-selection' study using a SNP array platform in which 255 cleavage- or blastocyst-stage embryos were evaluated by PGT-A, but results were only unblinded after clinical outcomes were known [150]. They observed a high predictive value for aneuploid results, with 96% of embryos designated as aneuploid failing to sustain implantation, while embryos classified as euploid resulted in sustained implantation 41% of times, which was significantly higher than the 28.2% overall rate of all embryos transferred.

In 2013, Scott and colleagues performed an RCT using qPCR and fresh embryo transfers, showing that the 134 blastocysts in the PGT-A group had a significantly higher sustained implantation rate compared to the 163 blastocysts in the control group (66.4% vs. 47.9%, respectively), as well as higher delivery rates from the group of embryos that implanted (84.7% vs 67.5%) [151].

Forman and colleagues published a noninferiority RCT in 2013, comparing the transfer of 89 single euploid blastocyst evaluated by qPCR compared with transfer of 86 pairs of unscreened blastocysts [152]. Ongoing pregnancy rates were comparable between the two arms (60.7% vs. 65.1%, respectively), but importantly the PGT-A arm did not experience any multiple pregnancies compared to the 53.4% incidence observed in the control arm, thereby demonstrating that an important complication of IVF could be eliminated without compromising success rates.

In 2015, two separate meta-analyses performed by the teams of Dahdouh [153] and Chen [154] evaluated the three blastocyst-stage RCTs detailed above and eight observational studies, clearly demonstrating the global positive impact of 24-chromosome PGT-A on clinical outcomes. Since then, a noteworthy large observational-cohort study in AMA patients published in 2019 by Sacchi and colleagues included the comparison of a blastocyst-stage qPCR PGT-A group (n = 201) with a blastocyst-stage group without PGT-A (n = 1,147), showing significantly increased live birth rate per transfer with PGT-A (40.3% vs. 23.4%, respectively) and lower miscarriage rate (3.6% vs. 23.4%, respectively) [155].

Furthermore, 24-chromosome PGT-A has also shown substantial benefits at non-blastocyst stages. An RCT published in 2017 on cleavage stage embryos conducted by Rubio and colleagues included 100 AMA patients in the aCGH PGT-A arm and 105 AMA patients in the control arm, and showed overall improved outcomes in the PGT-A group, including lower miscarriage rates (2.7% vs. 39% for control) and increased rate of delivery after first transfer attempt per patient (36.0% vs. 21.9%), significantly decreasing the number of transfers needed and time to pregnancy [156]. In a randomized clinical trial from 2018, Verpoest and colleagues showed benefits of aCGH PGT-A of PBs [157]. In total, 249 embryos with associated PB evaluation resulted in 50 live births (20.1%), compared to 440 of embryos with no PB evaluation resulting in 45 live births (10.2%). These findings are particularly important for countries that forbid culturing embryos to the blastocyst stage [7].

It has become evident that the transfer of a chromosomally normal embryo does not guarantee a favorable outcome, as other factors (e.g. maternal, environmental) influence its fate. Still, by 2019 the preponderance of data from 24-chromosome PGT-A had shown that excluding aneuploid embryos from transfer improved rates of positive outcome. The most recently published RCT used NGS technology [50]; however, it did not reveal any benefit to the overall patient population in the study. Those findings are discussed next.

5.3. A Note on the STAR Study

The much anticipated 'Single Embryo Transfer of Euploid Embryo' (STAR) study [50], a multicenter RCT, utilized a technical platform (NGS) and timepoint of biopsy collection (blastocyst stage) that, by current standards, should in principle exhibit the maximal benefit of PGT-A. Considering the overwhelmingly positive results from the previous 24-chromosome PGT-A RCTs (with perhaps less favorable conditions), the overall findings of the STAR study were unexpected: there was no general benefit in the euploidy plus morphology group compared to morphology assessment alone. Nevertheless, it must be emphasized that the STAR study focused on a singular, quite narrow question: Is PGT-A beneficial to good prognosis patients in the first, single embryo transfer?

In total, 34 clinics and 9 testing laboratories in the US, UK, Canada, and Australia contributed data from freeze-all cycles of patients aged 25–40 with at least two blastocysts available for transfer. IVF clinics operated independently, with no standardization regarding protocols of ovarian stimulation or embryo transfer. The PGT-A arm (euploidy plus morphology) comprised 330 patients, of which 274 ultimately received a transfer, while the control group (morphology only) comprised 331 patients, of which 313 ultimately received a transfer. Primary outcome of the study was ongoing pregnancy rate (OPR) at 20 week's gestation. Regarding intention to treat (ITT), there was no significant difference in OPR between the two arms (41.8% vs. 43.5%, respectively; $p = 0.65$). Importantly, in the PGT-A arm, 42 patients had produced no euploid embryos and were automatically counted as producing no pregnancy. When analyzing results on a 'per embryo transfer' level, again the authors did not observe a statistical difference in OPR (50.0% vs. 45.7%, respectively; $p = 0.32$). However, post hoc analysis of patients in the 35–40 age group showed a statistically significant benefit of PGT-A on a per embryo transfer level (50.8% vs. 37.2%, respectively; $p = 0.035$).

It is nonetheless surprising that for this good prognosis patient group at first transfer no overall benefit was observed. Data show that a well-executed TE biopsy collection does not significantly affect blastocyst viability [90], but a poorly performed procedure will undoubtedly have a negative effect. Because of the multi-center nature of the STAR study, there was possibly variation in the expertise of TE biopsy procedure between clinics. Those with inexperienced technicians might have harmed embryos and reduced their viability, potentially annulling the benefits of PGT-A selection. To really assess this, a third study arm could have comprised biopsied embryos that are not tested, although it is evident that obtaining IRB approval and patient consent for that purpose would be problematic.

It must be clearly noted that the findings of the STAR study cannot be extrapolated to other patient groups. For example, no patients over 40 years old or with obvious clinical indications (RIF, RPL) were included in the study, which are the populations with highest incidence of embryonic aneuploidy [27], and therefore with most to gain from chromosomal evaluation. At least seven RCTs assessing PGT-A in different populations are currently registered at ClinicalTrials.gov, and will continue to provide valuable information on the matter.

5.4. Which Patients and Embryos Should Be Offered PGT-A?

While evidence from RCTs and observational studies for different patient categories continues to grow over time, PGT-A has historically been offered preferentially to patient groups believed to produce a high incidence of embryonic aneuploidy. For example, PGT-A follows the law of increasing returns with a gradually aging patient population because of the associated elevated incidence of aneuploidy [11,27]. Hence, the most common referral categories have been patients with indication of advanced maternal age (AMA, often defined as > 35 years), prior recurrent pregnancy loss (RPL, defined as 2 or more miscarriages prior to 20 weeks of gestation), prior recurrent implantation failures (RIF, commonly defined as three or more failures), and severe male factor (MF) infertility [11,158].

However, some fertility clinics elect to test every embryo [159]. The following two premises provide a rationale for offering PGT-A to all patients: (1) Whole chromosome aneuploidies in the TE are excellent predictors of aneuploidy in the ICM/remaining embryo (see Section 5.1), and (2) Aneuploid cells retain their ploidy status over time [58]. In fact, proposed intracellular self-corrective mechanisms, where aneuploid cell become euploid, have not been convincingly demonstrated in human embryos [45,46]. If the two above statements are correct, then a uniform (non-mosaic) aneuploid embryo identified by PGT-A will invariably retain its aneuploid condition, and fail implantation, miscarry, or result in congenital syndromes. Performing a large study with transfers of embryos classified as aneuploid by PGT-A is close to unimaginable at present, considering the need to obtain IRB approval and patient consent. Nonetheless, Munné and colleagues report ten instances of patients opting to transfer embryos with aneuploid results from 24-chromsome PGT-A, since no euploid or mosaic embryos were available to them [38]. The ten transfers resulted in one ongoing pregnancy resulting in an affected newborn that died at 6 weeks after birth. The lowest incidences of aneuploidy are observed in patients of ages 26–30, with the average percent of aneuploid embryos hovering around 25% [26,27]. This translates into a 1 in 4 chance of randomly selecting an aneuploid embryo for transfer if no PGT-A is performed, as there is only a moderate correlation between embryo morphology and ploidy [5,160]. Thus, even in the most favorable patient population with lowest incidence of aneuploidy, PGT-A can hypothetically have considerable impact. In spite of the STAR study results (discussed above), there is evidence from observational studies that PGT-A is beneficial in young, good-prognosis patients: It improved outcomes with young oocytes from egg donation cycles [161], and increased live birth rates per cycle in a statistically significant fashion in patients younger than 35 [162].

Needless to say, there are substantial costs associated with evaluation of chromosomal status in preimplantation embryos, most notably biopsy procedure, testing expenses, and genetic counseling. However, numerous studies have shown cost-effectiveness for various patient populations when compared to transfers without PGT-A [163–165]. The cost of performing the test is offset by savings from factors that accompany transfers of untested embryos, such as increased number of cycles, miscarriages, multiple gestations, and neonatal/ongoing aneuploidy-related conditions. Those factors also add non-tangible costs and the emotional toll to patients.

6. Refinement of PGT-A Categories

6.1. Management of Mosaic Embryos in the Clinic

In 2015, Greco and colleagues reported the clinical transfer of embryos classified as mosaic by PGT-A for the first time [36]. Eighteen consenting patients with no available euploid embryos opted for this treatment strategy, resulting in six healthy births. Up until that point, 'mosaic' embryos were largely grouped with uniform aneuploids in an 'abnormal group'. Clinics and patients were understandably apprehensive of transferring embryos containing a proportion of aneuploid cells. Since then, several reports from different groups using NGS-based PGT-A (currently the most appropriate method to identify mosaicism) have described their experience of transferring mosaic embryos [35–40]. All studies coincided in one observation: Mosaic embryos had lower rates of implantation and higher likelihood of miscarriage than euploid embryos, but led to births with no overt medical conditions. This highly reproduced data in a combined > 800 transfers provide compelling evidence for mosaic embryos being considered for transfer as second priority after euploid embryos.

How can a mosaic blastocyst result in a healthy baby? What happens to the aneuploid cells? The described self-corrective mechanisms in mixed euploid and aneuploid cells (see Section 3.2) are likely responsible conversions of mosaic embryos into entirely euploid ones during development. In some instances, residual aneuploid cells might become diluted to the point of being medically negligible. In cases where aneuploid cells are confined to the TE lineage and persist through development, the potential consequence is CPM. Human placentas often contain islands of aneuploid cells, and are thought to be uniquely capable of adapting to chromosomal abnormalities, much more so than fetal tissues [166]. While most cases of CPM result in healthy babies [61], occasionally and depending on the aneuploidy involved and percent abnormal cells, the condition can result in miscarriage [167] (which, as noted, is more common after transfer of mosaic embryos than euploid embryos [123,168]).

However, it must be noted that mosaicism observed in TE biopsies by PGT-A has not been observed in matching CVS or NIPT samples (which test placental DNA) in existing publications [39,40]. Together, these models provide a framework of how blastocysts with intra-biopsy mosaicism can result in healthy babies.

Another putative alternative to the fate of embryonic mosaicism is its persistence in fetal tissues through gestation, resulting in true fetal mosaicism (TFM) [169]. Some of the > 800 mosaic embryo transfers reported to date had matching amniocentesis information (which tests fetal DNA), from patients that opted to share results [36,39,40]. In the overwhelming majority of cases amniocentesis results were normal, and if an abnormality was detected it was independent of the mosaicism observed during PGT-A.

To date, there has been a singular instance of TE mosaicism matching the results of amniocentesis, reported by Kahraman and colleagues [170]. Interestingly, the authors observed a 35% mosaic loss of Chr 2 with PGT-A, and upon transfer, a reciprocal Chr 2 mosaic gain was detected at amniocentesis in 2% of cells. No pathological features were determined in detailed ultrasonography with normal fetal growth and no signs of IUGR. Birth of a healthy baby followed, in which peripheral blood chromosome analysis validated with fluorescence in situ hybridization showed 2% mosaic monosomy in Chr 2. Epithelial cells in a buccal smear were euploid. The patterns of reciprocal Chr 2 mosaicisms indicate a mitotic non-disjunction event early in embryogenesis, before or during segregation of embryonic (fetal) and extraembryonic (uterine) lineages. Hence, even though the newborn presented no symptoms, this first confirmed case of embryonic mosaicism persisting through gestation to birth emphasizes the need of prenatal testing, particularly amniocentesis, in pregnancies from mosaic embryo transfers.

Recommendations for transfer based on parameters of mosaicism (level, type, chromosome involvement) have been issued before, but those are based on limited experimental data and are therefore largely conceptual [125,171]. A risk scoring system for mosaic embryo transfers has been proposed, basing its rationale on mosaicism and aneuploidies observed in chorionic villus sampling (CVS) data and products of conceptions (POCs) from miscarriages [23]. However, the precise extent to which mosaicism in TE cells reflects placental or fetal mosaicism remains unestablished, and the matched TE biopsy/amniocentesis data mentioned above suggest there is very little correlation. While there is consensus that mosaic embryos have a different set of outcomes than euploids, there is still no agreement among published studies on the specific mosaic features that affect implantation and miscarriage. Conflicting data exist on whether level of mosaicism in the TE biopsy (the percent aneuploid cells) is predictive of outcome [39,40], or whether the type of mosaic (involving segmental, versus whole chromosome, versus complex abnormalities) has an effect [35,37,40]. These reported discrepancies exist even when the same PGT-A platform and guidelines to define mosaicism were used [37,39,40]. The likeliest cause for these inconsistencies is the small sample sizes of the individual studies, making findings of sub-analyses questionable. One report of amassed data from different centers to increase power of analysis has made the following observations evaluating 822 mosaic embryo transfers: There was significant correlation between clinical outcome and level of mosaicism (low level mosaics perform better), as well as type of mosaicism (segmental mosaics perform better than whole chromosome mosaics, and complex mosaics perform worst of all) [168]. This is a rapidly developing topic, and as more clinics become inclined to transfer mosaic embryos in the absence of euploids, expanding data will further clarify these points.

As mentioned above, transfer of mosaic blastocysts should be accompanied by patient counsel with emphasis on prenatal testing (particularly amniocentesis), because data on the exact risk to fetuses are still forthcoming [55,172]. A recent study by Besser and colleagues describing the experience in their center showed that approximately 30% of counselled patients opted for transfer of a mosaic embryo rather than pursuing an additional treatment cycle [173]. The likelihood of undergoing mosaic embryo transfer grew considerably with increasing patient age or number of prior retrievals. Of the patients opting for mosaic embryo transfer, 54.5% pursued amniocentesis.

In summary, the available data indicate that mosaic embryos are viable and can result in seemingly healthy births, albeit with lower success rates than euploids. Ongoing studies will permit further refined ranking of embryos within the mosaic category. The next set of studies should focus on obstetrical and neonatal outcome data from mosaic embryo transfers to obtain a more thorough understanding of their chromosomal and physiological health.

6.2. Why Segmental Abnormality Should Be Managed Differently

Recent observations have noted the poor concordance of segmental copy number variations between TE biopsy and ICM (see Section 5.1). The data oblige the field to re-evaluate the category of segmental abnormality, which until now was combined with the conventional aneuploid group and deselected from transfer. This practice likely leads to discarding potentially competent embryos, as a segmental abnormality in a TE biopsy was shown to be predictive of the ICM only ~50% of the time [75,136,137]. Conversely, the transfer of a segmental abnormality embryo should not be performed heedlessly given the fact that ~50% of such embryo profiles do indeed reflect the presence of the same segmental loss or gain in the ICM, and an estimated ~32% of segmental abnormality are meiotic in nature and present throughout the cells of the remaining blastocyst [75]. This would result in failed implantation, miscarriage, or possibly liveborn congenital syndromes if carried to term.

How then should embryos presumed to harbor segmental abnormalities be managed in the clinic? Should some patients treat transfer of an embryo with segmental abnormality as a final alternative, subject to their tolerance for risk and inclination to perform prenatal testing? Interestingly, data indicate that collecting a second TE biopsy of such embryos may facilitate the clinical decision [75,136,137]. Experiments of multifocal biopsies in 31 blastocysts by Navratil and colleagues showed that approximately half of the time a segmental abnormality in the original TE biopsy was discordant with a second TE biopsy and remaining embryo, but in case of concordance between the two TE biopsies, the profile of the remaining embryo reflected the segmental abnormality 94% of the time [137]. In similar experiments analyzing 53 blastocysts, Girardi and colleagues observed that when two TE biopsies were discordant for a segmental abnormality, the likelihood of the ICM containing the segmental abnormality was 21%, but when the two TE biopsies were concordant, the ICM contained the segmental abnormality 84% of the time [75]. Although re-analyzing an embryo in the clinic demands a second freeze-thaw cycle and biopsy as well as another round of PGT-A, it might be the only way to appropriately prioritize embryos within the segmental abnormality category. At least one study has shown that a second round of TE biopsy collection and cryopreservation did not markedly affect implantation outcome or the likelihood of pregnancy complications [118].

Further studies are required in order to evaluate this approach. For now, the data should compel us to differentiate segmental abnormality embryos from whole chromosome aneuploids as two separate categories of PGT-A. A consensus for the clinical management of segmental abnormality embryos is yet to be elaborated.

6.3. Refinement of the PGT-A Category System: Is it Necessary?

Expansion of PGT-A categories might admittedly not be an easy change to integrate in medical practice. Clinicians and patients have become accustomed to a binary classification (normal/abnormal). The associated genetic counseling is straightforward, and so is the identification of embryos available for transfer. As a consequence, some have regarded the higher dynamic range and resolution of PGT-A by NGS and its ability to identify mosaicism and segmental abnormality as a nuisance at best and disadvantage at worst.

The strength of the more fragmented classification system lies in better predictability of outcome for each specific embryo. As mentioned above, the observation that blastocysts in the mosaic category have lower implantation potential than euploids has been replicated numerous times [35,37–40]. To retain the classical binary system means that either mosaic embryos become merged with the normal group, resulting in a lower implantation rate overall, or they become merged with the abnormal group, in which case they will be discarded even though competent. Either option is evidently disadvantageous. Furthermore, if indeed one kind of mosaic blastocyst has higher implantation rates than another, as recent data suggest, it is clearly advantageous to prioritize transfer of the former when the choice is presented. If no other embryos are available, embryos with segmental abnormality could undergo a second round of biopsy collection and PGT-A to identify those with increased potential to result in a healthy birth. This could provide a new opportunity to patients that would otherwise need to resort to further treatment cycles.

Hence, expanding the PGT-A categorization system seeks to: (1) increase overall rates of positive clinical outcome, and (2) identify potentially competent embryos that otherwise would have been deselected. Such clinical benefits should clearly outweigh the increased complexity in the system and associated burden of genetic counseling.

7. Current Developments and Future Directions of PGT for Chromosomal Abnormalities

7.1. Mitochondrial DNA Quantitation During PGT-A: Where Are We Now

The human genome in its entirety comprises autosomes, sex chromosomes, and the chromosome contained in mitochondria. The mitochondrial chromosome is a 16.5 kb circular double stranded multicopy DNA molecule encoding numerous essential genes for mitochondrial function. Each mitochondrion contains multiple replicas of mitochondrial DNA (mtDNA), and each cell contains numerous mitochondrial organelles. Since those numbers are not static and can fluctuate in response to energetic demands of the host tissue, there is substantial variation in the copy number of mtDNA present in each cell of the human body.

Two independent studies first raised the possibility that quantitation of mtDNA could serve as a biomarker of embryo viability [174,175]. They indicated that blastocysts with PGT-A that failed to implant tended on average to have higher mtDNA content in the TE biopsy, compared to successfully implanted blastocysts. In addition, the studies described a threshold of mtDNA copy number, that always led to failed implantation if it was surpassed.

Since then, the field of mtDNA quantitation in embryology has been turbulent and equivocal. Some studies have supported the initial reports [176–178], but many others have refuted them [179–183], showing no predictive power of mtDNA quantitation in TE biopsies regarding clinical outcome. An interesting observation to come out of this debate is that some clinics produce no embryos with substantially elevated mtDNA levels (about half of the 37 participating clinics in one study), whereas some clinics generate upwards of 20% of blastocysts with very high mtDNA copy number [176]. The underlying biological explanation remains to be confirmed, but is very likely tied to embryo staging and morphology. Several studies have reported an inverse correlation between mtDNA levels and embryo cellularity/developmental progression/expansion [179,180,184]. This is reasonable given that no mtDNA replication occurs between zygote and blastocyst stage, and the initial pool of mtDNA molecules becomes diluted between dividing cells [185–187]. Therefore, embryos that develop slower will retain more mtDNA copies per cell. If mtDNA copy number quantitation only reflects the embryo's developmental stage, it is an impractical tool when many clinics perform morphological assessment of embryos and eliminate poorly developing samples from consideration for transfer. Hence, the precise role of mtDNA quantitation in the fertility clinic is still being evaluated, but its routine and universal use to deselect embryos for transfer remains unsubstantiated, particularly after the recent report that blastocysts with disproportionally high mtDNA copy number can result in healthy births [181].

7.2. Variations and Add-Ons to Conventional PGT-A

A snapshot of today's PGT-A landscape reveals WGA-based low-pass/shallow NGS as the workhorse of the industry. The technique has found a balance between three key factors: cost, ease of use, and quality of information generated. Nonetheless, numerous alterations to the standard PGT-A platform have recently emerged or are currently in development.

One is the aforementioned targeted amplification-sequencing method [104], which increases sequencing depth in specific locations of the genome, but usually at the expense of breadth of genome coverage. Recent versions of this technique have taken advantage of repetitive sequences that are spread across the genome, permitting amplification using few primer pairs [188]. Some families of repetitive elements contain appreciable sequence variation, meaning that using a single primer pair in the reaction (reagent savings, added simplicity) potentially provides widely distributed mapping of reads across the genome after bioinformatic analysis. The depth of sequencing is adequate to perform SNP analysis, in addition to quantitation. Allelic ratio analysis can improve confidence of aneuploidy calling, and can provide information regarding haploidy, triploidy, and UPD [189].

There is substantial interest in developing methods to harness the sequence information gathered during NGS, aside from the usual copy number information. For example, Voet, Vermeesch and colleagues have developed haplarithmisis, a method that quantifies sequencing reads to perform PGT-A, but additionally uses the SNP information contained in the sequencing reads to determine haplotypes [190,191]. This can be used to identify embryos with haplotypes carrying disease alleles, but it also reinforces confidence in calling of copy number changes, and reveals the parental and mechanistic origin of chromosomal abnormalities.

Several efforts are underway to combine PGT for chromosomal abnormalities and monogenic conditions (PGT-A/-M) in a single reaction. For example, Zimmerman and colleagues have described a qPCR method to perform simultaneous aneuploidy analysis and single gene testing [192]. Farmer and colleagues have shown that combining a WGA reaction and specific primers targeting the 23 most common mutations in *CFTR* do not compromise NGS analysis of chromosomal abnormalities, and can simultaneously provide accurate single nucleotide variant (SNV) and small indel information for the *CFTR* gene [193]. Such a technique can be adapted to any mutation using appropriate primer spike-ins. Del Rey and colleagues have successfully combined NGS copy number analysis with large panels of common single gene conditions [194]. Alcaraz and colleagues reported a technique that combines chromosomal copy number calling with a SNP-based analysis of a mutation specific to a patient's genetic profile, showing its feasibility in over 150 different mutations [195].

Handyside and colleagues have developed a technique called karyomapping [196]. It relies on SNP arrays, which aside from providing copy number data, also harness the information contained in near 300,000 SNPs distributed in the genome, permitting linkage analysis for virtually any region of interest. Testing of the subject's relatives reveals the segregation patterns of mutated loci and flanking informative SNPs, which subsequently provide the framework for linkage analysis in tested embryos. The universal applicability of the technology to virtually any single gene mutation is potentially very advantageous to classical analysis of monogenic conditions in embryos, where each mutation requires a specific assay. In addition to combining PGT-A and -M [197,198], karyomapping allows detection of haploidy and triploidy, as well as UPD.

A recent array-based technology developed by Treff and colleagues combines copy number and SNP analysis, and can simultaneously perform PGT-A, -SR, -M, as well as testing for polygenic (-P) conditions [199,200]. A polygenic risk score (PRS) is calculated for a panel of diseases, estimating the relative likelihood of an embryo to develop conditions such as diabetes or heart disease.

In an effort to improve ease-of-use and lower costs, Wei and colleagues have recently adapted nanopore technology in a MinION instrument (Oxford Nanopore) [201] to PGT-A [202]. While thorough validation is still pending, pilot experiments have shown it can detect aneuploidy and, to some degree, mosaicism in TE biopsies. Compared to standard NGS methods, this technology is estimated to increase sequencing speed by 15,000-fold, has a 99X lower capital equipment cost (~USD 1000), and an instrument footprint the size of a deck of cards.

The limited amount of genetic material in a TE biopsy renders 'true' whole genome sequencing a formidable task. However, there have been valiant efforts at obtaining a much broader genome coverage than with standard approaches, typically by coupling high-level sequencing with bioinformatic methods for linkage analysis with familial genomic data. Kumar and colleagues have described a method to infer the entire genome of an embryo from a TE biopsy without performing deep sequencing, instead using SNP linkage analysis with familial genome information [203]. Two studies by Peters et al. [204] and Murphy et al. [205] have shown that detailed assessment of a TE biopsy by high-pass sequencing and linkage analysis can identify new, potentially disease-causing SNPs, in addition to producing copy number and single gene data (PGT-A/-M).

In summary, add-ons to PGT-A can provide valuable supplementary information and/or decrease costs, but should do so without compromising the very core question PGT-A seeks to answer: Are aneuploidies present in the sample? Many of the above tests still need to produce data that convincingly show their copy number analysis is as powerful as conventional WGA-based PGT-A, especially regarding mosaicism and segmental abnormalities.

7.3. The Prospect of Non-Invasive PGT-A

A method of PGT-A that does not require physical isolation of cells from the embryo would revolutionize the field. With the decreasing cost of sequencing, the most expensive component of PGT-A has become biopsy isolation, which requires hi-tech laser equipment and greatly skilled embryologists to perform the microsurgery. These hurdles likely prevent some clinics from adopting a PGT-A program. Even though studies have suggested negligible effect on blastocyst viability when TE biopsy isolation is performed correctly [90,118], there is still risk of poorly executed, harmful, or botched procedures and other more nuanced detrimental effects, such as those associated with prolonged temperature and gas fluctuations during the procedure. Furthermore, some embryos do not get tested because poor morphology precludes TE biopsy collection, and a non-invasive method could increase the pool of assessed embryos.

The concepts of minimally invasive (mi-), or non-invasive (ni-)PGT-A became plausible after discovery of (presumably embryo-derived) DNA in blastocoel fluid (BF) [206], and spent culture medium (SCM) [207]. The ensuing question was whether those fluids contained sufficient good quality DNA to evaluate chromosomal copy number. The option involving BF was explored first.

BF is isolated by 'blastocentesis' [208], in which a fine needle is inserted through the zona pellucida and between TE cell junctions into the blastocoel cavity, and fluid (< 1 µL) is aspirated. This collapses the blastocyst, which can subsequently be vitrified or left to re-expand. Gianaroli and colleagues have made an extensive exploration on the subject of concordance between BF and embryonic cells, publishing three studies based on WGA and aCGH technology [208–210]. The latest, published in 2018, is their largest analysis ($n = 256$ embryos), reporting 94% ploidy concordance between BF and a TE biopsy, and 66% full karyotype concordance [209]. Nevertheless, BF amplification failed in 29% of cases, and of those that amplified a further 13% did not produce an informative chromosome copy number result. An interesting observation was that euploid embryos were significantly more likely to fail BF amplification, possibly pointing at a biological mechanism. The authors hypothesized that DNA in BF is likely to originate from cell apoptosis, which is more frequent in aneuploidy [209]. Therefore, the quantity of DNA in BF might have some prognostic value regarding blastocyst competence.

Studies from other groups, one based on WGA and aCGH [211] and two based on WGA and NGS [127,212], have reported lower concordance of ploidy between BF and TE/ICM biopsy, between 62%–75%, as well as decreased full karyotype concordance, between 38%–48%. Crucially, failed amplification rates for BF showed a large range, between 13%–65%, possibly reflecting different approaches to blastocentesis, BF storage, and amplification chemistry [127,211,212], but also differences in blastocyst population analyzed and true incidence of euploidy, mosaicism, and aneuploidy.

Several groups have recently explored the alternative method (which would be truly non-invasive): analysis of SCM. DNA contamination has been an obvious concern, since some media formulations contain foreign DNA, and there is potential for carryover maternal DNA in the culture drop. However, the observation that the total amount of DNA increases with developmental progression [213,214] would indicate that the bulk DNA derives from the embryo. The first notable SCM study was performed by Shamonki and colleagues in 2016, reporting that their system (Qiagen's Repli-G kit for amplification and aCGH) produced suboptimal data for 96% of the 56 samples analyzed [215]. This confirmed that chemistries designed for chromosomal evaluation from cellular biopsy would unlikely be transferable to niPGT-A in their current formats. A series of studies followed, testing different methods of DNA amplification (MALBAC or SurePlex/PicoPlex, with various modifications), analysis (aCGH or NGS), and culturing protocols, expertly detailed by Leaver and Wells [216].

The biggest caveat in many of the publications to date is that embryos were subjected to some form of manipulation before SCM was collected [217–221]. Putting embryos through Day 3/4 assisted hatching, a freeze-thaw cycle, and/or a cellular biopsy prior to SCM collection provides a source of added DNA in the medium, confounding the subsequent analysis of amplification rate and concordance to the embryo. While it should not entirely invalidate such studies, these shortcomings must be carefully considered.

For the most part, studies with no embryo manipulation prior to SCM collection will be discussed here, as they can give a true sense of whether niPGT-A is applicable in the clinic. Liu and colleagues evaluated 88 SCM samples after continuous culture between Days 1–5, using MALBAC amplification (Yikon Genomics) and NGS on a HiSeq 2500 (Illumina) instrument, reporting a 91% amplification rate [222]. Ploidy concordance with a TE biopsy was observed in 84% of cases (although mosaic and aneuploid results were conflated into one 'abnormal' group), and full karyotype concordance was 65%. Only later studies revealed that maternal DNA contamination from the oocyte retrieval procedure is a significant concern, and the uninterrupted culture from zygote to blastocyst stage likely maximizes that problem. The same testing method, namely MALBAC amplification (Yikon Genomics) and NGS on a HiSeq 2500 instrument (Illumina), was used in a study by Fang and colleagues, this time washing embryos at Day 3 of culture and moving to new media drops until Day 5 or 6 [223]. The study reports a 97% amplification rate in the 170 samples analyzed. The authors did not collect a TE biopsy to perform concordance analysis, and instead embryos were transferred in the clinic, selecting them according to the result of the test (which they call 'NICS', for noninvasive chromosome screening). In total, 52 blastocysts that had been classified as normal were transferred to 50 patients, resulting in 30 implantations (58% rate), 3 miscarriages (10% rate), and 27 births (52% rate per embryo transfer). Those results could be regarded as favorable rates of positive clinical outcome, but unfortunately the study did not have a control arm, making the results difficult to evaluate. Are those outcomes better than if no niPGT-A had been performed? And would TE biopsy PGT-A have resulted in better outcomes? Two ongoing trials, in which NICS is compared to morphology assessment alone (ClinicalTrials.gov ID: NCT04339166) or to conventional PGT-A (ID: NCT03879265) will shed light on these questions.

A study by Vera-Rodriguez and colleagues [214] explored three important issues concerning niPGT-A: (1) Amount of DNA, (2) Maternal DNA contamination, and (3) Embryonic mosaicism. To explore those concepts, the authors used a high-performance DNA quantitation method, SNP analysis to discern maternal from embryonic DNA, and FISH to evaluate each cell in a subset of blastocysts. The authors analyzed 56 SCM samples collected at Day 5 of culture (after having performed a media change at Day 3). Detailed DNA quantitation showed a median 6.7 pg DNA, which is approximately equivalent to the DNA content of one diploid cell- with half of the samples containing fewer amounts. In comparison, no-embryo control drops contained a median 1.4 pg. It must be stressed that this particular study did perform assisted hatching at Day 3, meaning that a truly non-invasive protocol might result in lower amounts of DNA per SCM. There was no difference in the amount of DNA between euploid and aneuploid embryos, in contrast to what was observed in BF studies [209]. Strikingly, SNP analysis revealed maternal DNA presence in all samples tested, on average constituting a remarkable 92% of all DNA in SCM, even though a media change had been performed at Day 3. To explore the ploidy of SCM, the authors employed a double WGA amplification technique of SurePlex WGA (Illumina), followed by a complete IonReproseq (ThermoFisher) protocol and sequencing on an Ion PGM instrument (ThermoFisher). Ninety-one percent of samples yielded a result, compared to 100% using TE biopsies. FISH analysis of complete blastocyst cellular makeup revealed that SCM samples poorly reflected the status of embryos that were mosaics, and TE biopsy mosaicism was a far superior predictor of mosaicism in the remaining blastocyst. This was attributed to the possibility that in a mosaic context, cells with different ploidy release their DNA content into the SCM at different rates- rendering the SCM a poor representative of the embryo. Together, these findings clearly identified some of the hurdles that need to be addressed in developing niPGT-A for clinical use.

In 2019 the same group published a prospective blinded study, in which Rubio and colleagues analyzed 115 samples and showed a 95% amplification rate with 79% overall ploidy concordance to a TE biopsy and 64% full karyotype concordance (including segmental abnormalities) [224]. To perform niPGT-A, the group used a modified version of the IonReproseq protocol (ThermoFisher), followed by sequencing on an Ion S5TM XL system (ThermoFisher). Embryo culture did not involve assisted hatching, and embryos were thoroughly washed at Day 4 through three media drops in hopes of removing carryover maternal DNA and lingering cumulus cells. Each embryo was subsequently placed in a new reduced media drop of 10 µL (to ensure the entire sample could be included in a WGA reaction) and cultured to Day 5, 6, or 7, at which time SCM was collected. Sub-analysis showed that extended culture to Day 6 or 7 (≥48 h) improved results (compared to just 24 h), increasing the overall ploidy concordance with a TE biopsy to 84% and full karyotype concordance to 72%, as well as rate of amplification to 100%. This considerable enhancement clearly showed that extended time in culture increases the amount of embryo-representative DNA in the SCM. This study went on to show in a small sample group ($n = 29$) that embryos had an improved chance of implantation and lower miscarriage when TE biopsy and SCM concorded on euploidy status, compared to discordant cases for which TE biopsy indicated euploidy but SCM showed aneuploidy. If these results are replicated in a larger sample group, one could envision niPGT-A as an adjunct to conventional PGT-A to increase likelihood of favorable outcome. Two ongoing studies by this group (ClinicalTrials.gov IDs: NCT03520933 and NCT04000152) are further assessing the value of niPGT-A in the clinic.

A different approach altogether, combining BF and SCM, has so far been explored in a few studies that have all reported high rates of amplification 98%–100% [225–227]. Perhaps the most compelling are the efforts by Kuznyetsov and colleagues [226], since their protocol excluded freeze/thaw cycles prior to sample collection. In a publication from 2018, the Kuznyetsov group analyzed 19 fresh culture samples from 9 patients. Embryos were placed in new culture drops at Day 4 and left to grow until Day 5 or 6, at which point a TE biopsy was collected and the blastocyst was further collapsed with the use of lasers, allowing the BF to emanate into the SCM. The fact that a TE biopsy was collected prior to collection of fluids is a caveat, since the process likely releases DNA into the medium. An unspecified amount of the 25 µL combined BF and SCM sample was subsequently processed in one reaction by SurePlex amplification (Illumina) and VeriSeq NGS (Illumina) on a MiSeq instrument (Illumina) (the same protocol as the corresponding TE biopsies). The combined BF-SCM samples and corresponding TE biopsies had 100% ploidy concordance, and 100% full karyotype concordance for whole chromosome events (which decreased to 71% if segmental abnormalities and mosaicism were included).

Kuznyetsov and colleagues subsequently published a study in 2020 with a larger sample size ($n = 145$) excluding the prior TE biopsy collection, reporting a 100% amplification rate and a 97.8% concordance (euploid/aneuploid) with TE samples [228]. When mosaicism was considered (observed either in cell-free DNA or TE biopsy), rate of concordance declined. One parameter still required optimization: 88.2% of BF-SCM sample amplifications yielded informative NGS results, compared to 98% of TE biopsy amplifications. Overall, those are promising observations regarding the clinical application of this strategy. Since the protocol included assisted hatching at Day 4, an outstanding question is whether omitting this step (in an effort to further reduce the manipulations/invasiveness of the process) would influence the reaction. Other interesting findings from the study include that blastocyst morphology did not correlate with quantity of cell-free DNA, and the cell lysis step could be omitted from the WGA reaction (as it might contribute to maternal DNA contamination though carryover cumulus/corona cells).

There have also been efforts to quantify mtDNA levels in SCM samples. Stigliani and colleagues have reported that higher levels of cell-free mtDNA might be predictive of implantation in cleavage day embryo transfers [206]. Compared to embryos that failed to implant, they observed a threefold increase in mtDNA quantity (on average) in embryos that implanted, but these findings are yet to be replicated with a larger sample size ($n = 51$ not implanted, $n = 43$ implanted embryos, $p = 0.0452$). The same group also observed that higher quantities of cell-free mtDNA at Day 3 of culture have predictive power regarding the likelihood of reaching the blastocyst stage [229]. Whether cell free mtDNA quantitation may serve as a biomarker of implantation for blastocyst stage transfers remains to be explored.

Valuable lessons have been learned from the studies so far: (1) Manipulation of embryos prior to sample collection (freeze-thaw cycle, biopsy collection, assisted hatching) might release DNA into media, compromising a study's results regarding truly non-invasive PGT-A. Those manipulations should be avoided in future studies, (2) Fully euploid and aneuploid embryos might release similar amounts of DNA into the medium, but in a mosaic context, aneuploid cells might preferentially shed their content, adulterating the representativeness of the SCM in regards to the embryo, (3) The minute amounts of DNA require new adaptations of PGT-A chemistries and protocols that accommodate as much of the culture drop volume as possible, (4) Maternal DNA contamination is a big concern, (5) Longer cultures to Day 6 or 7 provide more cell-free (cf) DNA.

Still, several questions persist: (1) What is an acceptable rate of false or no results in niPGT-A (considering its many benefits)? (2) What is the biological mechanism that releases embryonic DNA into surrounding fluids? (3) Are SCM and/or BF better or worse representatives of the true ploidy status of the blastocyst, compared to a TE biopsy? (4) What is the capacity of niPGT to detect segmental abnormalities and mosaicism?

Together, the SCM and BF studies have revealed that the naturally small amount of DNA present in those fluids, possibly coupled with compromised integrity and maternal DNA contamination, present a real challenge in the development of niPGT-A. The reports have evidently pushed against the lower limits of detection of existing PGT-A platforms. There is however, cause for optimism; better cell-free DNA amplification chemistries and optimized bioinformatic analyses will bring us closer to an accurate niPGT-A screen suitable for routine clinical use.

8. Concluding Remarks

PGT-A is undergoing steady, global expansion; in 2019, the technology had a presence in at least 45 countries [7]. To illustrate its potential for growth, between 2014 and 2016 its utilization increased from 13% to 27% of all IVF cycles performed in the USA [230]. The methodology is constantly evolving, having undergone several rounds of transformative changes since its inception- even in name from PGS to PGD-A, to its current form, PGT-A. Each step has incorporated new approaches (chemistries, biopsy collection technique, bioinformatic tools) and has harnessed novel biological insights of aneuploidy (mosaicism, segmental abnormalities). Contemporary technologies make it possible to identify chromosomal abnormalities in greater detail than ever before, and clinical data call for an expansion of the PGT-A grouping system to include the categories of mosaicism and segmental abnormalities.

The current enthusiastic pursuit of niPGT-A may bear fruit in the near future. Time will tell whether its many benefits might come at the expense of data quality and genome resolution, or whether technical advances will be able to bridge those gaps. In parallel, numerous ongoing and ambitious efforts are developing ways to retrieve an ever-increasing amount of information from a single biopsy in order to achieve a more complete genomic profile and enhanced prognostic assessment of the embryo.

PGT-A is inherently limited because it does not (and probably never will) reflect the chromosomal state of the entire embryo with 100% accuracy, and cannot perfectly predict an embryo's clinical outcome. However, in many settings, its demonstrated capability to improve likelihood of positive outcome is undeniable and tremendously valuable. Thousands of past, current, and future infertility patients would certainly agree.

Funding: This research was funded by the Zouves Foundation for Reproductive Medicine.

Acknowledgments: I would like to thank Christo Zouves, Frank Barnes, Andrea Victor, and Alan Brake for thoughtful conversations in preparation of this review.

Conflicts of Interest: The authors declare no conflict of interest.

References

1. Bromer, J.G.; Ata, B.; Seli, M.; Lockwood, C.J.; Seli, E. Preterm deliveries that result from multiple pregnancies associated with assisted reproductive technologies in the USA: A cost analysis. *Curr. Opin. Obs. Gynecol.* **2011**, *23*, 168–173. [CrossRef]
2. Murray, S.R.; Norman, J.E. Multiple pregnancies following assisted reproductive technologies—A happy consequence or double trouble? *Semin. Fetal Neonatal Med.* **2014**, *19*, 222–227. [CrossRef]
3. Hill, G.A.; Freeman, M.; Bastias, M.C.; Rogers, B.J.; Herbert, C.M., 3rd; Osteen, K.G.; Wentz, A.C. The influence of oocyte maturity and embryo quality on pregnancy rate in a program for in vitro fertilization-embryo transfer. *Fertil. Steril.* **1989**, *52*, 801–806.
4. Gardner, D.K.; Schoolcraft, W.B. In vitro culture of human blastocysts. In *Towards Reproductive Certainty: Fertility and Genetics Beyond*; Jansen, R., Mortimer, D., Eds.; Parthenon Publishing: Nashville, TN, USA, 1999; pp. 378–388.
5. Capalbo, A.; Rienzi, L.; Cimadomo, D.; Maggiulli, R.; Elliott, T.; Wright, G.; Nagy, Z.P.; Ubaldi, F.M. Correlation between standard blastocyst morphology, euploidy and implantation: An observational study in two centers involving 956 screened blastocysts. *Hum. Reprod.* **2014**, *29*, 1173–1181. [CrossRef]
6. Handyside, A.H.; Kontogianni, E.H.; Hardy, K.; Winston, R.M. Pregnancies from biopsied human preimplantation embryos sexed by Y-specific DNA amplification. *Nature* **1990**, *344*, 768–770.
7. International Federation of Fertility Societies' Surveillance (IFFS) 2019: Global Trends in Reproductive Policy and Practice, 8th Edition. *Glob. Reprod. Health* **2019**, *4*, e29. [CrossRef]
8. Gruhn, J.R.; Zielinska, A.P.; Shukla, V.; Blanshard, R.; Capalbo, A.; Cimadomo, D.; Nikiforov, D.; Chan, A.C.; Newnham, L.J.; Vogel, I.; et al. Chromosome errors in human eggs shape natural fertility over reproductive life span. *Science* **2019**, *365*, 1466–1469.
9. Hawkes, K.; Smith, K.R. Do women stop early? Similarities in fertility decline in humans and chimpanzees. *Ann. N. Y. Acad. Sci.* **2010**, *1204*, 43–53. [CrossRef]
10. Franasiak, J.M.; Forman, E.J.; Hong, K.H.; Werner, M.D.; Upham, K.M.; Treff, N.R.; Scott, R.T. Aneuploidy across individual chromosomes at the embryonic level in trophectoderm biopsies: Changes with patient age and chromosome structure. *J. Assist. Reprod. Genet.* **2014**, *31*, 1501–1509.
11. Rubio, C.; Rodrigo, L.; Garcia-Pascual, C.; Peinado, V.; Campos-Galindo, I.; Garcia-Herrero, S.; Simon, C. Clinical application of embryo aneuploidy testing by next-generation sequencing. *Biol. Reprod.* **2019**, *101*, 1083–1090. [CrossRef]
12. Taylor, T.H.; Gitlin, S.A.; Patrick, J.L.; Crain, J.L.; Wilson, J.M.; Griffin, D.K. The origin, mechanisms, incidence and clinical consequences of chromosomal mosaicism in humans. *Hum. Reprod. Update* **2014**, *20*, 571–581. [CrossRef] [PubMed]
13. Bond, D.J.; Chandley, A.C. Aneuploidy: The Origins and Causes of Aneuploidy in Experimental Organisms. In *Aneuploidy*; Bond, D.J., Chandley, A.C., Eds.; Oxford University Press: Oxford, UK, 1983; pp. 27–54.
14. Irani, M.; Zaninovic, N.; Rosenwaks, Z.; Xu, K. Does maternal age at retrieval influence the implantation potential of euploid blastocysts? *Am. J. Obs. Gynecol.* **2019**, *220*, 379 e1–379 e7. [CrossRef]
15. Harton, G.L.; Munné, S.; Surrey, M.; Grifo, J.; Kaplan, B.; McCulloh, D.H.; Griffin, D.K.; Wells, D.; Group, P.G.D.P. Diminished effect of maternal age on implantation after preimplantation genetic diagnosis with array comparative genomic hybridization. *Fertil. Steril.* **2013**, *100*, 1695–1703. [CrossRef] [PubMed]
16. Nagaoka, S.I.; Hassold, T.J.; Hunt, P.A. Human aneuploidy: Mechanisms and new insights into an age-old problem. *Nat. Rev. Genet.* **2012**, *13*, 493–504. [CrossRef] [PubMed]

17. Kubicek, D.; Hornak, M.; Horak, J.; Navratil, R.; Tauwinklova, G.; Rubes, J.; Vesela, K. Incidence and origin of meiotic whole and segmental chromosomal aneuploidies detected by karyomapping. *Reprod. Biomed. Online* **2019**, *38*, 330–339. [CrossRef] [PubMed]
18. Konstantinidis, M.; Ravichandran, K.; Gunes, Z.; Prates, R.; Goodall, N.N.; Roman, B.; Ribustello, L.; Shanmugam, A.; Colls, P.; Munne, S.; et al. Aneuploidy and recombination in the human preimplantation embryo. Copy number variation analysis and genome-wide polymorphism genotyping. *Reprod. Biomed. Online* **2020**, *40*, 479–493. [CrossRef] [PubMed]
19. Capalbo, A.; Bono, S.; Spizzichino, L.; Biricik, A.; Baldi, M.; Colamaria, S.; Ubaldi, F.M.; Rienzi, L.; Fiorentino, F. Sequential comprehensive chromosome analysis on polar bodies, blastomeres and trophoblast: Insights into female meiotic errors and chromosomal segregation in the preimplantation window of embryo development. *Hum. Reprod.* **2013**, *28*, 509–518.
20. Ottolini, C.S.; Newnham, L.; Capalbo, A.; Natesan, S.A.; Joshi, H.A.; Cimadomo, D.; Griffin, D.K.; Sage, K.; Summers, M.C.; Thornhill, A.R.; et al. Genome-wide maps of recombination and chromosome segregation in human oocytes and embryos show selection for maternal recombination rates. *Nat. Genet.* **2015**, *47*, 727–735. [CrossRef]
21. Martin, R.H.; Rademaker, A. The frequency of aneuploidy among individual chromosomes in 6,821 human sperm chromosome complements. *Cytogenet. Cell Genet.* **1990**, *53*, 103–107. [CrossRef]
22. Templado, C.; Vidal, F.; Estop, A. Aneuploidy in human spermatozoa. *Cytogenet. Genome Res.* **2011**, *133*, 91–99.
23. Grati, F.R.; Gallazzi, G.; Branca, L.; Maggi, F.; Simoni, G.; Yaron, Y. An evidence-based scoring system for prioritizing mosaic aneuploid embryos following preimplantation genetic screening. *Reprod. Biomed. Online* **2018**, *36*, 442–449. [CrossRef] [PubMed]
24. Hassold, T.; Abruzzo, M.; Adkins, K.; Griffin, D.; Merrill, M.; Millie, E.; Saker, D.; Shen, J.; Zaragoza, M. Human aneuploidy: Incidence, origin, and etiology. *Env. Mol. Mutagen.* **1996**, *28*, 167–175. [CrossRef]
25. Munné, S.; Alikani, M.; Ribustello, L.; Colls, P.; Martinez-Ortiz, P.A.; McCulloh, D.H.; Referring Physician, G. Euploid rates in donor egg cycles significantly differ between fertility centers. *Hum. Reprod.* **2017**, *32*, 743–749. [CrossRef] [PubMed]
26. Demko, Z.P.; Simon, A.L.; McCoy, R.C.; Petrov, D.A.; Rabinowitz, M. Effects of maternal age on euploidy rates in a large cohort of embryos analyzed with 24-chromosome single-nucleotide polymorphism-based preimplantation genetic screening. *Fertil. Steril.* **2016**, *105*, 1307–1313. [CrossRef] [PubMed]
27. Franasiak, J.M.; Forman, E.J.; Hong, K.H.; Werner, M.D.; Upham, K.M.; Treff, N.R.; Scott, R.T., Jr. The nature of aneuploidy with increasing age of the female partner: A review of 15,169 consecutive trophectoderm biopsies evaluated with comprehensive chromosomal screening. *Fertil. Steril.* **2014**, *101*, 656–663. [CrossRef]
28. Irani, M.; Canon, C.; Robles, A.; Maddy, B.; Gunnala, V.; Qin, X.; Zhang, C.; Xu, K.; Rosenwaks, Z. No effect of ovarian stimulation and oocyte yield on euploidy and live birth rates: An analysis of 12 298 trophectoderm biopsies. *Hum. Reprod.* **2020**. [CrossRef] [PubMed]
29. Chiang, T.; Schultz, R.M.; Lampson, M.A. Meiotic origins of maternal age-related aneuploidy. *Biol. Reprod.* **2012**, *86*, 1–7. [CrossRef]
30. Capalbo, A.; Hoffmann, E.R.; Cimadomo, D.; Ubaldi, F.M.; Rienzi, L. Human female meiosis revised: New insights into the mechanisms of chromosome segregation and aneuploidies from advanced genomics and time-lapse imaging. *Hum. Reprod. Update* **2017**, *23*, 706–722. [CrossRef]
31. Carrasquillo, R.J.; Kohn, T.P.; Cinnioglu, C.; Rubio, C.; Simon, C.; Ramasamy, R.; Al-Asmar, N. Advanced paternal age does not affect embryo aneuploidy following blastocyst biopsy in egg donor cycles. *J. Assist. Reprod. Genet.* **2019**, *36*, 2039–2045. [CrossRef]
32. Baart, E.B.; Martini, E.; Eijkemans, M.J.; Van Opstal, D.; Beckers, N.G.; Verhoeff, A.; Macklon, N.S.; Fauser, B.C. Milder ovarian stimulation for in-vitro fertilization reduces aneuploidy in the human preimplantation embryo: A randomized controlled trial. *Hum. Reprod.* **2007**, *22*, 980–988. [CrossRef]
33. Rubio, C.; Mercader, A.; Alama, P.; Lizan, C.; Rodrigo, L.; Labarta, E.; Melo, M.; Pellicer, A.; Remohi, J. Prospective cohort study in high responder oocyte donors using two hormonal stimulation protocols: Impact on embryo aneuploidy and development. *Hum. Reprod.* **2010**, *25*, 2290–2297. [CrossRef]
34. Sheltzer, J.M.; Amon, A. The aneuploidy paradox: Costs and benefits of an incorrect karyotype. *Trends Genet.* **2011**, *27*, 446–453. [CrossRef]

35. Fragouli, E.; Alfarawati, S.; Spath, K.; Babariya, D.; Tarozzi, N.; Borini, A.; Wells, D. Analysis of implantation and ongoing pregnancy rates following the transfer of mosaic diploid-aneuploid blastocysts. *Hum. Genet.* **2017**, *136*, 805–819. [CrossRef]
36. Greco, E.; Minasi, M.G.; Fiorentino, F. Healthy Babies after Intrauterine Transfer of Mosaic Aneuploid Blastocysts. *N. Engl. J. Med.* **2015**, *373*, 2089–2090. [CrossRef]
37. Munné, S.; Blazek, J.; Large, M.; Martinez-Ortiz, P.A.; Nisson, H.; Liu, E.; Tarozzi, N.; Borini, A.; Becker, A.; Zhang, J.; et al. Detailed investigation into the cytogenetic constitution and pregnancy outcome of replacing mosaic blastocysts detected with the use of high-resolution next-generation sequencing. *Fertil. Steril.* **2017**, *108*, 62–71. [CrossRef]
38. Munné, S.; Spinella, F.; Grifo, J.; Zhang, J.; Beltran, M.P.; Fragouli, E.; Fiorentino, F. Clinical outcomes after the transfer of blastocysts characterized as mosaic by high resolution Next Generation Sequencing-further insights. *Eur. J. Med. Genet.* **2020**, *63*, 103741. [CrossRef]
39. Spinella, F.; Fiorentino, F.; Biricik, A.; Bono, S.; Ruberti, A.; Cotroneo, E.; Baldi, M.; Cursio, E.; Minasi, M.G.; Greco, E. Extent of chromosomal mosaicism influences the clinical outcome of in vitro fertilization treatments. *Fertil. Steril.* **2018**, *109*, 77–83. [CrossRef]
40. Victor, A.R.; Tyndall, J.C.; Brake, A.J.; Lepkowsky, L.T.; Murphy, A.E.; Griffin, D.K.; McCoy, R.C.; Barnes, F.L.; Zouves, C.G.; Viotti, M. One hundred mosaic embryos transferred prospectively in a single clinic: Exploring when and why they result in healthy pregnancies. *Fertil. Steril.* **2019**, *111*, 280–293. [CrossRef]
41. Vazquez-Diez, C.; FitzHarris, G. Causes and consequences of chromosome segregation error in preimplantation embryos. *Reproduction* **2018**, *155*, R63–R76. [CrossRef]
42. Victor, A.; Ogur, C.; Thornhill, A.; Griffin, D. Preimplantation Genetic Testing for Aneuploidies: Where We Are and Where We're Going. In *Preimplantation Genetic Testing: Recent Advances in Reproductive Medicine*, 2020 ed.; Griffin, D., Harton, G., Eds.; Taylor & Francis Group: Abingdon, UK, 2020.
43. Coonen, E.; Derhaag, J.G.; Dumoulin, J.C.; van Wissen, L.C.; Bras, M.; Janssen, M.; Evers, J.L.; Geraedts, J.P. Anaphase lagging mainly explains chromosomal mosaicism in human preimplantation embryos. *Hum. Reprod.* **2004**, *19*, 316–324. [CrossRef]
44. Ioannou, D.; Fonseka, K.G.; Meershoek, E.J.; Thornhill, A.R.; Abogrein, A.; Ellis, M.; Griffin, D.K. Twenty-four chromosome FISH in human IVF embryos reveals patterns of post-zygotic chromosome segregation and nuclear organisation. *Chromosome Res.* **2012**, *20*, 447–460. [CrossRef] [PubMed]
45. McCoy, R.C. Mosaicism in Preimplantation Human Embryos: When Chromosomal Abnormalities Are the Norm. *Trends Genet.* **2017**, *33*, 448–463. [CrossRef] [PubMed]
46. Li, X.; Hao, Y.; Elshewy, N.; Zhu, X.; Zhang, Z.; Zhou, P. The mechanisms and clinical application of mosaicism in preimplantation embryos. *J. Assist. Reprod. Genet.* **2020**, *37*, 497–508. [PubMed]
47. Delhanty, J.D.; Griffin, D.K.; Handyside, A.H.; Harper, J.; Atkinson, G.H.; Pieters, M.H.; Winston, R.M. Detection of aneuploidy and chromosomal mosaicism in human embryos during preimplantation sex determination by fluorescent in situ hybridisation, (FISH). *Hum. Mol. Genet.* **1993**, *2*, 1183–1185. [CrossRef] [PubMed]
48. Evsikov, S.; Verlinsky, Y. Mosaicism in the inner cell mass of human blastocysts. *Hum. Reprod.* **1998**, *13*, 3151–3155. [CrossRef]
49. Popovic, M.; Dhaenens, L.; Boel, A.; Menten, B.; Heindryckx, B. Chromosomal mosaicism in human blastocysts: The ultimate diagnostic dilemma. *Hum. Reprod. Update* **2020**, *26*, 313–334. [CrossRef]
50. Munné, S.; Kaplan, B.; Frattarelli, J.L.; Child, T.; Nakhuda, G.; Shamma, F.N.; Silverberg, K.; Kalista, T.; Handyside, A.H.; Katz-Jaffe, M.; et al. Preimplantation genetic testing for aneuploidy versus morphology as selection criteria for single frozen-thawed embryo transfer in good-prognosis patients: A multicenter randomized clinical trial. *Fertil. Steril.* **2019**, *112*, 1071–1079.
51. Munné, S.; Wells, D. Detection of mosaicism at blastocyst stage with the use of high-resolution next-generation sequencing. *Fertil. Steril.* **2017**, *107*, 1085–1091. [CrossRef]
52. Tsuiko, O.; Catteeuw, M.; Zamani Esteki, M.; Destouni, A.; Bogado Pascottini, O.; Besenfelder, U.; Havlicek, V.; Smits, K.; Kurg, A.; Salumets, A.; et al. Genome stability of bovine in vivo-conceived cleavage-stage embryos is higher compared to in vitro-produced embryos. *Hum. Reprod.* **2017**, *32*, 2348–2357. [CrossRef]
53. Zamani Esteki, M.; Viltrop, T.; Tsuiko, O.; Tiirats, A.; Koel, M.; Noukas, M.; Zilina, O.; Teearu, K.; Marjonen, H.; Kahila, H.; et al. In vitro fertilization does not increase the incidence of de novo copy number alterations in fetal and placental lineages. *Nat. Med.* **2019**, *25*, 1699–1705.

54. McCoy, R.C.; Demko, Z.P.; Ryan, A.; Banjevic, M.; Hill, M.; Sigurjonsson, S.; Rabinowitz, M.; Petrov, D.A. Evidence of Selection against Complex Mitotic-Origin Aneuploidy during Preimplantation Development. *PLoS Genet.* **2015**, *11*, e1005601. [CrossRef]
55. Vera-Rodriguez, M.; Rubio, C. Assessing the true incidence of mosaicism in preimplantation embryos. *Fertil. Steril.* **2017**, *107*, 1107–1112. [CrossRef] [PubMed]
56. Bolton, H.; Graham, S.J.; Van der Aa, N.; Kumar, P.; Theunis, K.; Fernandez Gallardo, E.; Voet, T.; Zernicka-Goetz, M. Mouse model of chromosome mosaicism reveals lineage-specific depletion of aneuploid cells and normal developmental potential. *Nat. Commun.* **2016**, *7*, 11165. [CrossRef] [PubMed]
57. Mashiko, D.; Ikeda, Z.; Yao, T.; Tokoro, M.; Fukunaga, N.; Asada, Y.; Yamagata, K. Chromosome segregation error during early cleavage in mouse pre-implantation embryo does not necessarily cause developmental failure after blastocyst stage. *Sci. Rep.* **2020**, *10*, 854. [PubMed]
58. Popovic, M.; Dhaenens, L.; Taelman, J.; Dheedene, A.; Bialecka, M.; De Sutter, P.; Chuva de Sousa Lopes, S.M.; Menten, B.; Heindryckx, B. Extended in vitro culture of human embryos demonstrates the complex nature of diagnosing chromosomal mosaicism from a single trophectoderm biopsy. *Hum. Reprod.* **2019**, *34*, 758–769. [CrossRef] [PubMed]
59. Kuliev, A.; Verlinsky, Y. Meiotic and mitotic nondisjunction: Lessons from preimplantation genetic diagnosis. *Hum. Reprod. Update* **2004**, *10*, 401–407. [CrossRef]
60. Gueye, N.A.; Devkota, B.; Taylor, D.; Pfundt, R.; Scott, R.T., Jr.; Treff, N.R. Uniparental disomy in the human blastocyst is exceedingly rare. *Fertil. Steril.* **2014**, *101*, 232–236. [CrossRef]
61. Fryburg, J.S.; Dimaio, M.S.; Yang-Feng, T.L.; Mahoney, M.J. Follow-up of pregnancies complicated by placental mosaicism diagnosed by chorionic villus sampling. *Prenat. Diagn.* **1993**, *13*, 481–494.
62. Kalousek, D.K.; Dill, F.J. Chromosomal mosaicism confined to the placenta in human conceptions. *Science* **1983**, *221*, 665–667. [CrossRef]
63. Leschot, N.J.; Schuring-Blom, G.H.; Van Prooijen-Knegt, A.C.; Verjaal, M.; Hansson, K.; Wolf, H.; Kanhai, H.H.; Van Vugt, J.M.; Christiaens, G.C. The outcome of pregnancies with confined placental chromosome mosaicism in cytotrophoblast cells. *Prenat. Diagn.* **1996**, *16*, 705–712.
64. Iourov, I.Y.; Vorsanova, S.G.; Yurov, Y.B. Chromosomal mosaicism goes global. *Mol. Cytogenet.* **2008**, *1*, 26. [CrossRef] [PubMed]
65. Acuna-Hidalgo, R.; Veltman, J.A.; Hoischen, A. New insights into the generation and role of de novo mutations in health and disease. *Genome Biol.* **2016**, *17*, 241. [CrossRef]
66. Yurov, Y.B.; Iourov, I.Y.; Vorsanova, S.G.; Liehr, T.; Kolotii, A.D.; Kutsev, S.I.; Pellestor, F.; Beresheva, A.K.; Demidova, I.A.; Kravets, V.S.; et al. Aneuploidy and confined chromosomal mosaicism in the developing human brain. *PLoS ONE* **2007**, *2*, e558. [CrossRef] [PubMed]
67. Fiorentino, F.; Biricik, A.; Bono, S.; Spizzichino, L.; Cotroneo, E.; Cottone, G.; Kokocinski, F.; Michel, C.E. Development and validation of a next-generation sequencing-based protocol for 24-chromosome aneuploidy screening of embryos. *Fertil. Steril.* **2014**, *101*, 1375–1382. [CrossRef] [PubMed]
68. Yin, X.; Tan, K.; Vajta, G.; Jiang, H.; Tan, Y.; Zhang, C.; Chen, F.; Chen, S.; Zhang, C.; Pan, X.; et al. Massively parallel sequencing for chromosomal abnormality testing in trophectoderm cells of human blastocysts. *Biol. Reprod.* **2013**, *88*, 69. [CrossRef] [PubMed]
69. Zheng, H.; Jin, H.; Liu, L.; Liu, J.; Wang, W.H. Application of next-generation sequencing for 24-chromosome aneuploidy screening of human preimplantation embryos. *Mol. Cytogenet.* **2015**, *8*, 38. [CrossRef] [PubMed]
70. Babariya, D.; Fragouli, E.; Alfarawati, S.; Spath, K.; Wells, D. The incidence and origin of segmental aneuploidy in human oocytes and preimplantation embryos. *Hum. Reprod.* **2017**, *32*, 2549–2560. [CrossRef]
71. Mehta, A.; Haber, J.E. Sources of DNA double-strand breaks and models of recombinational DNA repair. *Cold Spring Harb. Perspect. Biol.* **2014**, *6*, a016428. [CrossRef]
72. Richardson, C.; Horikoshi, N.; Pandita, T.K. The role of the DNA double-strand break response network in meiosis. *DNA Repair* **2004**, *3*, 1149–1164. [CrossRef]
73. Aguilera, A.; Garcia-Muse, T. Causes of genome instability. *Annu. Rev. Genet.* **2013**, *47*, 1–32. [CrossRef]
74. Escriba, M.J.; Vendrell, X.; Peinado, V. Segmental aneuploidy in human blastocysts: A qualitative and quantitative overview. *Reprod. Biol. Endocrinol.* **2019**, *17*, 76. [CrossRef] [PubMed]

75. Girardi, L.; Serdarogullari, M.; Patassini, C.; Poli, M.; Fabiani, M.; Caroselli, S.; Coban, O.; Findikli, N.; Boynukalin, F.K.; Bahceci, M.; et al. Incidence, Origin, and Predictive Model for the Detection and Clinical Management of Segmental Aneuploidies in Human Embryos. *Am. J. Hum. Genet.* **2020**, *106*, 525–534. [CrossRef] [PubMed]
76. Vera-Rodriguez, M.; Michel, C.E.; Mercader, A.; Bladon, A.J.; Rodrigo, L.; Kokocinski, F.; Mateu, E.; Al-Asmar, N.; Blesa, D.; Simon, C.; et al. Distribution patterns of segmental aneuploidies in human blastocysts identified by next-generation sequencing. *Fertil. Steril.* **2016**, *105*, 1047–1055. [PubMed]
77. Martinez, M.C.; Mendez, C.; Ferro, J.; Nicolas, M.; Serra, V.; Landeras, J. Cytogenetic analysis of early nonviable pregnancies after assisted reproduction treatment. *Fertil. Steril.* **2010**, *93*, 289–292.
78. Wellesley, D.; Dolk, H.; Boyd, P.A.; Greenlees, R.; Haeusler, M.; Nelen, V.; Garne, E.; Khoshnood, B.; Doray, B.; Rissmann, A.; et al. Rare chromosome abnormalities, prevalence and prenatal diagnosis rates from population-based congenital anomaly registers in Europe. *Eur. J. Hum. Genet.* **2012**, *20*, 521–526.
79. Shaffer, L.G.; Lupski, J.R. Molecular mechanisms for constitutional chromosomal rearrangements in humans. *Annu. Rev. Genet.* **2000**, *34*, 297–329. [CrossRef]
80. Chow, J.F.C.; Cheng, H.H.Y.; Lau, E.Y.L.; Yeung, W.S.B.; Ng, E.H.Y. Distinguishing between carrier and noncarrier embryos with the use of long-read sequencing in preimplantation genetic testing for reciprocal translocations. *Genomics* **2020**, *112*, 494–500. [CrossRef]
81. Treff, N.R.; Thompson, K.; Rafizadeh, M.; Chow, M.; Morrison, L.; Tao, X.; Garnsey, H.; Reda, C.V.; Metzgar, T.L.; Neal, S.; et al. SNP array-based analyses of unbalanced embryos as a reference to distinguish between balanced translocation carrier and normal blastocysts. *J. Assist. Reprod. Genet.* **2016**, *33*, 1115–1119.
82. Wang, L.; Shen, J.; Cram, D.S.; Ma, M.; Wang, H.; Zhang, W.; Fan, J.; Gao, Z.; Zhang, L.; Li, Z.; et al. Preferential selection and transfer of euploid noncarrier embryos in preimplantation genetic diagnosis cycles for reciprocal translocations. *Fertil. Steril.* **2017**, *108*, 620–627.
83. Xu, J.; Zhang, Z.; Niu, W.; Yang, Q.; Yao, G.; Shi, S.; Jin, H.; Song, W.; Chen, L.; Zhang, X.; et al. Mapping allele with resolved carrier status of Robertsonian and reciprocal translocation in human preimplantation embryos. *Proc. Natl. Acad. Sci. USA* **2017**, *114*, E8695–E8702. [CrossRef]
84. Ferfouri, F.; Bernicot, I.; Schneider, A.; Haquet, E.; Hedon, B.; Anahory, T. Is the resulting phenotype of an embryo with balanced X-autosome translocation, obtained by means of preimplantation genetic diagnosis, linked to the X inactivation pattern? *Fertil. Steril.* **2016**, *105*, 1035–1046. [CrossRef] [PubMed]
85. Griffin, D.K.; Wilton, L.J.; Handyside, A.H.; Atkinson, G.H.; Winston, R.M.; Delhanty, J.D. Diagnosis of sex in preimplantation embryos by fluorescent in situ hybridisation. *BMJ* **1993**, *306*, 1382. [PubMed]
86. Munné, S.; Lee, A.; Rosenwaks, Z.; Grifo, J.; Cohen, J. Diagnosis of major chromosome aneuploidies in human preimplantation embryos. *Hum. Reprod.* **1993**, *8*, 2185–2191. [CrossRef] [PubMed]
87. Schrurs, B.M.; Winston, R.M.; Handyside, A.H. Preimplantation diagnosis of aneuploidy using fluorescent in-situ hybridization: Evaluation using a chromosome 18-specific probe. *Hum. Reprod.* **1993**, *8*, 296–301. [PubMed]
88. Munné, S.; Fragouli, E.; Colls, P.; Katz-Jaffe, M.; Schoolcraft, W.; Wells, D. Improved detection of aneuploid blastocysts using a new 12-chromosome FISH test. *Reprod. Biomed. Online* **2010**, *20*, 92–97. [CrossRef] [PubMed]
89. Griffin, D.K.; Ogur, C. Chromosomal analysis in IVF: Just how useful is it? *Reproduction* **2018**, *156*, F29–F50. [CrossRef]
90. Scott, R.T., Jr.; Upham, K.M.; Forman, E.J.; Zhao, T.; Treff, N.R. Cleavage-stage biopsy significantly impairs human embryonic implantation potential while blastocyst biopsy does not: A randomized and paired clinical trial. *Fertil. Steril.* **2013**, *100*, 624–630. [CrossRef]
91. Verlinsky, Y.; Ginsberg, N.; Lifchez, A.; Valle, J.; Moise, J.; Strom, C.M. Analysis of the first polar body: Preconception genetic diagnosis. *Hum. Reprod.* **1990**, *5*, 826–829.
92. Salvaggio, C.N.; Forman, E.J.; Garnsey, H.M.; Treff, N.R.; Scott, R.T., Jr. Polar body based aneuploidy screening is poorly predictive of embryo ploidy and reproductive potential. *J. Assist. Reprod. Genet.* **2014**, *31*, 1221–1226. [CrossRef]
93. Levin, I.; Almog, B.; Shwartz, T.; Gold, V.; Ben-Yosef, D.; Shaubi, M.; Amit, A.; Malcov, M. Effects of laser polar-body biopsy on embryo quality. *Fertil. Steril.* **2012**, *97*, 1085–1088.
94. Mastenbroek, S.; Twisk, M.; van der Veen, F.; Repping, S. Preimplantation genetic screening: A systematic review and meta-analysis of RCTs. *Hum. Reprod. Update* **2011**, *17*, 454–466. [CrossRef] [PubMed]

95. Gawad, C.; Koh, W.; Quake, S.R. Single-cell genome sequencing: Current state of the science. *Nat. Rev. Genet.* **2016**, *17*, 175–188. [CrossRef] [PubMed]
96. Deleye, L.; De Coninck, D.; Christodoulou, C.; Sante, T.; Dheedene, A.; Heindryckx, B.; Van den Abbeel, E.; De Sutter, P.; Menten, B.; Deforce, D.; et al. Whole genome amplification with SurePlex results in better copy number alteration detection using sequencing data compared to the MALBAC method. *Sci. Rep.* **2015**, *5*, 11711. [PubMed]
97. Wells, D.; Delhanty, J.D. Comprehensive chromosomal analysis of human preimplantation embryos using whole genome amplification and single cell comparative genomic hybridization. *Mol. Hum. Reprod.* **2000**, *6*, 1055–1062.
98. Schoolcraft, W.B.; Fragouli, E.; Stevens, J.; Munné, S.; Katz-Jaffe, M.G.; Wells, D. Clinical application of comprehensive chromosomal screening at the blastocyst stage. *Fertil. Steril.* **2010**, *94*, 1700–1706. [CrossRef]
99. Hellani, A.; Abu-Amero, K.; Azouri, J.; El-Akoum, S. Successful pregnancies after application of array-comparative genomic hybridization in PGS-aneuploidy screening. *Reprod. Biomed. Online* **2008**, *17*, 841–847. [CrossRef]
100. Gutierrez-Mateo, C.; Colls, P.; Sanchez-Garcia, J.; Escudero, T.; Prates, R.; Ketterson, K.; Wells, D.; Munne, S. Validation of microarray comparative genomic hybridization for comprehensive chromosome analysis of embryos. *Fertil. Steril.* **2011**, *95*, 953–958. [CrossRef]
101. Treff, N.R.; Su, J.; Tao, X.; Levy, B.; Scott, R.T., Jr. Accurate single cell 24 chromosome aneuploidy screening using whole genome amplification and single nucleotide polymorphism microarrays. *Fertil. Steril.* **2010**, *94*, 2017–2021.
102. Wells, D.; Kaur, K.; Grifo, J.; Glassner, M.; Taylor, J.C.; Fragouli, E.; Munné, S. Clinical utilisation of a rapid low-pass whole genome sequencing technique for the diagnosis of aneuploidy in human embryos prior to implantation. *J. Med. Genet.* **2014**, *51*, 553–562.
103. Treff, N.R.; Tao, X.; Ferry, K.M.; Su, J.; Taylor, D.; Scott, R.T., Jr. Development and validation of an accurate quantitative real-time polymerase chain reaction-based assay for human blastocyst comprehensive chromosomal aneuploidy screening. *Fertil. Steril.* **2012**, *97*, 819–824.
104. Zimmerman, R.S.; Tao, X.; Marin, D.; Werner, M.D.; Hong, K.H.; Lonczak, A.; Landis, J.; Taylor, D.; Zhan, Y.; Scott, R.T., Jr.; et al. Preclinical validation of a targeted next generation sequencing-based comprehensive chromosome screening methodology in human blastocysts. *Mol. Hum. Reprod.* **2018**, *24*, 37–45. [CrossRef] [PubMed]
105. Dokras, A.; Sargent, I.L.; Ross, C.; Gardner, R.L.; Barlow, D.H. Trophectoderm biopsy in human blastocysts. *Hum. Reprod.* **1990**, *5*, 821–825. [CrossRef] [PubMed]
106. Capalbo, A.; Romanelli, V.; Cimadomo, D.; Girardi, L.; Stoppa, M.; Dovere, L.; Dell'Edera, D.; Ubaldi, F.M.; Rienzi, L. Implementing PGD/PGD-A in IVF clinics: Considerations for the best laboratory approach and management. *J. Assist. Reprod. Genet.* **2016**, *33*, 1279–1286. [CrossRef] [PubMed]
107. McArthur, S.J.; Leigh, D.; Marshall, J.T.; de Boer, K.A.; Jansen, R.P. Pregnancies and live births after trophectoderm biopsy and preimplantation genetic testing of human blastocysts. *Fertil. Steril.* **2005**, *84*, 1628–1636. [CrossRef] [PubMed]
108. Taylor, T.H.; Stankewicz, T.; Katz, S.L.; Patrick, J.L.; Johnson, L.; Griffin, D.K. Preliminary assessment of aneuploidy rates between the polar, mid and mural trophectoderm. *Zygote* **2019**, 1–4. [CrossRef]
109. Romanelli, V.; Poli, M.; Capalbo, A. Preimplantation genetic testing in assisted reproductive technology. *Panminerva Med.* **2019**, *61*, 30–41. [CrossRef]
110. Rubino, P.; Tapia, L.; Ruiz de Assin Alonso, R.; Mazmanian, K.; Guan, L.; Dearden, L.; Thiel, A.; Moon, C.; Kolb, B.; Norian, J.M.; et al. Trophectoderm biopsy protocols can affect clinical outcomes: Time to focus on the blastocyst biopsy technique. *Fertil. Steril.* **2020**, *113*, 981–989. [CrossRef]
111. Cimadomo, D.; Rienzi, L.; Capalbo, A.; Rubio, C.; Innocenti, F.; Garcia-Pascual, C.M.; Ubaldi, F.M.; Handyside, A. The dawn of the future: 30 years from the first biopsy of a human embryo. The detailed history of an ongoing revolution. *Hum. Reprod. Update* **2020**. [CrossRef]
112. Marek, D.; Langley, M.; Gardner, D.K.; Confer, N.; Doody, K.M.; Doody, K.J. Introduction of blastocyst culture and transfer for all patients in an in vitro fertilization program. *Fertil. Steril.* **1999**, *72*, 1035–1040. [CrossRef]
113. Quinn, P. Enhanced results in mouse and human embryo culture using a modified human tubal fluid medium lacking glucose and phosphate. *J. Assist. Reprod. Genet.* **1995**, *12*, 97–105. [CrossRef]

114. Kuwayama, M. Highly efficient vitrification for cryopreservation of human oocytes and embryos: The Cryotop method. *Theriogenology* **2007**, *67*, 73–80. [CrossRef] [PubMed]
115. Harton, G.L.; De Rycke, M.; Fiorentino, F.; Moutou, C.; SenGupta, S.; Traeger-Synodinos, J.; Harper, J.C.; European Society for Human, R.; Embryology, P.G.D.C. ESHRE PGD consortium best practice guidelines for amplification-based PGD. *Hum. Reprod.* **2011**, *26*, 33–40. [CrossRef] [PubMed]
116. Capalbo, A.; Ubaldi, F.M.; Rienzi, L.; Scott, R.; Treff, N. Detecting mosaicism in trophectoderm biopsies: Current challenges and future possibilities. *Hum. Reprod.* **2017**, *32*, 492–498. [CrossRef] [PubMed]
117. Fragouli, E.; Lenzi, M.; Ross, R.; Katz-Jaffe, M.; Schoolcraft, W.B.; Wells, D. Comprehensive molecular cytogenetic analysis of the human blastocyst stage. *Hum. Reprod.* **2008**, *23*, 2596–2608. [CrossRef] [PubMed]
118. Cimadomo, D.; Rienzi, L.; Romanelli, V.; Alviggi, E.; Levi-Setti, P.E.; Albani, E.; Dusi, L.; Papini, L.; Livi, C.; Benini, F.; et al. Inconclusive chromosomal assessment after blastocyst biopsy: Prevalence, causative factors and outcomes after re-biopsy and re-vitrification. A multicenter experience. *Hum. Reprod.* **2018**, *33*, 1839–1846. [CrossRef]
119. Chaubey, A.; Shenoy, S.; Mathur, A.; Ma, Z.; Valencia, C.A.; Reddy Nallamilli, B.R.; Szekeres, E., Jr.; Stansberry, L.; Liu, R.; Hegde, M.R. Low-Pass Genome Sequencing: Validation and Diagnostic Utility from 409 Clinical Cases of Low-Pass Genome Sequencing for the Detection of Copy Number Variants to Replace Constitutional Microarray. *J. Mol. Diagn.* **2020**, *20*, 1525–1578. [CrossRef]
120. Ruttanajit, T.; Chanchamroen, S.; Cram, D.S.; Sawakwongpra, K.; Suksalak, W.; Leng, X.; Fan, J.; Wang, L.; Yao, Y.; Quangkananurug, W. Detection and quantitation of chromosomal mosaicism in human blastocysts using copy number variation sequencing. *Prenat. Diagn.* **2016**, *36*, 154–162. [CrossRef]
121. Friedenthal, J.; Maxwell, S.M.; Munné, S.; Kramer, Y.; McCulloh, D.H.; McCaffrey, C.; Grifo, J.A. Next generation sequencing for preimplantation genetic screening improves pregnancy outcomes compared with array comparative genomic hybridization in single thawed euploid embryo transfer cycles. *Fertil. Steril.* **2018**, *109*, 627–632. [CrossRef]
122. Friedenthal, J.; Maxwell, S.M.; Tiegs, A.W.; Besser, A.G.; McCaffrey, C.; Munné, S.; Noyes, N.; Grifo, J.A. Clinical error rates of next generation sequencing and array comparative genomic hybridization with single thawed euploid embryo transfer. *Eur. J. Med. Genet.* **2020**, *63*, 103852. [CrossRef]
123. Maxwell, S.M.; Colls, P.; Hodes-Wertz, B.; McCulloh, D.H.; McCaffrey, C.; Wells, D.; Munné, S.; Grifo, J.A. Why do euploid embryos miscarry? A case-control study comparing the rate of aneuploidy within presumed euploid embryos that resulted in miscarriage or live birth using next-generation sequencing. *Fertil. Steril.* **2016**, *106*, 1414–1419. [CrossRef]
124. Deleye, L.; Dheedene, A.; De Coninck, D.; Sante, T.; Christodoulou, C.; Heindryckx, B.; Van den Abbeel, E.; De Sutter, P.; Deforce, D.; Menten, B.; et al. Shallow whole genome sequencing is well suited for the detection of chromosomal aberrations in human blastocysts. *Fertil. Steril.* **2015**, *104*, 1276–1285. [CrossRef] [PubMed]
125. Cram, D.S.; Leigh, D.; Handyside, A.; Rechitsky, L.; Xu, K.; Harton, G.; Grifo, J.; Rubio, C.; Fragouli, E.; Kahraman, S.; et al. PGDIS Position Statement on the Transfer of Mosaic Embryos 2019. *Reprod. Biomed. Online* **2019**, *39*, e1–e4. [CrossRef] [PubMed]
126. Popovic, M.; Dheedene, A.; Christodoulou, C.; Taelman, J.; Dhaenens, L.; Van Nieuwerburgh, F.; Deforce, D.; Van den Abbeel, E.; De Sutter, P.; Menten, B.; et al. Chromosomal mosaicism in human blastocysts: The ultimate challenge of preimplantation genetic testing? *Hum. Reprod.* **2018**, *33*, 1342–1354. [CrossRef] [PubMed]
127. Tsuiko, O.; Zhigalina, D.I.; Jatsenko, T.; Skryabin, N.A.; Kanbekova, O.R.; Artyukhova, V.G.; Svetlakov, A.V.; Teearu, K.; Trosin, A.; Salumets, A.; et al. Karyotype of the blastocoel fluid demonstrates low concordance with both trophectoderm and inner cell mass. *Fertil. Steril.* **2018**, *109*, 1127–1134. [CrossRef] [PubMed]
128. Scott, R.T., Jr.; Galliano, D. The challenge of embryonic mosaicism in preimplantation genetic screening. *Fertil. Steril.* **2016**, *105*, 1150–1152.
129. Cuman, C.; Beyer, C.E.; Brodie, D.; Fullston, T.; Lin, J.I.; Willats, E.; Zander-Fox, D.; Mullen, J. Defining the limits of detection for chromosome rearrangements in the preimplantation embryo using next generation sequencing. *Hum. Reprod.* **2018**, *33*, 1566–1576. [CrossRef]
130. Theisen, A.; Shaffer, L.G. Disorders caused by chromosome abnormalities. *Appl. Clin. Genet.* **2010**, *3*, 159–174.
131. Hardy, K.; Handyside, A.H.; Winston, R.M. The human blastocyst: Cell number, death and allocation during late preimplantation development in vitro. *Development* **1989**, *107*, 597–604.

132. Capalbo, A.; Rienzi, L. Mosaicism between trophectoderm and inner cell mass. *Fertil. Steril.* **2017**, *107*, 1098–1106.
133. Huang, J.; Yan, L.; Lu, S.; Zhao, N.; Qiao, J. Re-analysis of aneuploidy blastocysts with an inner cell mass and different regional trophectoderm cells. *J. Assist. Reprod. Genet.* **2017**, *34*, 487–493.
134. Sachdev, N.M.; McCulloh, D.H.; Kramer, Y.; Keefe, D.; Grifo, J.A. The reproducibility of trophectoderm biopsies in euploid, aneuploid, and mosaic embryos using independently verified next-generation sequencing (NGS): A pilot study. *J. Assist. Reprod. Genet.* **2020**, *37*, 559–571. [CrossRef] [PubMed]
135. Lawrenz, B.; El Khatib, I.; Linan, A.; Bayram, A.; Arnanz, A.; Chopra, R.; De Munck, N.; Fatemi, H.M. The clinicians dilemma with mosaicism-an insight from inner cell mass biopsies. *Hum. Reprod.* **2019**, *34*, 998–1010. [PubMed]
136. Victor, A.R.; Griffin, D.K.; Brake, A.J.; Tyndall, J.C.; Murphy, A.E.; Lepkowsky, L.T.; Lal, A.; Zouves, C.G.; Barnes, F.L.; McCoy, R.C.; et al. Assessment of aneuploidy concordance between clinical trophectoderm biopsy and blastocyst. *Hum. Reprod.* **2019**, *34*, 181–192. [PubMed]
137. Navratil, R.; Horak, J.; Hornak, M.; Kubicek, D.; Balcova, M.; Tauwinklova, G.; Travnik, P.; Vesela, K. Concordance of various chromosomal errors among different parts of the embryo and the value of re-biopsy in embryos with segmental aneuploidies. *Mol. Hum. Reprod.* **2020**, *26*. [CrossRef]
138. Ou, Z.; Chen, Z.; Yin, M.; Deng, Y.; Liang, Y.; Wang, W.; Yao, Y.; Sun, L. Re-analysis of whole blastocysts after trophectoderm biopsy indicated chromosome aneuploidy. *Hum. Genom.* **2020**, *14*, 3.
139. Van der Aa, N.; Cheng, J.; Mateiu, L.; Zamani Esteki, M.; Kumar, P.; Dimitriadou, E.; Vanneste, E.; Moreau, Y.; Vermeesch, J.R.; Voet, T. Genome-wide copy number profiling of single cells in S-phase reveals DNA-replication domains. *Nucleic Acids Res.* **2013**, *41*, e66. [CrossRef]
140. Demczuk, A.; Gauthier, M.G.; Veras, I.; Kosiyatrakul, S.; Schildkraut, C.L.; Busslinger, M.; Bechhoefer, J.; Norio, P. Regulation of DNA replication within the immunoglobulin heavy-chain locus during B cell commitment. *PLoS Biol.* **2012**, *10*, e1001360.
141. Dimitriadou, E.; Van der Aa, N.; Cheng, J.; Voet, T.; Vermeesch, J.R. Single cell segmental aneuploidy detection is compromised by S phase. *Mol. Cytogenet.* **2014**, *7*, 46.
142. Ramos, L.; del Rey, J.; Daina, G.; Martinez-Passarell, O.; Rius, M.; Tunon, D.; Campillo, M.; Benet, J.; Navarro, J. Does the S phase have an impact on the accuracy of comparative genomic hybridization profiles in single fibroblasts and human blastomeres? *Fertil. Steril.* **2014**, *101*, 488–495. [CrossRef]
143. Munné, S.; Sultan, K.M.; Weier, H.U.; Grifo, J.A.; Cohen, J.; Rosenwaks, Z. Assessment of numeric abnormalities of X, Y, 18, and 16 chromosomes in preimplantation human embryos before transfer. *Am. J. Obs. Gynecol.* **1995**, *172*, 1191–1199.
144. Rubio, C.; Rodrigo, L.; Perez-Cano, I.; Mercader, A.; Mateu, E.; Buendia, P.; Remohi, J.; Simon, C.; Pellicer, A. FISH screening of aneuploidies in preimplantation embryos to improve IVF outcome. *Reprod. Biomed. Online* **2005**, *11*, 497–506. [PubMed]
145. Verlinsky, Y.; Cieslak, J.; Freidine, M.; Ivakhnenko, V.; Wolf, G.; Kovalinskaya, L.; White, M.; Lifchez, A.; Kaplan, B.; Moise, J.; et al. Pregnancies following pre-conception diagnosis of common aneuploidies by fluorescent in-situ hybridization. *Hum. Reprod.* **1995**, *10*, 1923–1927. [CrossRef] [PubMed]
146. Vidal, F.; Gimenez, C.; Rubio, C.; Simon, C.; Pellicer, A.; Santalo, J.; Egozcue, J. FISH preimplantation diagnosis of chromosome aneuploidy in recurrent pregnancy wastage. *J. Assist. Reprod. Genet.* **1998**, *15*, 310–313. [CrossRef] [PubMed]
147. Fragouli, E.; Munné, S.; Wells, D. The cytogenetic constitution of human blastocysts: Insights from comprehensive chromosome screening strategies. *Hum. Reprod. Update* **2019**, *25*, 15–33. [CrossRef] [PubMed]
148. Rubio, C.; Bellver, J.; Rodrigo, L.; Bosch, E.; Mercader, A.; Vidal, C.; De los Santos, M.J.; Giles, J.; Labarta, E.; Domingo, J.; et al. Preimplantation genetic screening using fluorescence in situ hybridization in patients with repetitive implantation failure and advanced maternal age: Two randomized trials. *Fertil. Steril.* **2013**, *99*, 1400–1407. [PubMed]
149. Yang, Z.; Liu, J.; Collins, G.S.; Salem, S.A.; Liu, X.; Lyle, S.S.; Peck, A.C.; Sills, E.S.; Salem, R.D. Selection of single blastocysts for fresh transfer via standard morphology assessment alone and with array CGH for good prognosis IVF patients: Results from a randomized pilot study. *Mol. Cytogenet.* **2012**, *5*, 24.
150. Scott, R.T., Jr.; Ferry, K.; Su, J.; Tao, X.; Scott, K.; Treff, N.R. Comprehensive chromosome screening is highly predictive of the reproductive potential of human embryos: A prospective, blinded, nonselection study. *Fertil. Steril.* **2012**, *97*, 870–875. [CrossRef]

151. Scott, R.T., Jr.; Upham, K.M.; Forman, E.J.; Hong, K.H.; Scott, K.L.; Taylor, D.; Tao, X.; Treff, N.R. Blastocyst biopsy with comprehensive chromosome screening and fresh embryo transfer significantly increases in vitro fertilization implantation and delivery rates: A randomized controlled trial. *Fertil. Steril.* **2013**, *100*, 697–703.
152. Forman, E.J.; Hong, K.H.; Ferry, K.M.; Tao, X.; Taylor, D.; Levy, B.; Treff, N.R.; Scott, R.T., Jr. In vitro fertilization with single euploid blastocyst transfer: A randomized controlled trial. *Fertil. Steril.* **2013**, *100*, 100–107. [CrossRef]
153. Dahdouh, E.M.; Balayla, J.; Garcia-Velasco, J.A. Comprehensive chromosome screening improves embryo selection: A meta-analysis. *Fertil. Steril.* **2015**, *104*, 1503–1512.
154. Chen, M.; Wei, S.; Hu, J.; Quan, S. Can Comprehensive Chromosome Screening Technology Improve IVF/ICSI Outcomes? A Meta-Analysis. *PLoS ONE* **2015**, *10*, e0140779. [CrossRef] [PubMed]
155. Sacchi, L.; Albani, E.; Cesana, A.; Smeraldi, A.; Parini, V.; Fabiani, M.; Poli, M.; Capalbo, A.; Levi-Setti, P.E. Preimplantation Genetic Testing for Aneuploidy Improves Clinical, Gestational, and Neonatal Outcomes in Advanced Maternal Age Patients Without Compromising Cumulative Live-Birth Rate. *J. Assist. Reprod. Genet.* **2019**, *36*, 2493–2504. [CrossRef] [PubMed]
156. Rubio, C.; Bellver, J.; Rodrigo, L.; Castillon, G.; Guillen, A.; Vidal, C.; Giles, J.; Ferrando, M.; Cabanillas, S.; Remohi, J.; et al. In vitro fertilization with preimplantation genetic diagnosis for aneuploidies in advanced maternal age: A randomized, controlled study. *Fertil. Steril.* **2017**, *107*, 1122–1129. [CrossRef] [PubMed]
157. Verpoest, W.; Staessen, C.; Bossuyt, P.M.; Goossens, V.; Altarescu, G.; Bonduelle, M.; Devesa, M.; Eldar-Geva, T.; Gianaroli, L.; Griesinger, G.; et al. Preimplantation genetic testing for aneuploidy by microarray analysis of polar bodies in advanced maternal age: A randomized clinical trial. *Hum. Reprod.* **2018**, *33*, 1767–1776. [CrossRef] [PubMed]
158. Zegers-Hochschild, F.; Adamson, G.D.; Dyer, S.; Racowsky, C.; de Mouzon, J.; Sokol, R.; Rienzi, L.; Sunde, A.; Schmidt, L.; Cooke, I.D.; et al. The International Glossary on Infertility and Fertility Care, 2017. *Fertil. Steril.* **2017**, *108*, 393–406. [CrossRef] [PubMed]
159. Sermon, K.; Capalbo, A.; Cohen, J.; Coonen, E.; De Rycke, M.; De Vos, A.; Delhanty, J.; Fiorentino, F.; Gleicher, N.; Griesinger, G.; et al. The why, the how and the when of PGS 2.0: Current practices and expert opinions of fertility specialists, molecular biologists, and embryologists. *Mol. Hum. Reprod.* **2016**, *22*, 845–857. [CrossRef]
160. Minasi, M.G.; Colasante, A.; Riccio, T.; Ruberti, A.; Casciani, V.; Scarselli, F.; Spinella, F.; Fiorentino, F.; Varricchio, M.T.; Greco, E. Correlation between aneuploidy, standard morphology evaluation and morphokinetic development in 1730 biopsied blastocysts: A consecutive case series study. *Hum. Reprod.* **2016**, *31*, 2245–2254. [CrossRef]
161. Coates, A.; Bankowski, B.J.; Kung, A.; Griffin, D.K.; Munné, S. Differences in pregnancy outcomes in donor egg frozen embryo transfer (FET) cycles following preimplantation genetic screening (PGS): A single center retrospective study. *J. Assist. Reprod. Genet.* **2017**, *34*, 71–78. [CrossRef]
162. Anderson, R.E.; Whitney, J.B.; Schiewe, M.C. Clinical benefits of preimplantation genetic testing for aneuploidy (PGT-A) for all in vitro fertilization treatment cycles. *Eur. J. Med. Genet.* **2020**, *63*, 103731. [CrossRef]
163. Neal, S.A.; Morin, S.J.; Franasiak, J.M.; Goodman, L.R.; Juneau, C.R.; Forman, E.J.; Werner, M.D.; Scott, R.T., Jr. Preimplantation genetic testing for aneuploidy is cost-effective, shortens treatment time, and reduces the risk of failed embryo transfer and clinical miscarriage. *Fertil. Steril.* **2018**, *110*, 896–904. [CrossRef]
164. Somigliana, E.; Busnelli, A.; Paffoni, A.; Vigano, P.; Riccaboni, A.; Rubio, C.; Capalbo, A. Cost-effectiveness of preimplantation genetic testing for aneuploidies. *Fertil. Steril.* **2019**, *111*, 1169–1176. [PubMed]
165. Collins, S.C.; Xu, X.; Mak, W. Cost-effectiveness of preimplantation genetic screening for women older than 37 undergoing in vitro fertilization. *J. Assist. Reprod. Genet.* **2017**, *34*, 1515–1522. [CrossRef] [PubMed]
166. Yuen, R.K.; Robinson, W.P. Review: A high capacity of the human placenta for genetic and epigenetic variation: Implications for assessing pregnancy outcome. *Placenta* **2011**, *32*, S136–S141. [CrossRef] [PubMed]
167. Kalousek, D.K.; Barrett, I. Confined placental mosaicism and stillbirth. *Pediatr. Pathol.* **1994**, *14*, 151–159.
168. Viotti, M.; Victor, A.R.; Barnes, F.L.; Zouves, C.G.; Besser, A.G.; Grifo, J.; Cheng, E.H.; Lee, M.S.; Greco, E.; Minasi, M.G.; et al. Mosaic embryos—A comprehensive and powered analysis of clinical outcomes. *Fertil. Steril.* **2019**, *112*, e33. [CrossRef]
169. Grati, F.R. Chromosomal Mosaicism in Human Feto-Placental Development: Implications for Prenatal Diagnosis. *J. Clin. Med.* **2014**, *3*, 809–837. [CrossRef]

170. Kahraman, S.; Cetinkaya, M.; Yuksel, B.; Yesil, M.; Pirkevi Cetinkaya, C. The birth of a baby with mosaicism resulting from a known mosaic embryo transfer: A case report. *Hum. Reprod.* **2020**, *35*, 727–733. [CrossRef]
171. COGEN Position Statement on Chromosomal Mosaicism Detected in Preimplantation Blastocyst Biopsies. Available online: https://ivf-worldwide.com/cogen/oep/publications/cogen-position-statement-on-chromosomal-mosaicism-detected-in-preimplantation-blastocyst-biopsies.html (accessed on 28 May 2020).
172. Besser, A.G.; Mounts, E.L. Counselling considerations for chromosomal mosaicism detected by preimplantation genetic screening. *Reprod. Biomed. Online* **2017**, *34*, 369–374. [CrossRef]
173. Besser, A.G.; McCulloh, D.H.; Grifo, J.A. What are patients doing with their mosaic embryos? Decision making after genetic counseling. *Fertil. Steril.* **2019**, *111*, 132–137. [CrossRef]
174. Diez-Juan, A.; Rubio, C.; Marin, C.; Martinez, S.; Al-Asmar, N.; Riboldi, M.; Diaz-Gimeno, P.; Valbuena, D.; Simon, C. Mitochondrial DNA content as a viability score in human euploid embryos: Less is better. *Fertil. Steril.* **2015**, *104*, 534–541. [CrossRef]
175. Fragouli, E.; Spath, K.; Alfarawati, S.; Kaper, F.; Craig, A.; Michel, C.E.; Kokocinski, F.; Cohen, J.; Munné, S.; Wells, D. Altered levels of mitochondrial DNA are associated with female age, aneuploidy, and provide an independent measure of embryonic implantation potential. *PLoS Genet.* **2015**, *11*, e1005241.
176. Ravichandran, K.; McCaffrey, C.; Grifo, J.; Morales, A.; Perloe, M.; Munné, S.; Wells, D.; Fragouli, E. Mitochondrial DNA quantification as a tool for embryo viability assessment: Retrospective analysis of data from single euploid blastocyst transfers. *Hum. Reprod.* **2017**, *32*, 1282–1292. [CrossRef]
177. Fragouli, E.; McCaffrey, C.; Ravichandran, K.; Spath, K.; Grifo, J.A.; Munné, S.; Wells, D. Clinical implications of mitochondrial DNA quantification on pregnancy outcomes: A blinded prospective non-selection study. *Hum. Reprod.* **2017**, *32*, 2340–2347. [CrossRef] [PubMed]
178. Lledo, B.; Ortiz, J.A.; Morales, R.; Garcia-Hernandez, E.; Ten, J.; Bernabeu, A.; Llacer, J.; Bernabeu, R. Comprehensive mitochondrial DNA analysis and IVF outcome. *Hum. Reprod. Open* **2018**, *2018*, hoy023.
179. Klimczak, A.M.; Pacheco, L.E.; Lewis, K.E.; Massahi, N.; Richards, J.P.; Kearns, W.G.; Saad, A.F.; Crochet, J.R. Embryonal mitochondrial DNA: Relationship to embryo quality and transfer outcomes. *J. Assist. Reprod. Genet.* **2018**, *35*, 871–877.
180. Treff, N.R.; Zhan, Y.; Tao, X.; Olcha, M.; Han, M.; Rajchel, J.; Morrison, L.; Morin, S.J.; Scott, R.T., Jr. Levels of trophectoderm mitochondrial DNA do not predict the reproductive potential of sibling embryos. *Hum. Reprod.* **2017**, *32*, 954–962. [PubMed]
181. Victor, A.; Griffin, D.; Dardner, K.G.; Brake, A.; Zouves, C.; Barnes, F.; Viotti, M. Births from embryos with highly elevated levels of mitochondrial DNA. *Reprod. Biomed. Online* **2019**, *39*, 403–412. [CrossRef]
182. Victor, A.R.; Brake, A.J.; Tyndall, J.C.; Griffin, D.K.; Zouves, C.G.; Barnes, F.L.; Viotti, M. Accurate quantitation of mitochondrial DNA reveals uniform levels in human blastocysts irrespective of ploidy, age, or implantation potential. *Fertil. Steril.* **2017**, *107*, 34–42. [CrossRef]
183. Lee, Y.X.; Chen, C.H.; Lin, S.Y.; Lin, Y.H.; Tzeng, C.R. Adjusted mitochondrial DNA quantification in human embryos may not be applicable as a biomarker of implantation potential. *J. Assist. Reprod. Genet.* **2019**, *36*, 1855–1865.
184. de Los Santos, M.J.; Diez Juan, A.; Mifsud, A.; Mercader, A.; Meseguer, M.; Rubio, C.; Pellicer, A. Variables associated with mitochondrial copy number in human blastocysts: What can we learn from trophectoderm biopsies? *Fertil. Steril.* **2018**, *109*, 110–117. [CrossRef]
185. Piko, L.; Taylor, K.D. Amounts of mitochondrial DNA and abundance of some mitochondrial gene transcripts in early mouse embryos. *Dev. Biol.* **1987**, *123*, 364–374. [PubMed]
186. Hashimoto, S.; Morimoto, N.; Yamanaka, M.; Matsumoto, H.; Yamochi, T.; Goto, H.; Inoue, M.; Nakaoka, Y.; Shibahara, H.; Morimoto, Y. Quantitative and qualitative changes of mitochondria in human preimplantation embryos. *J. Assist. Reprod. Genet.* **2017**, *34*, 573–580.
187. St John, J. The control of mtDNA replication during differentiation and development. *Biochim. Biophys. Acta* **2014**, *1840*, 1345–1354. [CrossRef] [PubMed]
188. Kinde, I.; Papadopoulos, N.; Kinzler, K.W.; Vogelstein, B. FAST-SeqS: A simple and efficient method for the detection of aneuploidy by massively parallel sequencing. *PLoS ONE* **2012**, *7*, e41162. [CrossRef] [PubMed]
189. Marin, D.; Zimmerman, R.; Tao, X.; Zhan, Y.; Scott, R.T., Jr.; Treff, N.R. Validation of a targeted next generation sequencing-based comprehensive chromosome screening platform for detection of triploidy in human blastocysts. *Reprod. Biomed. Online* **2018**, *36*, 388–395. [PubMed]

190. Masset, H.; Zamani Esteki, M.; Dimitriadou, E.; Dreesen, J.; Debrock, S.; Derhaag, J.; Derks, K.; Destouni, A.; Drusedau, M.; Meekels, J.; et al. Multi-centre evaluation of a comprehensive preimplantation genetic test through haplotyping-by-sequencing. *Hum. Reprod.* **2019**, *34*, 1608–1619. [CrossRef]
191. Zamani Esteki, M.; Dimitriadou, E.; Mateiu, L.; Melotte, C.; Van der Aa, N.; Kumar, P.; Das, R.; Theunis, K.; Cheng, J.; Legius, E.; et al. Concurrent whole-genome haplotyping and copy-number profiling of single cells. *Am. J. Hum. Genet.* **2015**, *96*, 894–912. [CrossRef]
192. Zimmerman, R.S.; Jalas, C.; Tao, X.; Fedick, A.M.; Kim, J.G.; Pepe, R.J.; Northrop, L.E.; Scott, R.T., Jr.; Treff, N.R. Development and validation of concurrent preimplantation genetic diagnosis for single gene disorders and comprehensive chromosomal aneuploidy screening without whole genome amplification. *Fertil. Steril.* **2016**, *105*, 286–294. [CrossRef]
193. Kimura, Y.; Laliberte, J.; Kamberov, E.; Viotti, M.; Victor, A.R.; Brake, A.J.; Zouves, C.G.; Barnes, F.L.; Farmer, A. Novel approach enabling the simultaneous detection of snv and cnv for pgt-m and pgt-a using a single-tube assay. *Reprod. Biomed. Online* **2019**, *39*, E16–E17.
194. Del Rey, J.; Vidal, F.; Ramirez, L.; Borras, N.; Corrales, I.; Garcia, I.; Martinez-Pasarell, O.; Fernandez, S.F.; Garcia-Cruz, R.; Pujol, A.; et al. Novel Double Factor PGT strategy analyzing blastocyst stage embryos in a single NGS procedure. *PLoS ONE* **2018**, *13*, e0205692.
195. Alcaraz Mas, L.A.; Pérez, C.; González-Reig, S.; Brígido, P.; Amorós, D.; Penacho, V.; Blanca, H. Pgd-seq: Validation of a novel solution for pgt-m and pgt-sr based on target enrichment. *Reprod. Biomed. Online* **2019**, *39*, E62. [CrossRef]
196. Handyside, A.H.; Harton, G.L.; Mariani, B.; Thornhill, A.R.; Affara, N.; Shaw, M.A.; Griffin, D.K. Karyomapping: A universal method for genome wide analysis of genetic disease based on mapping crossovers between parental haplotypes. *J. Med. Genet.* **2010**, *47*, 651–658. [PubMed]
197. Natesan, S.A.; Handyside, A.H.; Thornhill, A.R.; Ottolini, C.S.; Sage, K.; Summers, M.C.; Konstantinidis, M.; Wells, D.; Griffin, D.K. Live birth after PGD with confirmation by a comprehensive approach (karyomapping) for simultaneous detection of monogenic and chromosomal disorders. *Reprod. Biomed. Online* **2014**, *29*, 600–605. [CrossRef] [PubMed]
198. Thornhill, A.R.; Handyside, A.H.; Ottolini, C.; Natesan, S.A.; Taylor, J.; Sage, K.; Harton, G.; Cliffe, K.; Affara, N.; Konstantinidis, M.; et al. Karyomapping-a comprehensive means of simultaneous monogenic and cytogenetic PGD: Comparison with standard approaches in real time for Marfan syndrome. *J. Assist. Reprod. Genet.* **2015**, *32*, 347–356. [CrossRef]
199. Treff, N.R.; Eccles, J.; Lello, L.; Bechor, E.; Hsu, J.; Plunkett, K.; Zimmerman, R.; Rana, B.; Samoilenko, A.; Hsu, S.; et al. Utility and First Clinical Application of Screening Embryos for Polygenic Disease Risk Reduction. *Front. Endocrinol.* **2019**, *10*, 845. [CrossRef]
200. Treff, N.R.; Zimmerman, R.; Bechor, E.; Hsu, J.; Rana, B.; Jensen, J.; Li, J.; Samoilenko, A.; Mowrey, W.; Van Alstine, J.; et al. Validation of concurrent preimplantation genetic testing for polygenic and monogenic disorders, structural rearrangements, and whole and segmental chromosome aneuploidy with a single universal platform. *Eur. J. Med. Genet.* **2019**, *62*, 103647. [CrossRef]
201. Jain, M.; Olsen, H.E.; Paten, B.; Akeson, M. The Oxford Nanopore MinION: Delivery of nanopore sequencing to the genomics community. *Genome Biol.* **2016**, *17*, 239. [CrossRef]
202. Wei, S.; Weiss, Z.R.; Gaur, P.; Forman, E.; Williams, Z. Rapid preimplantation genetic screening using a handheld, nanopore-based DNA sequencer. *Fertil. Steril.* **2018**, *110*, 910–916. [CrossRef]
203. Kumar, A.; Ryan, A.; Kitzman, J.O.; Wemmer, N.; Snyder, M.W.; Sigurjonsson, S.; Lee, C.; Banjevic, M.; Zarutskie, P.W.; Lewis, A.P.; et al. Whole genome prediction for preimplantation genetic diagnosis. *Genome Med.* **2015**, *7*, 35. [CrossRef]
204. Peters, B.A.; Kermani, B.G.; Alferov, O.; Agarwal, M.R.; McElwain, M.A.; Gulbahce, N.; Hayden, D.M.; Tang, Y.T.; Zhang, R.Y.; Tearle, R.; et al. Detection and phasing of single base de novo mutations in biopsies from human in vitro fertilized embryos by advanced whole-genome sequencing. *Genome Res.* **2015**, *25*, 426–434. [CrossRef]
205. Murphy, N.M.; Samarasekera, T.S.; Macaskill, L.; Mullen, J.; Rombauts, L.J.F. Genome sequencing of human in vitro fertilisation embryos for pathogenic variation screening. *Sci. Rep.* **2020**, *10*, 3795. [CrossRef] [PubMed]

206. Stigliani, S.; Persico, L.; Lagazio, C.; Anserini, P.; Venturini, P.L.; Scaruffi, P. Mitochondrial DNA in Day 3 embryo culture medium is a novel, non-invasive biomarker of blastocyst potential and implantation outcome. *Mol. Hum. Reprod.* **2014**, *20*, 1238–1246. [CrossRef] [PubMed]
207. Palini, S.; Galluzzi, L.; De Stefani, S.; Bianchi, M.; Wells, D.; Magnani, M.; Bulletti, C. Genomic DNA in human blastocoele fluid. *Reprod. Biomed. Online* **2013**, *26*, 603–610. [CrossRef]
208. Gianaroli, L.; Magli, M.C.; Pomante, A.; Crivello, A.M.; Cafueri, G.; Valerio, M.; Ferraretti, A.P. Blastocentesis: A source of DNA for preimplantation genetic testing. Results from a pilot study. *Fertil. Steril.* **2014**, *102*, 1692–1699. [CrossRef]
209. Magli, M.C.; Albanese, C.; Crippa, A.; Tabanelli, C.; Ferraretti, A.P.; Gianaroli, L. Deoxyribonucleic acid detection in blastocoelic fluid: A new predictor of embryo ploidy and viable pregnancy. *Fertil. Steril.* **2019**, *111*, 77–85. [CrossRef] [PubMed]
210. Magli, M.C.; Pomante, A.; Cafueri, G.; Valerio, M.; Crippa, A.; Ferraretti, A.P.; Gianaroli, L. Preimplantation genetic testing: Polar bodies, blastomeres, trophectoderm cells, or blastocoelic fluid? *Fertil. Steril.* **2016**, *105*, 676–683. [CrossRef] [PubMed]
211. Tobler, K.J.; Zhao, Y.; Ross, R.; Benner, A.T.; Xu, X.; Du, L.; Broman, K.; Thrift, K.; Brezina, P.R.; Kearns, W.G. Blastocoel fluid from differentiated blastocysts harbors embryonic genomic material capable of a whole-genome deoxyribonucleic acid amplification and comprehensive chromosome microarray analysis. *Fertil. Steril.* **2015**, *104*, 418–425. [CrossRef]
212. Capalbo, A.; Romanelli, V.; Patassini, C.; Poli, M.; Girardi, L.; Giancani, A.; Stoppa, M.; Cimadomo, D.; Ubaldi, F.M.; Rienzi, L. Diagnostic efficacy of blastocoel fluid and spent media as sources of DNA for preimplantation genetic testing in standard clinical conditions. *Fertil. Steril.* **2018**, *110*, 870–879. [CrossRef]
213. Hammond, E.R.; McGillivray, B.C.; Wicker, S.M.; Peek, J.C.; Shelling, A.N.; Stone, P.; Chamley, L.W.; Cree, L.M. Characterizing nuclear and mitochondrial DNA in spent embryo culture media: Genetic contamination identified. *Fertil. Steril.* **2017**, *107*, 220–228. [CrossRef]
214. Vera-Rodriguez, M.; Diez-Juan, A.; Jimenez-Almazan, J.; Martinez, S.; Navarro, R.; Peinado, V.; Mercader, A.; Meseguer, M.; Blesa, D.; Moreno, I.; et al. Origin and composition of cell-free DNA in spent medium from human embryo culture during preimplantation development. *Hum. Reprod.* **2018**, *33*, 745–756. [CrossRef]
215. Shamonki, M.I.; Jin, H.; Haimowitz, Z.; Liu, L. Proof of concept: Preimplantation genetic screening without embryo biopsy through analysis of cell-free DNA in spent embryo culture media. *Fertil. Steril.* **2016**, *106*, 1312–1318. [CrossRef] [PubMed]
216. Leaver, M.; Wells, D. Non-invasive preimplantation genetic testing (niPGT): The next revolution in reproductive genetics? *Hum. Reprod. Update* **2020**, *26*, 16–42. [CrossRef] [PubMed]
217. Xu, J.; Fang, R.; Chen, L.; Chen, D.; Xiao, J.P.; Yang, W.; Wang, H.; Song, X.; Ma, T.; Bo, S.; et al. Noninvasive chromosome screening of human embryos by genome sequencing of embryo culture medium for in vitro fertilization. *Proc. Natl. Acad. Sci. USA* **2016**, *113*, 11907–11912. [PubMed]
218. Feichtinger, M.; Vaccari, E.; Carli, L.; Wallner, E.; Madel, U.; Figl, K.; Palini, S.; Feichtinger, W. Non-invasive preimplantation genetic screening using array comparative genomic hybridization on spent culture media: A proof-of-concept pilot study. *Reprod. Biomed. Online* **2017**, *34*, 583–589. [CrossRef] [PubMed]
219. Ho, J.R.; Arrach, N.; Rhodes-Long, K.; Ahmady, A.; Ingles, S.; Chung, K.; Bendikson, K.A.; Paulson, R.J.; McGinnis, L.K. Pushing the limits of detection: Investigation of cell-free DNA for aneuploidy screening in embryos. *Fertil. Steril.* **2018**, *110*, 467–475.
220. Huang, L.; Bogale, B.; Tang, Y.; Lu, S.; Xie, X.S.; Racowsky, C. Noninvasive preimplantation genetic testing for aneuploidy in spent medium may be more reliable than trophectoderm biopsy. *Proc. Natl. Acad. Sci. USA* **2019**, *116*, 14105–14112. [CrossRef]
221. Yeung, Q.S.Y.; Zhang, Y.X.; Chung, J.P.W.; Lui, W.T.; Kwok, Y.K.Y.; Gui, B.; Kong, G.W.S.; Cao, Y.; Li, T.C.; Choy, K.W. A prospective study of non-invasive preimplantation genetic testing for aneuploidies (NiPGT-A) using next-generation sequencing (NGS) on spent culture media (SCM). *J. Assist. Reprod. Genet.* **2019**, *36*, 1609–1621. [CrossRef]
222. Liu, W.; Liu, J.; Du, H.; Ling, J.; Sun, X.; Chen, D. Non-invasive pre-implantation aneuploidy screening and diagnosis of beta thalassemia IVSII654 mutation using spent embryo culture medium. *Ann. Med.* **2017**, *49*, 319–328. [CrossRef]

223. Fang, R.; Yang, W.; Zhao, X.; Xiong, F.; Guo, C.; Xiao, J.; Chen, L.; Song, X.; Wang, H.; Chen, J.; et al. Chromosome screening using culture medium of embryos fertilised in vitro: A pilot clinical study. *J. Transl. Med.* **2019**, *17*, 73.
224. Rubio, C.; Rienzi, L.; Navarro-Sanchez, L.; Cimadomo, D.; Garcia-Pascual, C.M.; Albricci, L.; Soscia, D.; Valbuena, D.; Capalbo, A.; Ubaldi, F.; et al. Embryonic cell-free DNA versus trophectoderm biopsy for aneuploidy testing: Concordance rate and clinical implications. *Fertil. Steril.* **2019**, *112*, 510–519. [CrossRef]
225. Li, P.; Song, Z.; Yao, Y.; Huang, T.; Mao, R.; Huang, J.; Ma, Y.; Dong, X.; Huang, W.; Huang, J.; et al. Preimplantation Genetic Screening with Spent Culture Medium/Blastocoel Fluid for in Vitro Fertilization. *Sci. Rep.* **2018**, *8*, 9275. [PubMed]
226. Kuznyetsov, V.; Madjunkova, S.; Antes, R.; Abramov, R.; Motamedi, G.; Ibarrientos, Z.; Librach, C. Evaluation of a novel non-invasive preimplantation genetic screening approach. *PLoS ONE* **2018**, *13*, e0197262.
227. Jiao, J.; Shi, B.; Sagnelli, M.; Yang, D.; Yao, Y.; Li, W.; Shao, L.; Lu, S.; Li, D.; Wang, X. Minimally invasive preimplantation genetic testing using blastocyst culture medium. *Hum. Reprod.* **2019**, *34*, 1369–1379.
228. Kuznyetsov, V.; Madjunkova, S.; Abramov, R.; Antes, R.; Ibarrientos, Z.; Motamedi, G.; Zaman, A.; Kuznyetsova, I.; Librach, C.L. Minimally Invasive Cell-Free Human Embryo Aneuploidy Testing (miPGT-A) Utilizing Combined Spent Embryo Culture Medium and Blastocoel Fluid-Towards Development of a Clinical Assay. *Sci. Rep.* **2020**, *10*, 7244. [CrossRef] [PubMed]
229. Stigliani, S.; Orlando, G.; Massarotti, C.; Casciano, I.; Bovis, F.; Anserini, P.; Ubaldi, F.M.; Remorgida, V.; Rienzi, L.; Scaruffi, P. Non-invasive mitochondrial DNA quantification on Day 3 predicts blastocyst development: A prospective, blinded, multi-centric study. *Mol. Hum. Reprod.* **2019**, *25*, 527–537. [PubMed]
230. Theobald, R.; SenGupta, S.; Harper, J. The status of preimplantation genetic testing in the UK and USA. *Hum. Reprod.* **2020**, *35*, 986–998. [CrossRef] [PubMed]

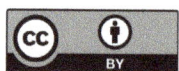

© 2020 by the author. Licensee MDPI, Basel, Switzerland. This article is an open access article distributed under the terms and conditions of the Creative Commons Attribution (CC BY) license (http://creativecommons.org/licenses/by/4.0/).

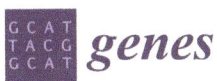

Article

Preimplantation Genetic Testing for Polygenic Disease Relative Risk Reduction: Evaluation of Genomic Index Performance in 11,883 Adult Sibling Pairs

Nathan R. Treff [1,2,*], Jennifer Eccles [1], Diego Marin [1], Edward Messick [1], Louis Lello [1,3], Jessalyn Gerber [4], Jia Xu [1] and Laurent C.A.M. Tellier [1,3]

1. Genomic Prediction Inc. 675 US Highway One, North Brunswick, NJ 08902, USA; jen@genomicprediction.com (J.E.); diego@genomicprediction.com (D.M.); ed@genomicprediction.com (E.M.); lou@genomicprediction.com (L.L.); jia@genomicprediction.com (J.X.); laurent@genomicprediction.com (L.C.A.M.T.)
2. Department of Obstetrics, Gynecology, and Reproductive Sciences, Rutgers University-Robert Wood Johnson Medical School, New Brunswick, NJ 08903, USA
3. Department of Physics and Astronomy, Hannah Administration Building, Michigan State University, 426 Auditorium Rd., East Lansing, MI 48824, USA
4. Department of Genetics, Rutgers University, Piscataway, NJ 08854, USA; jag607@dls.rutgers.edu
* Correspondence: nathan@genomicprediction.com

Received: 23 April 2020; Accepted: 10 June 2020; Published: 12 June 2020

Abstract: Preimplantation genetic testing for polygenic disease risk (PGT-P) represents a new tool to aid in embryo selection. Previous studies demonstrated the ability to obtain necessary genotypes in the embryo with accuracy equivalent to in adults. When applied to select adult siblings with known type I diabetes status, a reduction in disease incidence of 45–72% compared to random selection was achieved. This study extends analysis to 11,883 sibling pairs to evaluate clinical utility of embryo selection with PGT-P. Results demonstrate simultaneous relative risk reduction of all diseases tested in parallel, which included diabetes, cancer, and heart disease, and indicate applicability beyond patients with a known family history of disease.

Keywords: preimplantation genetic testing; PGT-P; polygenic risk scoring; genomic index; relative risk reduction

---

1. Introduction

In vitro fertilization (IVF) is the most effective treatment for infertility. As clinical and laboratory methods have improved, so has the efficiency of producing blastocysts suitable for intrauterine transfer. As a result, IVF patients and physicians are often faced with determining which specific embryo to transfer. The default strategy for choosing which embryo to transfer involves ranking embryos through careful microscopy-based characterization of development and morphology. However, preimplantation genetic testing (PGT) has become a routine method for embryo selection, now implemented in 40% of all in vitro fertilization (IVF) cycles in the United States [1]. PGT is most commonly applied to select euploid embryos for transfer, while avoiding those embryos designated as aneuploid (PGT-A). The primary objective of PGT-A is to improve the success of IVF in the first attempted embryo transfer [2,3]. Again, the default strategy for choosing which euploid embryo to transfer involves ranking embryos through careful microscopy-based characterization of development and morphology [4].

More recently, the opportunity to characterize the risk of polygenic disease in the preimplantation embryo has been made possible. Polygenic disorders, conditions influenced by genetic variants in multiple genes, account for a large percentage of premature deaths in humans [5,6]. These are largely contributed to by cancer, heart disease, and diabetes. There is a growing body of evidence that the risk of these diseases is higher in individuals seeking fertility treatments [7]. Despite the potential for environmental influence, polygenic disease risk can now be accurately predicted for several common diseases, including cancer, heart disease, and diabetes, using DNA alone [8,9]. We recently demonstrated the ability to achieve equivalent accuracy in genome-wide genotyping of DNA from a preimplantation embryo, as is already achieved when DNA is tested from adults. Therefore, the same performance in predicting polygenic disease in adults can now be achieved in preimplantation embryos [10].

Polygenic risk scoring in adults is often performed and evaluated in the context of entire populations of unrelated people [11]. In contrast, PGT involves evaluating genetic risks among sibling embryos within a single family. This was addressed previously by evaluating blinded DNA from 2601 adult sibling pair families with known type 1 diabetes status. Results demonstrated a 45–72% reduction in the incidence of type 1 diabetes when one sibling was chosen based on a polygenic risk score compared to when one sibling was chosen randomly. This study demonstrated clinical utility of PGT-P in a situation that is similar to PGT for monogenic disease, where intended parents have a known risk of passing on the disease [12].

Independent of fertility, polygenic conditions present in families at a much higher rate compared to monogenic disease, with most polygenic disorders manifesting in adulthood [6]. As such, while it is common for a couple to report a family history of polygenic disorders, it is rarer for a couple to present for PGT-P based on having a previously affected child. Exceptions to this involve polygenic disorders that present with early age of onset, such as type 1 diabetes. In this case, intended parents seeking IVF treatment may already be the parents of an affected child. As reported here, this very case is presented for PGT-P. Still, the spectrum of patients who may consider PGT-P could vary from those being affected or having an affected child to those having an unknown family history of any of the polygenic diseases being tested. In order to address whether PGT-P may apply to intended parents with unknown family history of polygenic disease, several thousand sibling pairs represented in the United Kingdom (UK) Biobank repository were evaluated using a blinded genomic disease index methodology. We also test whether preimplantation embryo genomic index values correlate with the extent of the embryos' family history.

2. Materials and Methods

2.1. PGT-P Case with First Degree Affected Family History

A couple with a family history of type 1 diabetes (T1D) presented to the Genomic Prediction Clinical Laboratory and was counseled for and consented to PGT-P as previously described [12]. The couple reported that their 5-year-old son was diagnosed with T1D at 3 years of age, and that two additional relatives, a paternal first cousin and a maternal second cousin, were diagnosed with T1D in their 20s (Figure 1). The patient reported two maternal relatives who were diagnosed with breast cancer. The couple otherwise denied a personal or family history of polygenic conditions that are included on the current PGT-P panel. The couple also reported three first trimester miscarriages with a normal karyotype. The couple denied a history of parental chromosome rearrangements and previous pregnancies or family history of aneuploidy. The couple declined a family history of additional genetic conditions that they wished to test for via PGT studies.

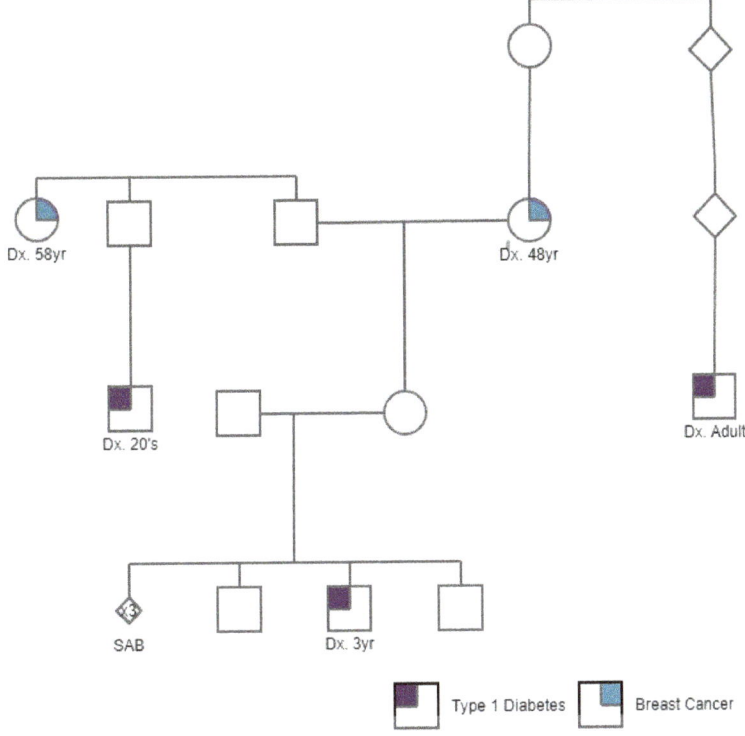

Figure 1. A pedigree of a case presenting for PGT-P with a family history of type 1 diabetes and breast cancer (shown in purple and turquoise, respectively).

2.2. PGT-P Case Series including Unknown Family History

To begin to evaluate the frequency of high-risk embryos across different degrees of family history, 24 consecutive PGT cases were analyzed and compared. PGT was performed using trophectoderm-biopsy-derived DNA, followed by whole-genome amplification and Axiom UKBB SNP-array-based analyses as previously described [10]. For each case, parental DNA was analyzed, and the ethnicity was predicted (Caucasian, Asian, African, other) with a pipeline built on a previously established supervised admixture methodology [13] and trained with 551 known ancestry samples [14]. The internal validation was performed on 229 samples from Coriell Cell Repository [15], resulting in an accuracy of 99.6% (228/229).

This consecutive PGT case series included couples who consented to research during genetic counseling for routine clinical use of PGT. Indications ranged from unknown family history to having 1st-degree relatives (i.e., the embryo's sibling or parent) affected with a polygenic disease. In all cases, PGT-A was performed in parallel and from the same biopsy, as previously described [10]. Risk of type 1 and 2 diabetes, breast, prostate, and testicular cancer, malignant melanoma, basal cell carcinoma, heart attack, coronary artery disease, hypercholesterolemia, and hypertension was tested in embryos with Caucasian ancestry, and risk of type 2 diabetes, hypercholesterolemia, and hypertension in embryos with Asian ancestry. High risk of polygenic disease was defined as previously described [12].

2.3. PGT-P in 11,883 Adult Sibling Pairs

A recent study reported that SNPs which are predictive of specific diseases do not overlap with one another [16]. This suggests that genetic selection to avoid one disease may not result in increasing another (pleiotropy). Instead, there may exist a positive effect of combining predictors into one "index" score. A genomic index algorithm, Equation (1), was developed by combining P_i (the absolute probability of getting the disease computed from SNP genotypes) with quality-adjusted life year QALY weights [17] determined by Q_i (the effect on life expectancy from each disease measured as lifespan impact years) and PA_i (the population average probability of getting the disease):

$$Gi = \sum_i (Qi(PAi - Pi)), \quad (1)$$

where i extends over all of the disease predictors, including type 1 and 2 diabetes, breast, prostate, and testicular cancer, malignant melanoma, basal cell carcinoma, heart attack, coronary artery disease, high cholesterol, and hypertension [18]. The genomic index = Gi is the sum of each of these contributions. Life expectancy effects Q_i are sourced from the medical literature [19–25].

Predictors were constructed from data obtained from the UK Biobank by first selecting the top 50,000 SNPs (by p-value) obtained from GWAS generated using the PLINK software (version 1.9, Cognitive Genomics Lab, Shenzhen, China) and then using the LASSO-path algorithm from the Python Scikit Learn package [26]. The UK Biobank identified all pairwise relationships stronger than 2nd cousins using the King kinship software. These results were used to identify all individuals who were within a sibling pair. This set of sibling pairs was further restricted to all individuals who self-reported their ethnic background to be "White, British, Irish or Any Other White Background" and was set aside as a final testing set [27]. The remaining non-sibling-paired self-reported white individuals were used as a training cohort. A small set of 500 cases/controls were withheld from the training cohort to tune the LASSO hyperparameter and select the final model—the value chosen is such that the AUC between cases/controls was maximized.

In order to validate the application of the genomic index to real sibling data, and to address the potential impact of pleiotropy upon PGT-P, a genomic index score was generated for same-sex sibling pairs from the genome-wide genotyping data of the UK Biobank [27]. In each pair, one of the two siblings was assigned to the cohort of "higher-risk sibling" (worse index score sibling), and one to "lower-risk sibling" (better index score sibling). Then, the prevalence of disease was calculated among the two cohorts. The prevalence of disease in the lower-risk sibling selected cohort was compared to the randomly selected cohort using binomial testing. Sex-specific relative risk reductions for diseases which affect both sexes were averaged.

Finally, genomic indexing was tested on blastocysts from the consecutive case series cohort described in Section 2.2, and with respect to the extent of family history of polygenic disease. Family history of polygenic disease was divided into three main categories with respect to the tested embryos: (1) having one or more first-degree affected relatives, for example an affected parent or an existing affected sibling; (2) having one or more second-degree or higher affected relatives, such as a grandparent or cousin; and (3) unknown or not reported by the patient. A two-tailed pairwise t-test was computed to compare the average genomic index of embryos among the three family history categories.

3. Results

3.1. PGT-P Case with First-Degree Affected Family History

Four euploid embryos were evaluated for polygenic disease risk and this resulted in identification of two at high risk for T1D (Figure 2).

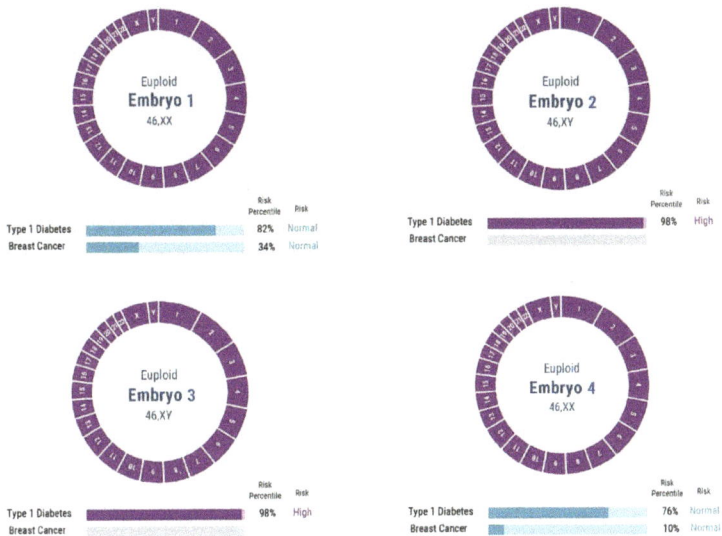

Figure 2. Type 1 diabetes case PGT-P results. Risk percentile indicates the predicted risk in terms of the computed polygenic risk score with respect to the distribution of risk scores from the UK Biobank cohort. Risk is classified as high when the embryo polygenic risk score is in the top 2% when compared to the average population-matched sample; otherwise, it is classified as normal risk.

3.2. PGT-P Case Series Including Unknown Family History

Based upon these results, involving a case where the embryos had a first-degree relative affected by a polygenic disease, and prior results where embryos had a more distant relative (second-degree relative or higher) affected by a polygenic disease [12], we investigated the potential for correlation between the frequency of high-risk embryos produced and the extent of an embryo's family history of polygenic disease in a larger cohort of cases. A consecutive series of 24 PGT cases with 181 embryos was evaluated by PGT-P analysis. The mean maternal age was 34.5. Thirty-seven percent of the embryos were aneuploid (67/181). Ten couples were predicted as Asian and 14 as Caucasian. There were no high-risk embryos identified from the Asian euploid embryo cohort (0/28 with no known history, and 0/3 with a more distant affected relative). Among Caucasian cases, 3 out of 51 euploid embryos (6%) were identified as high risk from couples with no known or reported family history, 3 out of 28 (11%) in cases with a more distant relative, and 4 out of 4 (100%) in a case with a first-degree affected relative.

3.3. Genomic Index Selection in 11,883 Adult Sibling Pairs

A cohort of 11,883 sibling pairs was available for analysis from the UK Biobank. The intent of evaluating genomic indexing in this cohort was to model application of PGT-P in families with no known history of disease. However, the prevalence of disease in this cohort was often lower than what has been reported for the general population, which would bias the results of PGT-P in the direction of finding no reduction in risk. For instance, the prevalence of breast cancer in this UK Biobank cohort was 8.0%, while it has been reported as a 12.3% lifetime risk in the general population [28]. Likewise, 7.4% of individuals in the UK Biobank adult sibling cohort were affected with type 2 diabetes, whereas a prevalence of 9.8% has been estimated in the United States [29]. Nonetheless, these sibling pairs were used to compare the relative risk of disease with either random selection or blinded genetic selection of one of the two siblings. Results indicate a relative risk reduction for all diseases tested (Figure 3) (Table 1).

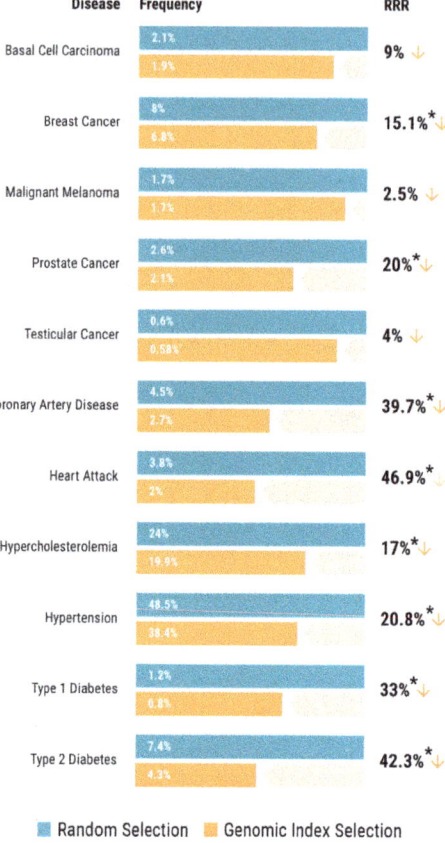

Figure 3. Relative risk reduction (RRR) across 11 diseases using genomic index selection compared to random selection within 11,883 sibling pairs. The frequency of disease with random selection is shown in blue, while the frequency of disease with genomic index selection is shown in orange. These data show a clear benefit from genetic selection of one of only two siblings with an unknown family history of disease. * p-value < 0.05 (Table 1).

Table 1. Binomial test p-values for relative disease risk reduction between random selection and genomic index selection of 11,883 sibling pairs.

Disease.	Male	Female
Basal Cell Carcinoma	0.0224	0.2655
Breast Cancer		0.0001
Malignant Melanoma	0.3518	0.4661
Prostate Cancer	0.0224	
Testicular Cancer	0.5	
Coronary Artery Disease	9.53×10^{-16}	3.09×10^{-7}
Heart Attack	7.31×10^{-22}	1.24×10^{-6}
Hypercholesterolemia	4.73×10^{-10}	1.21×10^{-11}
Hypertension	3.03×10^{-25}	3.08×10^{-33}
Type 1 Diabetes	0.0019	0.0083
Type 2 Diabetes	1.64×10^{-17}	2.09×10^{-21}

Genomic indexing was also performed on embryos evaluated in the PGT-P case series described in Section 3.2. Each embryo was classified based on the aforementioned categories of family history Results indicate that embryos with a first-degree affected relative have a higher genomic risk index compared to embryos with a more distant affected relative ($p = 0.0132$, $t = 3.09$, $df = 9$, $a = 0.05$) or with unknown family history ($p = 0.0015$, $t = 4.34$, $df = 10$, $a = 0.05$). Likewise, even embryos with at least one distant affected relative presented a higher average genomic index compared to those with unknown family history ($p = 0.0129$, $t = 2.55$, $df = 66$, $a = 0.05$) (Figure 4).

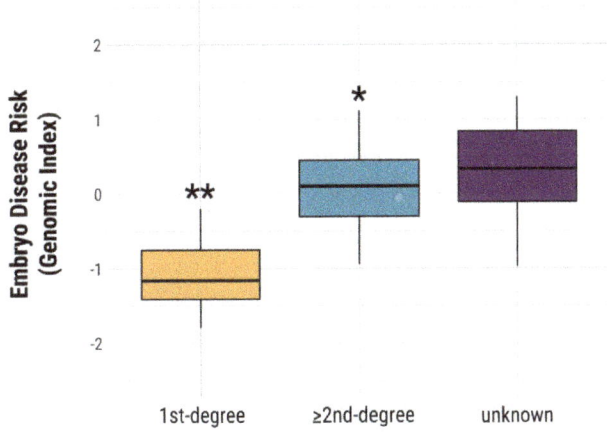

Figure 4. Preimplantation embryo genomic index versus family history. Embryos with a 1st degree affected relative have a significantly higher risk of polygenic disease than embryos with an unknown family history of polygenic disease. ** $p = 0.0015$ vs unknown. * $p = 0.0129$ vs unknown.

4. Discussion

This study extends the validity of PGT-P to reduce disease risk beyond families with a known history of disease. While many patients may elect to utilize PGT-P specifically because of a personal or family history of disease, the data presented here demonstrates utility in a more general application to routine embryo selection. One unique feature of this method is that PGT-A results are obtained in parallel with PGT-P [10], allowing patients to elect for additional information after knowing how many euploid embryos are suitable for transfer. In other words, instead of choosing which embryo to transfer based on morphology, choosing based upon PGT-P provides an option for patients to reduce the risk of polygenic disease, even when only two euploid embryos are available to choose from and when the intended parents have no known family history of polygenic disease.

In the case series reported here, 114 of 181 embryos tested were chromosomally normal (63%). Among the euploid embryos, only ten (5%) were identified as having a high risk of a polygenic disease. With this information, patients would still be faced with deciding which euploid normal risk embryo to choose for embryo transfer. Additional empirical analyses with the use of genomic indexing demonstrated relative risk reduction in all diseases tested, thereby providing additional criteria for patients to choose which embryo to transfer. Again, risk reduction was demonstrated with only two siblings to select from. Based upon a previous study, the availability of more than two siblings will further improve the relative risk reductions observed here [12].

Another important consideration relates to the potential for pleiotropy, the genetic effect of a single gene on multiple phenotypic traits [30]. With respect to PGT-P, avoiding high risk of one disease may lead to increased risk of another. The present study also demonstrated that negative pleiotropy was not observed. That is, selection with PGT-P resulted in a reduction in risk for all diseases in parallel. In support of this observation, a recent study [16] reported that SNP sets used to predict the risk of different diseases were largely disjoint.

Although the present study clearly demonstrates the utility of PGT-P-based sibling selection to reduce the relative risk of disease, several improvements may still be possible. The current metric of the impact of each disease used in the genomic index was limited to reported years of lost life. Several studies on the burden of disease have incorporated more comprehensive metrics, including reduced quality of life [6,31,32]. More validation can be performed and optimized on the genomic index by testing it on the life span and quality-of-life outcome data from the UKBB. In addition, patients may have unique interests in reducing the risk of certain diseases over others. More careful curation of these metrics will likely improve the utility of PGT-P.

While the clinical utility of tracing monogenic disorders through detailed pedigree analysis is well established [33], family history alone has been shown to be less effective as a single predictor of polygenic disease [34]. The results presented here may also have implications similar to when expanded carrier screening was introduced to contemporary genetic testing strategies [35]. Just as ethnicity and family history cannot be completely relied on to identify couples at risk for recessive disease, family history and ethnicity cannot be relied on alone to predict polygenic risk. That is, there is clear benefit to PGT-P in situations where "no known family history" exists, given that this status may only indicate that there was no reported history or no confirmed history, and that most families have a relative with at least one of the polygenic diseases tested by PGT-P [6,7]. This also may further benefit couples who have no known history because they know very little about their family tree, were adopted, or are using gamete donation.

5. Conclusions

In conclusion, PGT-P provides an additional method for embryo selection beyond conventional aneuploidy screening and morphological assessment and is applicable to prospective parents whose embryos have family histories ranging from an affected first-degree relative to no known history. At each level of embryonic family history evaluated, and in consideration of reducing the risk of polygenic disease through selection, this study demonstrates a measurable reduction in disease risk. Future work will involve incorporating additional quality-of-life metrics and DNA repository datasets, additional disease predictors, analysis of correlation with embryonic morphological characteristics, and relative risk reduction with more than two siblings to select from. The ability of genomic indexing to reduce risk of multiple diseases in parallel may allow an indirect reduction in risk of diseases where direct genomic predictors are not yet available.

Author Contributions: Conceptualization, N.R.T., J.E., J.X., and L.C.A.M.T. formal analysis, writing—original draft preparation, writing—review and editing, N.R.T., J.E., L.C.A.M.T., D.M., J.X., E.M. and L.L.; data curation, J.G. All authors have read and agreed to the published version of the manuscript.

Funding: This research received no external funding.

Acknowledgments: This study has been performed with UK Biobank data under application 15326.

Conflicts of Interest: N.R.T., J.E., L.C.A.M.T., D.M., J.X., E.M., and L.L. are employees and or shareholders of Genomic Prediction.

References

1. SART. Preliminary National Summary Report for 2018. Available online: https://www.sartcorsonline.com/rptCSR_PublicMultYear.aspx?reportingYear=2018 (accessed on 14 April 2020).
2. Forman, E.J.; Hong, K.H.; Ferry, K.M.; Tao, X.; Taylor, D.; Levy, B.; Treff, N.R.; Jr, R.T.S. In vitro fertilization with single euploid blastocyst transfer: A randomized controlled trial. *Fertil. Steril.* **2013**, *100*, 100–107. [CrossRef] [PubMed]
3. Juneau, C.; Franasiak, J.; Treff, N. Challenges facing contemporary preimplantation genetic screening. *Curr. Opin. Obstet. Gynecol.* **2016**, *28*, 151–157. [CrossRef] [PubMed]

4. Gardner, D.K.; Meseguer, M.; Rubio, C.; Treff, N.R. Diagnosis of human preimplantation embryo viability. *Hum. Reprod. Updat.* **2015**, *21*, 727–747. [CrossRef]
5. World Health Organization. *Global Status Report on Roncommunicable Riseases 2014*; World Health Organization: Geneva, Switzerland, 2014.
6. Forouzanfar, M.H.; Afshin, A.; Alexander, L.T.; Anderson, H.R.; A Bhutta, Z.; Biryukov, S.; Brauer, M.; Burnett, R.; Cercy, K.; Charlson, F.J.; et al. Global, regional, and national comparative risk assessment of 79 behavioural, environmental and occupational, and metabolic risks or clusters of risks, 1990–2015: A systematic analysis for the Global Burden of Disease Study 2015. *Lancet* **2016**, *388*, 1659–1724. [CrossRef]
7. Cedars, M.I.; Taymans, S.E.; DePaolo, L.V.; Warner, L.; Moss, S.B.; Eisenberg, M.L. The sixth vital sign: What reproduction tells us about overall health. Proceedings from a NICHD/CDC workshop. *Hum. Reprod. Open* **2017**, *2017*, hox008. [CrossRef]
8. Khera, A.V.; Chaffin, M.D.; Aragam, K.G.; Haas, M.E.; Roselli, C.; Choi, S.H.; Natarajan, P.; Lander, E.S.; Lubitz, S.A.; Ellinor, P.T.; et al. Genome-wide polygenic scores for common diseases identify individuals with risk equivalent to monogenic mutations. *Nat. Genet.* **2018**, *50*, 1219–1224. [CrossRef]
9. Torkamani, A.; E Wineinger, N.; Topol, E.J. The personal and clinical utility of polygenic risk scores. *Nat. Rev. Genet.* **2018**, *19*, 581–590. [CrossRef]
10. Treff, N.; Zimmerman, R.; Bechor, E.; Hsu, J.; Rana, B.; Jensen, J.; Li, J.; Samoilenko, A.; Mowrey, W.; Van Alstine, J.; et al. Validation of concurrent preimplantation genetic testing for polygenic and monogenic disorders, structural rearrangements, and whole and segmental chromosome aneuploidy with a single universal platform. *Eur. J. Med Genet.* **2019**, *62*, 103647. [CrossRef]
11. Duncan, L.; Shen, H.; Gelaye, B.; Meijsen, J.; Ressler, K.; Feldman, M.; Peterson, R.; Domingue, B.W. Analysis of polygenic risk score usage and performance in diverse human populations. *Nat. Commun.* **2019**, *10*, 3328. [CrossRef]
12. Treff, N.; Eccles, J.; Lello, L.; Bechor, E.; Hsu, J.; Plunkett, K.; Zimmerman, R.; Rana, B.; Samoilenko, A.; Hsu, S.; et al. Utility and First Clinical Application of Screening Embryos for Polygenic Disease Risk Reduction. *Front. Endocrinol.* **2019**, *10*, 845. [CrossRef]
13. Alexander, D.H.; Novembre, J.; Lange, K. Fast model-based estimation of ancestry in unrelated individuals. *Genome Res.* **2009**, *19*, 1655–1664. [CrossRef]
14. Gibbs, R.A.; Belmont, J.W.; Hardenbol, P.; Willis, T.D.; Yu, F.; Yang, H.; Ch'ang, L.-Y.; Huang, W.; Liu, B.; Shen, Y.; et al. The International HapMap Project. *Nature* **2003**, *426*, 789–796. [CrossRef]
15. Packer, B.R. SNP500Cancer: A public resource for sequence validation, assay development, and frequency analysis for genetic variation in candidate genes. *Nucleic Acids Res.* **2006**, *34*, 617–621. [CrossRef]
16. Yong, S.Y.; Raben, T.; Lello, L.; Hsu, S.D.H. Genetic Architecture of Complex Traits and Disease Risk Predictors. *bioRxiv* **2020**. [CrossRef]
17. Torrance, G.W.; Feeny, D. Utilities and Quality-Adjusted Life Years. *Int. J. Technol. Assess. Heal. Care* **1989**, *5*, 559–575. [CrossRef]
18. Lello, L.; Raben, T.; Yong, S.Y.; Tellier, L.C.A.M.; Hsu, S.D.H. Genomic Prediction of 16 Complex Disease Risks Including Heart Attack, Diabetes, Breast and Prostate Cancer. *Sci. Rep.* **2019**, *9*, 1–16. [CrossRef]
19. Franco, O.H.; Peeters, A.; Bonneux, L.; De Laet, C. Blood Pressure in Adulthood and Life Expectancy With Cardiovascular Disease in Men and Women. *Hypertens.* **2005**, *46*, 280–286. [CrossRef]
20. Yang, J.; Liu, Y.N.; Liu, J.M.; Zeng, X.Y.; Zhao, Y.F.; Wang, Z.Q.; Zhou, M.G. The effect of high total cholesterol on life expectancy in 2013 in China. *Zhonghua Liu Xing Bing Xue Za Zhi* **2017**, *38*, 1017–1021. [CrossRef]
21. Grundtvig, M.; Hagen, T.P.; Amrud, E.S.; Reikvam, Å. Reduced life expectancy after an incident hospital diagnosis of acute myocardial infarction — Effects of smoking in women and men. *Int. J. Cardiol.* **2013**, *167*, 2792–2797. [CrossRef]
22. Capocaccia, R.; Gatta, G.; Maso, L.D. Life expectancy of colon, breast, and testicular cancer patients: An analysis of US-SEER population-based data. *Ann. Oncol.* **2015**, *26*, 1263–1268. [CrossRef]
23. Livingstone, S.J.; Levin, D.; Looker, H.C.; Lindsay, R.S.; Wild, S.H.; Joss, N.; Leese, G.; Leslie, P.; McCrimmon, R.J.; Metcalfe, W.; et al. Estimated life expectancy in a Scottish cohort with type 1 diabetes, 2008-2010. *JAMA* **2015**, *313*, 37–44. [CrossRef] [PubMed]
24. Syriopoulou, E.; Bower, H.; Andersson, T.M.-L.; Lambert, P.C.; Rutherford, M.A. Estimating the impact of a cancer diagnosis on life expectancy by socio-economic group for a range of cancer types in England. *Br. J. Cancer* **2017**, *117*, 1419–1426. [CrossRef] [PubMed]

25. Hollestein, L.M.; De Vries, E.; Aarts, M.J.; Schroten, C.; Nijsten, T.E. Burden of disease caused by keratinocyte cancer has increased in The Netherlands since 1989. *J. Am. Acad. Dermatol.* **2014**, *71*, 896–903. [CrossRef]
26. Chang, C.C.; Chow, C.C.; Tellier, L.C.A.M.; Vattikuti, S.; Purcell, S.M.; Lee, J.J. Second-generation PLINK: Rising to the challenge of larger and richer datasets. *GigaScience* **2015**, *4*, 7. [CrossRef] [PubMed]
27. Bycroft, C.; Freeman, C.; Petkova, D.; Band, G.; Elliott, L.T.; Sharp, K.; Motyer, A.; Vukcevic, D.; Delaneau, O.; O'Connell, J.; et al. The UK Biobank resource with deep phenotyping and genomic data. *Nature* **2018**, *562*, 203–209. [CrossRef]
28. Rojas, K.; Stuckey, A. Breast Cancer Epidemiology and Risk Factors. *Clin. Obstet. Gynecol.* **2016**, *59*, 651–672. [CrossRef]
29. Hariri, S.; Yoon, P.W.; Qureshi, N.; Valdez, R.; Scheuner, M.T.; Khoury, M.J. Family history of type 2 diabetes: A population-based screening tool for prevention? *Genet. Med.* **2006**, *8*, 102–108. [CrossRef]
30. Watanabe, K.; Stringer, S.; Frei, O.; Mirkov, M.U.; De Leeuw, C.A.; Polderman, T.J.; Van Der Sluis, S.; Andreassen, O.A.; Neale, B.M.; Posthuma, D. A global overview of pleiotropy and genetic architecture in complex traits. *Nat. Genet.* **2019**, *51*, 1339–1348. [CrossRef]
31. Murray, C.J.; Lopez, A. Measuring the Global Burden of Disease. *N. Engl. J. Med.* **2013**, *369*, 448–457. [CrossRef]
32. Devleesschauwer, B.; De Noordhout, C.M.; Smit, S.; Duchateau, L.; Dorny, P.; Stein, C.; Van Oyen, H.; Speybroeck, N. Quantifying burden of disease to support public health policy in Belgium: Opportunities and constraints. *BMC Public Heal.* **2014**, *14*, 1196. [CrossRef]
33. Badano, J.; Katsanis, N. Beyond Mendel: An evolving view of human genetic disease transmission. *Nat. Rev. Genet.* **2002**, *3*, 779–789. [CrossRef] [PubMed]
34. Do, C.B.; Hinds, D.A.; Francke, U.; Eriksson, N. Comparison of Family History and SNPs for Predicting Risk of Complex Disease. *PLoS Genet.* **2012**, *8*, e1002973. [CrossRef] [PubMed]
35. Lazarin, G.A.; Haque, I.S.; Nazareth, S.; Iori, K.; Patterson, A.S.; Jacobson, J.L.; Marshall, J.R.; Seltzer, W.K.; Patrizio, P.; Evans, E.A.; et al. An empirical estimate of carrier frequencies for 400+ causal Mendelian variants: Results from an ethnically diverse clinical sample of 23,453 individuals. *Genet. Med.* **2012**, *15*, 178–186. [CrossRef] [PubMed]

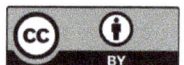

© 2020 by the authors. Licensee MDPI, Basel, Switzerland. This article is an open access article distributed under the terms and conditions of the Creative Commons Attribution (CC BY) license (http://creativecommons.org/licenses/by/4.0/).

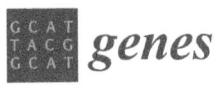

Article

Combined Preimplantation Genetic Testing for Autosomal Dominant Polycystic Kidney Disease: Consequences for Embryos Available for Transfer

Pere Mir Pardo [1,*], José Antonio Martínez-Conejero [1], Julio Martín [1,2], Carlos Simón [1,2,3,4] and Ana Cervero [1]

1. Igenomix, 46980 Valencia, Spain; joseantonio.conejero@igenomix.com (J.A.M.-C.); julio.martin@igenomix.com (J.M.); Carlos.simon@igenomix.com (C.S.); ana.cervero@igenomix.com (A.C.)
2. Igenomix Foundation-INCLIVA, 46010 Valencia, Spain
3. Department of Obstetrics and Gynecology, BIDMC, Harvard University, Boston, MA 02215, USA
4. Department of Pediatrics, Obstetrics & Gynecology, University of Valencia, 46010 Valencia, Spain
* Correspondence: pere.mir@igenomix.com

Received: 1 June 2020; Accepted: 22 June 2020; Published: 24 June 2020

Abstract: Autosomal dominant polycystic kidney disease (ADPKD) is the most common hereditary kidney disease and presents with genetic and clinical heterogeneity. ADPKD can also manifest extra-renally, and seminal cysts have been associated with male infertility in some cases. ADPKD-linked male infertility, along with female age, have been proposed as factors that may influence the clinical outcomes of preimplantation genetic testing (PGT) for monogenic disorders (PGT-M). Large PGT for aneuploidy assessment (PGT-A) studies link embryo aneuploidy to increasing female age; other studies suggest that embryo aneuploidy is also linked to severe male-factor infertility. We aimed to assess the number of aneuploid embryos and the number of cycles with transferable embryos in ADPKD patients after combined-PGT. The combined-PGT protocol, involving PGT-M by PCR and PGT-A by next-generation sequencing, was performed in single trophectoderm biopsies from 289 embryos in 83 PGT cycles. Transferable embryos were obtained in 69.9% of cycles. The number of aneuploid embryos and cycles with transferable embryos did not differ when the male or female had the ADPKD mutation. However, a significantly higher proportion of aneuploid embryos was found in the advanced maternal age (AMA) group, but not in the male factor (MF) group, when compared to non-AMA and non-MF groups, respectively. Additionally, no significant differences in the percentage of cycles with transferable embryos were found in any of the groups. Our results indicate that AMA couples among ADPKD patients have an increased risk of aneuploid embryos, but ADPKD-linked male infertility does not promote an increased aneuploidy rate.

Keywords: combined preimplantation genetic testing; Preimplantation genetic testing for monogenic disorders (PGT-M); Preimplantation genetic testing for aneuploidy assessment (PGT-A); Autosomal dominant polycystic kidney disease (ADPKD); male infertility; advanced maternal age; aneuploidy

1. Introduction

Autosomal dominant polycystic kidney disease (ADPKD) is the most common hereditary kidney disease, with an estimated prevalence of 1:1000 to 1:2500 individuals [1]. ADPKD is a genetically heterogeneous disorder attributed to two main genes: *PKD1* (located at chromosome 16p13.3) and *PKD2* (located at chromosome 4q21–q23). Mutations in *PKD1* account for most (78–85%) ADPKD cases, but more than 1500 different mutations in *PKD1* or *PKD2* have been identified in patients with ADPKD [1,2]. In addition, six pseudogenes with a high homology to *PKD1* have been identified on chromosome 16. Consequently, only 3.5 kb of the 14 kb of the *PKD1* transcript is single copy [1,3].

Mutations in *PKD1* generally cause more severe nephropathy than mutations in *PKD2*, and the age of onset varies within and between families. ADPKD is clinically heterogeneous, but generally characterized by cysts that develop in one or both kidneys and increase in number over time, leading to nephromegaly and chronic renal failure [1]. ADPKD can also have extra-renal manifestations, with cysts in the liver (70–90%), the seminal tract (10–35%), and more rarely in the pancreas (5–10%), as well as with non-cystic manifestations, such as intracranial aneurysms (9–12%) [1–3]. The presence of cysts in seminal vesicles and ejaculatory ducts may be associated with infertility or subfertility [4,5], though not always [6]. On the other hand, fertility does not appear to be affected in women with ADPKD mutations, but pregnant women with a compromised kidney function must be monitored for the development of complications such as hypertension and preeclampsia, which could affect reproductive outcomes [5].

The offspring of individuals affected by ADPKD have a 50% chance of inheriting the causal mutation. To avert the inheritance of the disorder, either prenatal (PND) or preimplantation genetic testing for monogenic disorders (PGT-M) can be offered [5–9]. PND uses DNA obtained from the fetus, usually collected from amniotic fluid or chorionic villus sampling, to inform medical termination of the pregnancy in cases with confirmed genetic abnormality. In contrast, regardless of the fertility status, PGT-M requires assisted reproductive techniques (ART) such as in-vitro fertilization (IVF) or intracytoplasmic sperm injection to assess embryonic DNA, and only genetically normal embryos for the analyzed condition will be candidates for transfer to the maternal uterus. This difference, combined with the variability in the expression of the disease and age of onset, means that most patients would prefer PGT-M over PND [5,7,10].

PGT-M is most often performed via a polymerase chain reaction (PCR) [11] to directly amplify specific DNA sequences from an embryo biopsy, as is applied to ADPKD couples [7,8,12]. While next-generation sequencing (NGS) has been clinically applied for PGT-M [13], this method has not yet been used for ADPKD cases. In familial ADPKD, the genetic and clinical heterogeneity can obscure the causal mutation in some cases, but a family history of the disease is known in one, two, or even three different generations [14]. This phenomenon facilitates performing PGT-M by PCR through linkage analysis [2,7,12]. This strategy can be complemented with an analysis of the specific mutation, but is not necessarily applied for familial ADPKD cases.

A recent paper successfully applied PGT-M for ADPKD in day-3 embryo biopsies, resulting in 27 healthy live births. The report also evaluated the impact of parental ADPKD on the clinical outcome, showing a lower clinical pregnancy rate and live birth rate in couples with the male partner affected compared with couples with the female partner affected [12]. However, the authors concluded that their multivariate logistic regression analysis only identified an association of an increased maternal age with a lower live birth rate [12]. Embryo aneuploidy rates are widely reported to increase with increasing female age [15–17] and to cause a lower pregnancy and delivery rate [17]. In contrast, the relationship between aneuploidy rates and male infertility factors is less clear; some studies found no difference in aneuploidy rates between male-factor (MF) infertility and normal sperm patients [18], while others only reported higher aneuploidy rates in severe infertility cases, suggesting that PGT aneuploidy assessment (PGT-A) may be advisable for these patients [19,20].

Increasingly, PGT-M and PGT-A are performed in the same embryo [21–23]. However, few instances of combined testing have been reported for ADPKD. Indeed, we identified only two reports of combined-PGT for ADPKD: a case report of two ART cycles from a woman with ADPKD in a couple with no reported fertility issues [8], and a series of seven cycles from seven couples with reported ADPKD-linked male infertility [24]. Importantly, combining PGT-A with PGT-M could reduce the number of transferable embryos (i.e., neither genetically abnormal nor aneuploid embryos would be considered for transfer) and may result in a higher number of ART cycles without a transferable embryo. To date, the data reported for combined-PGT in ADPKD are limited. With 37 embryos analyzed across the two reports, 18.2% (2/11) [8] and 46.2% (12/26) [24] of embryos were transferable.

To help guide clinical application, we aimed to ascertain the impact on the number of cycles with transferable embryos after introducing PGT-A into routine PGT-M for ADPKD. For this purpose, we assessed the percentages of aneuploid embryos, transferable embryos, and cycles with transferable embryos after combined-PGT in (i) overall ADPKD cases; (ii) cycles where the male carried the mutation compared to when the female carried the mutation; and (iii) patients grouped as those with an expected higher aneuploidy rate: advanced maternal age (AMA) or male-factor infertility (MF).

2. Materials and Methods

2.1. Patient Demography

This retrospective analysis included 74 couples affected by ADPKD that underwent at least one combined-PGT (PGT-M for ADPKD along with PGT-A for 24-chromosomes) from October 2016 to April 2020; nine of these couples underwent two combined-PGT cycles, for a total of 83 combined-PGT cycles. Most cases were associated with *PKD1* (83.1%) mutations, and the remainder (16.9%) with *PKD2* mutations. All 13 *PKD2* cases and 53/61 (86.4%) *PKD1* cases had a mutation identified.

Couples were ascertained from 39 IVF clinics in 10 countries. The top contributors were Spain (37 cases, 46 cycles), the USA (18 cases, 18 cycles), and Brazil (9 cases, 9 cycles).

2.2. Combined-PGT Protocol

All patients underwent genetic counseling and were requested to provide a report showing the causal mutation for ADPKD in any of the two progenitors or other family members, and/or a clinical report confirming the diagnosis of ADPKD before beginning PGT. Then, written informed consent for both PGT-M and PGT-A was obtained for all couples. Combined-PGT comprised four main steps: (1) PGT-M work-up; (2) an IVF procedure (controlled ovarian stimulation, ovum pick-up, fertilization, and embryo culture) to obtain trophectoderm biopsies from viable embryos; (3) the shipment of biopsies to our facilities; and (4) PGT-M and PGT-A protocols. Once the PGT-M work-up was approved by the staff of our company (Igenomix, Valencia, Spain), the IVF procedure was the responsibility of each IVF center. After the embryo biopsy, Igenomix handled the shipment of samples, analysis, and reporting. All trophectoderm biopsies were obtained on day 5 or 6 of embryo culture, and each biopsy was collected and shipped in a PCR tube containing 2 µL of phosphate-buffered saline as transport medium. Sample preparation for testing included whole genome amplification (WGA) using the Ion ReproSeq PGS Kit (ThermoFisher Scientific, Waltham, MA, USA). The same WGA product was used for both PGT-M and PGT-A. PGT-M was performed by PCR following a laboratory-developed protocol, and PGT-A was performed by a semi-automated protocol by NGS (ThermoFisher Scientific, Waltham, MA, USA).

2.3. PGT-M Work-Up

A preclinical work-up was required for all couples before undergoing PGT-M. Informativity for several polymorphic genetic markers (short tandem repeats (STR)) and segregation analysis were assessed for every family in genomic DNA from blood or buccal cells. Additionally, in cases in which the mutation in *PKD1* or *PKD2* was needed for PGT-M purposes, its analysis was also included in the work-up. Haplotyping analysis was assessed by fluorescence multiplex PCR using a minimum of 12 STR. Amplification was conducted using a T3000 thermocycler (Biometra, Goettingen, Germany) or similar equipment, and PCR products were analyzed in an AB3500 genetic analyzer (ThermoFisher Scientific, Waltham, MA, USA). After haplotyping analysis, a minimum of four informative STR, two upstream and two downstream, and all of them within 1–2 Mb, were required for approving the PGT-M work-up. The laboratory-developed protocol included the selected informative STR, as well as the *PKD* mutation when applicable.

2.4. PGT-M Protocol

PGT-M was performed on WGA products from trophectoderm biopsies using the same protocol selected in the PGT-M work-up. After PGT-M analysis, embryos were classified as (i) "normal", when a paternal and a maternal haplotype were present, confirming the presence of the haplotype unlinked to the PKD mutation, and the mutation was not detected; (ii) "abnormal", when a paternal and maternal haplotype were present, confirming the presence of the haplotype linked to the PKD mutation, and/or the mutation was detected; or (iii) "non-informative" or inconclusive results, when any paternal or maternal information was missing. For "non-informative" cases, it was not possible to specifically classify the embryo as normal or abnormal. In such cases, a trophectoderm re-biopsy was recommended, but clinics made the ultimate decision on whether to send a new biopsy.

2.5. PGT-A Protocol

For aneuploidy assessment, DNA barcoding was performed during the WGA process using the Ion ReproSeq PGS Kit (ThermoFisher Scientific, Waltham, MA, USA). Ion Chef equipment was used for library preparation, and samples were sequenced in batches of 24 or 96 samples (using 520 and 530 chips, respectively) in an S5 XL sequencer (ThermoFisher Scientific, Waltham, MA, USA), as previously described [25].

After PGT-A analysis, embryos were classified as (i) "euploid", when no aneuploidy was found; (ii) "aneuploid", when at least one aneuploidy was found; or (iii) "non-informative" or inconclusive, when the pattern obtained did not enable a definitive classification of the embryo as euploid or aneuploid. As for PGT-M, non-informative results prompted a recommendation for trophectoderm re-biopsy.

2.6. Combined-PGT Strategy

Only embryos both "normal" for PGT-M and "euploid" for PGT-A were considered to be "transferable" embryos. However, couples had several options in terms of electing a combined-PGT strategy: (i) to perform PGT-M and PGT-A in all embryos (elected for 29 cycles); (ii) to perform PGT-M first, and only apply PGT-A to embryos considered "normal" or "non-informative" (elected in 52 cycles); or (iii) to perform PGT-A first, and only apply PGT-M to embryos considered "euploid" or "non-informative" (elected in only two cycles). In total, PGT-M was performed in 432 embryos, PGT-A in 298 embryos, and combined-PGT in 289 embryos.

2.7. Analysis of Results

ADPKD results were divided into two groups, according to Berckmoes [12] classification, by whether the female (female-ADPKD) or the male (male-ADPKD) carried the ADPKD mutation. The main indicators analyzed were the (i) number of aneuploid embryos; (ii) number of transferable embryos; and (iii) number of cycles with transferable embryos after combined-PGT.

The same analysis was performed in patient subsets of AMA and MF, and compared with non-AMA and non-MF results, respectively. AMA was defined as 38 years old or above, and male patients with the ADPKD mutation that self-reported male infertility were considered for MF.

Statistical analyses for comparing the results of the different groups were conducted using Fisher's exact test for categorical variables. Comparisons of mean ages were performed using an unpaired t-test. Statistical significance was defined by a two-sided test with a p value of < 0.05.

3. Results

Overall, in 69.9% of combined-PGT cycles (58/83), there was at least one transferable embryo. By PGT-M, 94.0% of these cycles (78/83) had genetically normal embryos; by PGT-A, 74.7% of cycles (62/83) had euploid embryos. Additionally, no difference in the percentage of cycles with transferable embryos was found between female-ADPKD and male-ADPKD (Table 1).

Table 1. Results per cycle presented by cases where the female (female-autosomal dominant polycystic kidney disease (ADPKD)) or the male (male-ADPKD) carried the ADPKD mutation.

	Male-ADPKD	Female-ADPKD	Total	p-Value
No. couples	41	33	74	-
No. combined-PGT cycles	47	36	83	-
Female age, years (SD)	36.3 (3.9)	35.8 (4.3)	36.1 (4.1)	ns
Mean no. analyzed embryos per cycle (SD)	5.4 (3.4)	5.4 (3.3)	5.4 (3.4)	ns
Cycles with transfer, n (%)	31 (66.0)	27 (75.0)	58 (69.9)	ns
% cycles with euploid embryos	70.2	80.6	74.7	ns
% cycles with PGT-M normal embryos	95.7	91.7	94.0	ns

ns: not significant; SD: standard deviation.

For combined-PGT, 98.2% of embryos were informative for both techniques. The percentage of transferable embryos tended to be higher in the ADPKD-male group, but did not reach statistical significance (43.8% vs. 33.8% in ADPKD-female; $p = 0.0978$). There were no differences in the number of euploid embryos (PGT-A) or the number of genetically normal ones (PGT-M) (Table 2).

Table 2. Results per embryo presented by male-ADPKD and female-ADPKD cycles (% (n)).

EMBRYOS		Male-ADPKD	Female-ADPKD	TOTAL	p-Value
Combined PGT (n = 289)	Normal	43.8 (67)	33.8 (46)	39.1 (113)	ns
	Abnormal	54.2 (83)	64.7 (88)	59.2 (171)	
	NI	2.0 (3)	1.5 (2)	1.8 (5) *	
PGT-M (n = 432)	Normal	49.0 (123)	49.7 (90)	49.3 (213)	ns
	Abnormal	48.2 (121)	45.9 (83)	47.2 (204)	
	NI	2.8 (7)	4.4 (8)	3.5 (15)	
PGT-A (n = 298)	Normal	51.8 (84)	49.3 (67)	50.7 (151)	ns
	Abnormal	45.7 (74)	48.5 (66)	47.0 (140)	
	NI	2.5 (4)	2.3 (3)	2.3 (7)	

NI: non-informative embryos; ns: not significant; * final non-informative embryos. Seven embryos (three embryos in the male group and four in the female group) showed the presence of only one allele that was confirmed to be a monosomy for the corresponding chromosome after preimplantation genetic testing aneuploidy assessment (PGT-A) analysis. Therefore, they were initially classified as non-informative for PGT for monogenic disorders (PGT-M), but finally classified as chromosomally abnormal.

Combined-PGT results in the subsets of AMA and MF couples showed no differences in the percentage of cycles with transferable embryos compared with the overall results (Table 3). However, the comparison of PGT-A results per embryo showed a significantly higher percentage of aneuploid embryos in the AMA group when compared with non-AMA cases (Table 4). In contrast, the percentage of aneuploid embryos in the MF group did not significantly differ from the percentage in non-MF cases (Table 5).

Table 3. Results per cycle in the advanced maternal age (AMA) and male-factor infertility (MF) groups.

	AMA	MF	OVERALL	p-Value
No. couples	23	5	74	
No. combined-PGT cycles	32	6	83	
Female age, years (SD)	39.5 (1.3)	33.3 (2.2)	36.1 (4.1)	<0.0001 *
Mean no. analyzed embryos (SD)	4.9 (3.2)	5.2 (3.8)	5.4 (3.4)	ns
Cycles with euploid embryos, n (%)	20 (62.5)	5 (83.3)	62 (74.7)	ns
Combined-PGT cycles with transfer, n (%)	18 (56.3)	4 (66.7)	58 (69.9)	ns

ns: not significant; SD: standard deviation; * between AMA and MF.

Table 4. Comparison of results per embryo in AMA and non-AMA groups [% (n)].

		AMA	Non-AMA	p-Value
Combined PGT	Normal	28.0 (26)	44.4 (87)	
	Abnormal	69.9 (65)	54.1 (106)	ns
	NI	2.1 (2)	1.5 (3)	
PGT-M	Normal	46.1 (71)	50.4 (142)	
	Abnormal	47.4 (73)	47.8 (131)	ns
	NI	6.5 (10)	1.8 (5)	
PGT-A	Normal	33.3 (31)	58.5 (120)	
	Abnormal	64.5 (60)	39.0 (80)	<0.0001
	NI	2.2 (2)	2.5 (5)	

NI: non-informative embryos; ns: not significant.

Table 5. Comparison of results per embryo in MF and non-MF groups (% (n)).

		MF	Non-MF	p-Value
Combined PGT	Normal	64.7 (11)	37.5 (102)	
	Abnormal	25.3 (6)	60.7 (165)	ns
	NI	0	1.8 (5)	
PGT-M	Normal	54.8 (17)	48.6 (195)	
	Abnormal	45.2 (14)	47.6 (191)	ns
	NI	0	3.8 (15)	
PGT-A	Normal	70.6 (12)	49.5 (139)	
	Abnormal	29.4 (5)	48.0 (135)	ns
	NI	0	2.5 (7)	

NI: non-informative embryos; ns: not significant.

4. Discussion

This study provides detailed information to support the utility of combining PGT-M and PGT-A to guide embryo selection in couples affected by ADPKD who are undergoing ART. A larger study on PGT-M for ADPKD [12] reported 78 cycles and found that 35.7% of embryos were transferable (174/487), while 92.3% (72/78) of cycles had transferable embryos. These data can be compared with ours when only considering the PGT-M results; we found that 49.3% of embryos were transferable and 94.0% of cycles had transferable embryos. In our study, fewer cycles had transferable embryos after combined-PGT (94.0% of cycles with PGT-M vs. 69.9% with combined-PGT; $p = 0.0001$). This finding cannot be directly compared with previous publications due to limited data availability [8,24]. The percentage of transferable embryos we found after combined-PGT (39.1%) could be compared, but existing reports utilized small samples (2/11 or 18.2% [8]; 12/26 or 46.2% [24]).

Berckmoes et al. [12] suggested ADPKD-linked male infertility and female age as factors influencing the clinical outcome of PGT-M. In our data, when dividing cycles by male-ADPKD and female-ADPKD, results at the embryo level showed a similar percentage of (i) euploid embryos, (ii) genetically normal embryos, and (iii) transferable embryos after combined-PGT. Accordingly, no differences in the percentage of cycles with transferable embryos were detected between groups. Similarly, no differences were found when comparing MF versus non-MF cases. In contrast, the percentage of aneuploid embryos was significantly higher in the AMA group compared to the non-AMA group, but the number of cycles with transferable embryos was not statistically different.

In our study, ADPKD-linked male infertility was not associated with a higher aneuploidy rate or fewer cycles with transferable embryos; this finding was consistent across all male-ADPKD couples. Therefore, our data do not support that aneuploidy can be an influencing factor for poorer reproductive outcomes in male-ADPKD cases. These data align with recent reports on PGT-A results for MF patients, where significantly higher aneuploidy rates were only observed in severe cases [19,20], and not in overall MF patients [18]. However, in the present study, it was not possible to stratify the results by the severity of sperm parameters and, given the low number of cases of self-reported male infertility, any conclusions obtained for this group are limited.

On the other hand, AMA is established as a factor for higher aneuploidy rates [15–17]. Our data align with this phenomenon, and support the lower live birth rate associated with female age in Berckmoes et al. [12]. This higher aneuploidy rate will translate into a higher probability of transferring aneuploid embryos when PGT-A is not performed. For instance, aneuploid embryos still develop to the blastocyst stage and are responsible for lower probabilities of pregnancy, but a higher miscarriage likelihood [26]. Unfortunately, our study did not have access to data for pregnancy, miscarriage, or live birth rates, and Berckmoes et al. did not analyze PGT-M outcomes from the subset of patients categorized as AMA. However, in their data (see Table 2), the mean female age is significantly higher in the group of male-ADPKD compared with the female-ADPKD. Therefore, considering the information above, this feature may have had a negative impact on PGT-M outcomes for the male-ADPKD group.

5. Conclusions

In summary, we demonstrated a feasible approach for every ADPKD patient through a simultaneous analysis of PGT-M and PGT-A in the same embryo biopsy. The incorporation of combined-PGT helps in selecting euploid and genetically normal embryos, ensuring 70% of cycles with transferable embryos, and highlighting the impact of maternal age on embryo aneuploidy in this cohort. A similar approach could be available for every PGT-M case in the daily clinical routine.

Author Contributions: All authors contributed to conceptualizing the study and defining the objectives. P.M.P. built the database by gathering combined-PGT results. A.C. and J.A.M.-C. were involved in supervising and administering the project. The manuscript was written by P.M.P. and reviewed by J.A.M.-C., J.M., C.S., and A.C. All authors have read and agreed to the published version of the manuscript.

Funding: No funding was received for this study.

Acknowledgments: The authors would like to thank all of the Igenomix staff involved in these combined-PGT cycles around the world for sharing valuable data, as well as the staff who performed the embryo biopsies, ran the lab protocols, and analyzed the results. Special thanks to Mónica Clemente, our beloved statistician, who helped in reviewing the statistical analysis for this work.

Conflicts of Interest: All the authors are employees of Igenomix, the company where all combined-PGT analyses were performed.

References

1. Cornec-Le Gall, E.; Alam, A.; Perrone, R.D. Autosomal dominant polycystic kidney disease. *Lancet* **2019**, *393*, 919–935. [CrossRef]
2. Harris, P.C.; Torres, V.E. Polycystic kidney disease. *Annu. Rev. Med.* **2009**, *60*, 321–337. [CrossRef] [PubMed]
3. Boucher, C.; Sandford, R. Autosomal dominant polycystic kidney disease (ADPKD, MIM 173900, PKD1 and PKD2 genes, protein products known as polycystin-1 and polycystin-2). *Eur. J. Hum. Genet.* **2004**, *12*, 347–354. [CrossRef] [PubMed]
4. Peces, R.; Drenth., J.P.; Te Morsche, R.H.; González, P.; Peces, C. Autosomal dominant polycystic liver disease in a family without polycystic kidney disease associated with a novel missense protein kinase C substrate 80K-H mutation. *World J. Gastroenterol.* **2005**, *11*, 7690–7693. [CrossRef]
5. Vora, N.; Perrone, R.; Bianchi, D.W. Reproductive issues for adults with autosomal dominant polycystic kidney disease. *Am. J. Kidney Dis.* **2008**, *51*, 307–318. [CrossRef]
6. Torra, R.; Sarquella, J.; Calabia, J.; Martí, J.; Ars, E.; Fernández-Llama, P.; Ballarin, J. Prevalence of cysts in seminal tract and abnormal semen parameters in patients with autosomal dominant polycystic kidney disease. *Clin. J. Am. Soc. Nephrol.* **2008**, *3*, 790–793. [CrossRef]

7. Verlinsky, Y.; Rechitsky, S.; Verlinsky, O.; Ozen, S.; Beck, R.; Kuliev, A. Preimplantation genetic diagnosis for polycystic kidney disease. *Fertil Steril* **2004**, *82*, 926–929. [CrossRef]
8. Murphy, E.L.; Droher, M.L.; Di Maio, M.S.; Dahl, N.K.S.; Dahl, N.K. Preimplantation Genetic Diagnosis Counseling in Autosomal Dominant Polycystic Kidney Disease. *Am. J. Kidney Dis.* **2018**, *72*, 866–872. [CrossRef]
9. Torra, R.; Ars, E. Molecular diagnosis of autosomal dominant polycystic kidney disease. *Nefrologia* **2011**, *31*, 35–43. [CrossRef]
10. Swift, O.; Vilar, E.; Rahman, B.; Side, L.; Gale, D.P. Attitudes in Patients with Autosomal Dominant Polycystic Kidney Disease Toward Prenatal Diagnosis and Preimplantation Genetic Diagnosis. *Genet. Test. Mol. Biomark.* **2016**, *20*, 741–746. [CrossRef]
11. De Rycke, M.; Goossens, V.; Kokkali, G.; Meijer-Hoogeveen, M.; Coonen, E.; Moutou, C. ESHRE PGD Consortium data collection XIV-XV: Cycles from January 2011 to December 2012 with pregnancy follow-up to October 2013. *Hum. Reprod.* **2017**, *32*, 1974–1994. [CrossRef] [PubMed]
12. Berckmoes, V.; Verdyck, P.; De Becker, P.; De Vos, A.; Verheyen, G.; Van der Niepen, P.; Verpoest, W.; Liebaers, I.; Bonduelle, M.; Keymolen, K.; et al. Factors influencing the clinical outcome of preimplantation genetic testing for polycystic kidney disease. *Hum. Reprod.* **2019**, *34*, 949–958. [CrossRef] [PubMed]
13. Chamayou, S.; Sicali, M.; Lombardo, D.; Alecci, C.; Ragolia, C.; Maglia, E.; Liprino, A.; Cardea, C.; Storaci, G.; Romano, S.; et al. Universal strategy for preimplantation genetic testing for cystic fibrosis based on next generation sequencing. *J. Assist. Reprod. Genet.* **2020**, *37*, 213–222. [CrossRef] [PubMed]
14. Morales-García, A.I.; Martínez-Atienza, M.; García-Valverde, M.; Fontes-Jiménez, J.; Martínez-Morcillo, A.; Esteban de la Rosa, M.A.; de Diego Fernández, P.; García González, M.; Fernández Castillo, R.; Argüelles Toledo, I.; et al. Overview of autosomal dominant polycystic kidney disease in the south of Spain. *Nefrologia* **2018**, *38*, 190–196. [CrossRef]
15. Franasiak, J.M.; Forman, E.J.; Hong, K.H.; Werner, M.D.; Upham, K.M.; Treff, N.R.; Scott, R.T. The nature of aneuploidy with increasing age of the female partner: A review of 15,169 consecutive trophectoderm biopsies evaluated with comprehensive chromosomal screening. *Fertil. Steril.* **2014**, *101*, 656–663.e1. [CrossRef]
16. Rubio, C.; Rodrigo, L.; Garcia-Pascual, C.; Peinado, V.; Campos-Galindo, I.; Garcia-Herrero, S.; Simón, C. Clinical application of embryo aneuploidy testing by next-generation sequencing. *Biol. Reprod.* **2019**, *101*, 1083–1090. [CrossRef]
17. Reig, A.; Franasiak, J.; Scott, R.T.; Seli, E. The impact of age beyond ploidy: Outcome data from 8175 euploid single embryo transfers. *J. Assist. Reprod. Genet.* **2020**, *37*, 595–602. [CrossRef]
18. Kort, J.; McCoy, R.; Demko, Z.; Lathi, RB. Are blastocyst aneuploidy rates different between fertile and infertile populations? *J. Assist. Reprod. Genet.* **2018**, *35*, 403–408. [CrossRef]
19. Rodrigo, L.; Meseguer, M.; Mateu, E.; Mercader, A.; Peinado, V.; Bori, L.; Campos-Galindo, I.; Milán, M.; García-Herrero, S.; Simón, C.; et al. Sperm chromosomal abnormalities and their contribution to human embryo aneuploidy. *Biol. Reprod.* **2019**, *101*, 1091–1101. [CrossRef]
20. Kahraman, S.; Sahin, Y.; Yelke, H.; Kumtepe, Y.; Tufekci, M.; Yapan, C.; Yesil, M.; Cetinkaya, M. High rates of aneuploidy, mosaicism and abnormal morphokinetic development in cases with low sperm concentration. *J. Assist. Reprod. Genet.* **2020**, *37*, 629–640. [CrossRef]
21. Obradors, A.; Fernández, E.; Oliver-Bonet, M.; Rius, M.; de la Fuente, A.; Wells, D.; Benet, J.; Navarro, J. Birth of a healthy boy after a double factor PGD in a couple carrying a genetic disease and at risk for aneuploidy: Case report. *Hum. Reprod.* **2008**, *23*, 1949–1956. [CrossRef] [PubMed]
22. Minasi, M.G.; Fiorentino, F.; Ruberti, A.; Biricik, A.; Cursio, E.; Cotroneo, E.; Varricchio, M.T.; Surdo, M.; Spinella, F.; Greco, E. Genetic diseases and aneuploidies can be detected with a single blastocyst biopsy: A successful clinical approach. *Hum. Reprod.* **2017**, *32*, 1770–1777. [CrossRef] [PubMed]
23. Del Rey, J.; Vidal, F.; Ramírez, L.; Borràs, N.; Corrales, I.; Garcia, I.; Martinez-Pasarell, O.; Fernandez, S.F.; Garcia-Cruz, R.; Pujol, A.; et al. Novel Double Factor PGT strategy analyzing blastocyst stage embryos in a single NGS procedure. *PLoS ONE* **2018**, *13*, e0205692. [CrossRef]
24. Yang, X.Y.; Li, T.; Liu, X.J.; Shen, J.D.; Cui, Y.G.; Zhang, G.R.; Liu, J.Y. Preimplantation genetic diagnosis for infertile males with autosomal dominant polycystic kidney disease. *Zhonghua Nan Ke Xue* **2018**, *24*, 409–413. (In Chinese)

25. García-Pascual, C.M.; Navarro-Sánchez, L.; Navarro, R.; Martínez, L.; Jiménez, J.; Rodrigo, L.; Simón, C.; Rubio, C. Optimized NGS approach for detection of aneuploidies and mosaicism in PGT-A and PGT-SR. *Genes* **2020**, in press.
26. Neal, S.A.; Morin, S.J.; Franasiak, J.M.; Goodman, L.R.; Juneau, C.R.; Forman, E.J.; Werner, M.D.; Scott, R.T. Preimplantation genetic testing for aneuploidy is cost-effective, shortens treatment time, and reduces the risk of failed embryo transfer and clinical miscarriage. *Fert. Stert.* **2018**, *110*, 896–904. [CrossRef] [PubMed]

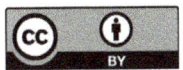

© 2020 by the authors. Licensee MDPI, Basel, Switzerland. This article is an open access article distributed under the terms and conditions of the Creative Commons Attribution (CC BY) license (http://creativecommons.org/licenses/by/4.0/).

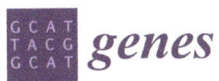

Article

Optimized NGS Approach for Detection of Aneuploidies and Mosaicism in PGT-A and Imbalances in PGT-SR

Carmen M. García-Pascual [1,2,*,†], Luis Navarro-Sánchez [1,†], Roser Navarro [1], Lucía Martínez [1], Jorge Jiménez [1], Lorena Rodrigo [1], Carlos Simón [1,3,4,5] and Carmen Rubio [1,2]

1. R&D Department, Igenomix, 46980 Valencia, Spain; luis.navarro@igenomix.com (L.N.-S.); roser.navarro@igenomix.com (R.N.); lucia.martinez@igenomix.com (L.M.); jorge.jimenez@igenomix.com (J.J.); lorena.rodrigo@igenomix.com (L.R.); carlos.simon@igenomix.com (C.S.); carmen.rubio@igenomix.com (C.R.)
2. Igenomix Foundation, 46980 Valencia, Spain
3. School of Medicine, University of Valencia/INCLIVA, Valencia 46106, Spain
4. Department of Obstetrics and Gynecology, School of Medicine, Stanford University, Stanford, CA 94305, USA
5. Department of Obstetrics and Gynecology, Baylor College of Medicine, Houston, TX 77030, USA
* Correspondence: carmen.garcia@igenomix.com; Tel.: +34-96-390-53-10
† Carmen M. García-Pascual and Luis Navarro-Sánchez have contributed equally.

Received: 19 May 2020; Accepted: 24 June 2020; Published: 29 June 2020

Abstract: The detection of chromosomal aneuploidies and mosaicism degree in preimplantation embryos may be essential for achieving pregnancy. The aim of this study was to determine the robustness of diagnosing homogenous and mosaic aneuploidies using a validated algorithm and the minimal resolution for de novo and inherited deletions and duplications (Del/Dup). Two workflows were developed and validated: (a,b) preimplantation genetic testing for uniform whole and segmental aneuploidies, plus mixtures of euploid/aneuploid genomic DNA to develop an algorithm for detecting mosaicism; and (c) preimplantation genetic testing for structural rearrangements for detecting Del/Dup ≥ 6 Mb. Next-generation sequencing (NGS) was performed with automatic library preparation and multiplexing up to 24–96 samples. Specificity and sensitivity for PGT-A were both 100% for whole chromosomes and segmentals. The thresholds stablished for mosaicism were: euploid embryos (<30% aneuploidy), low mosaic (from 30% to <50%), high mosaic (50–70%) or aneuploid (>70%). In the PGT-SR protocol, changes were made to increase the detection level to ≥6 Mb. This is the first study reporting an accurate assessment of semiautomated-NGS protocols using Reproseq on pools of cells. Both protocols allow for the analysis of homogeneous and segmental aneuploidies, different degrees of mosaicism, and small Del/Dup with high sensitivity and specificity.

Keywords: NGS; aneuploidy; mosaicism; segmental; translocations; PGT-A

---

1. Introduction

Aneuploidies underlie most reproductive failures in humans [1] and, based on large datasets, over half of the embryos produced through in vitro fertilization (IVF) are aneuploid [2,3]. Thus, preimplantation genetic testing for aneuploidy (PGT-A) was proposed to improve pregnancy rates per transfer and to decrease miscarriage mostly in advanced maternal age (AMA) patients [4–7]. Recently, PGT-A has been shown to offer shorter time for pregnancy with lower cost compared to conventional IVF for some subgroups of couples [8,9]. Currently, PGT-A includes the study of uniform aneuploidies, small deletions/duplications (Del/Dup ≥ 10 Mb), and mosaicism. Preimplantation genetic testing for structural rearrangements (PGT-SR) aims to detect smaller imbalances (≥6 Mb), mostly in embryos where at least one parent is a carrier of a balanced translocations and/or inversions.

The earliest technologies to assess all 24 chromosomes were comparative genome hybridization arrays (aCGH), single-nucleotide polymorphism (SNP) microarrays, and quantitative polymerase chain reaction (qPCR). These were applied to both PGT-A [10–13] and PGT-SR [14,15]. More recently, techniques have been developed based on next-generation sequencing (NGS). NGS has significant advantages. It is a versatile platform that can be used for detecting uniform/whole aneuploidies and Del/Dup [16] and, compared to aCGH, is a reliable high-throughput technology with higher resolution and a broader dynamic range facilitating mosaicism diagnosis [15,17]. It is also cheaper and requires less hands-on time. Current NGS protocols consist of (a) whole genome amplification (WGA) and barcoding; (b) library preparation, purification, and templating; (c) loading and sequencing; (d) alignment of sequenced reads to a human reference genome; and, finally, (e) data analysis and reporting. The templating preparation steps, chip loading, and data analysis can potentially be automated, which is strongly recommended to decrease technical and human errors and increase the robustness and reproducibility of results when processing large numbers of samples.

However, two important issues should be addressed before implementing NGS in a clinical diagnostic laboratory: (1) defining the sequencing parameters required for each application, the minimal resolution of each platform to detect Del/Dup and identify the presence of mosaicism; and (2) creating a bioinformatics pipeline and diagnostic algorithms best able to avoid the subjectivity linked to the visualization of sequencing plots. Del/Dup detection is limited by the minimal resolution of the platform, number of reads and signal/noise ratio affecting the minimal fragment size that can be detected [18–20]. Mosaicism detection is challenging since the degree of mosaicism is estimated from a single trophectoderm biopsy (TE) with an uncertain number of cells. As live births after the transfer of mosaic embryos have been reported [20–23] and the clinical outcome seems to be influenced by the level of mosaicism [24], the identity [25] and, the number [26] of affected chromosomes; a proper validation to define mosaicism thresholds is required for each platform to avoid overdiagnosis due to technical artefacts.

To address these issues, we sought to validate a semi-automated NGS protocol for PGT-A to detect uniform whole-chromosome aneuploidies and segmental aneuploidies ≥10 Mb, and a modified protocol to increase the resolution up to 6 Mb to detect imbalances in carriers of structural rearrangements (PGT-SR). Regarding mosaicism, we wanted to define thresholds for an accurate diagnosis and develop an algorithm to automatically detect its levels in TE samples, avoiding inter-individual and inter-laboratory subjectivity.

2. Materials and Methods

2.1. Experimental Design

This study was carried out in two phases from August 2017 to April 2018. Phase I, for PGT-A, was conducted from August 2017 to February 2018 to validate the detection of uniform aneuploidies, Del/Dup ≥ 10 Mb, and mosaic whole chromosome aneuploidies. Phase II, for PGT-SR, was carried out from February 2018 to April 2018 for the detection of imbalances ≥ 6 Mb. In all validation experiments, the tests were assessed using cell lines/DNA samples purchased from the NIGMS Human Genetic Cell Repository at the Coriell Institute for Medical Research (Camden, NJ, USA). All cell lines were grown in cell culture conditions established by the manufacturer. Before being collected, cells were passaged once. Then, confluent cells were detached using Tryple E [27] and resuspended in PBS (Gibco, Walthan, MA, USA). Cells were isolated under a dissecting microscope and placed in sterile PCR tubes (Eppendorf, Hamburg, Germany). All samples were analyzed at least in triplicate.

For phase I, three types of experiments were designed (Figure 1): (a) pools (n = 96 samples) of 4–6 cells mimicking TE biopsies from nine cell lines of known karyotype with aneuploidies in chromosomes 8, 9, 13, 18, 21, X0, XXX, XXY, and XYY as well as two with normal XX and XY karyotypes, hence

11 cell lines in total; and (b) mixes (n = 168 samples) of gDNA with different percentages of euploid (normal XX and normal XY) and aneuploid (0%, 30%, 50%, 70% or 100%) chromosomes (2, 8, 9, 13, 15, 18, 20 or 21). Once the algorithm was established, we tested its ability to correctly diagnose samples prepared to have 40%, 60%, or 100% mosaicism using two cell lines with trisomy in chromosome 8 or 9 (GM00425 and NA09287, respectively). To finalize the algorithm's testing, we applied the algorithm retrospectively to 14,108 TE biopsies analyzed in 10 different diagnostic laboratories from our group and estimated the percentage of mosaicism in these clinical TE biopsies.

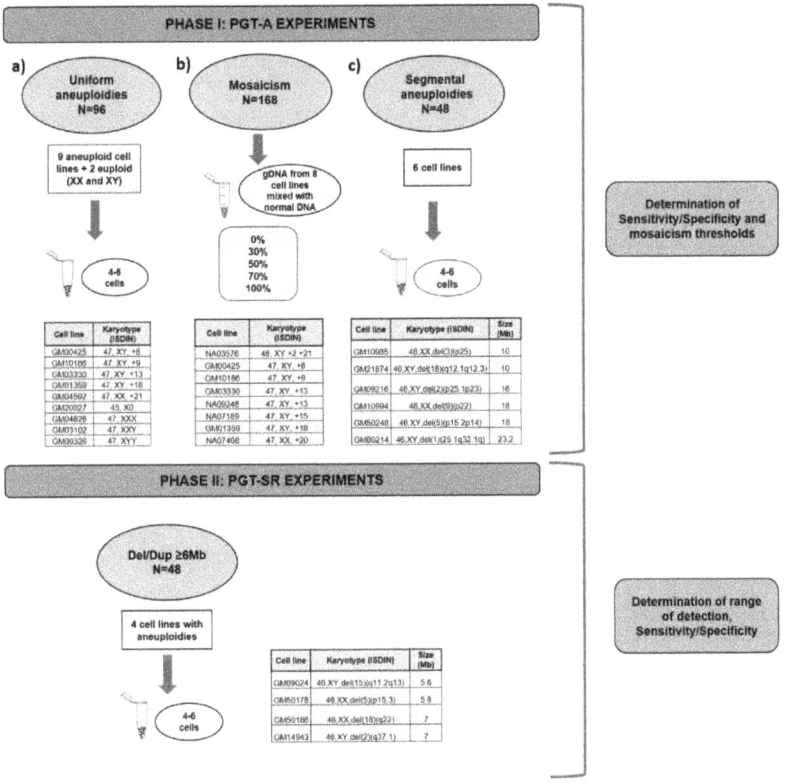

Figure 1. Experimental design for the validation of PGT-A and PGT-SR. Phase I: (a) PGT-A validation was divided in 3 experiments: (a) PGT-A for full aneuploidies, (b) PGT-A for mosaicism and, (c) PGT-A for segmental aneuploidies ≥ 10Mb. Phase II: PGT-SR for small rearrangements Del/Dupl ≥ 6Mb.

To establish the algorithm's ability to detect segmental aneuploidies ≥ 10 Mb, (c) pools (n = 48 samples) of 4–6 cells from six cell lines with Del/Dup ranging from 10 to 24 Mb were used.

Phase II experiments were designed to validate PGT-SR for imbalances ≥ 6 Mb in pools (n = 48) of 4–6 cells using four cell lines from carriers of segmental aneuploidies with sizes from 5.6 Mb to 7 Mb (Figure 1). This protocol was optimized to increase resolution, as explained below.

2.2. NGS Protocol for PGT-A and PGT-SR

The NGS platform validated in this study was a semiautomated protocol using the Ion Chef™ equipment for library preparation and the S5 XL sequencer (ThermoFisher Scientific, Walthan, MA, USA). Samples were tested in batches of 24 or 96 (520 and 530 chips, respectively) for PGT-A and batches of 12 (520 chips) for PGT-SR (ThermoFisher Scientific). WGA and DNA barcoding were performed using the Ion ReproSeq PGS Kit (ThermoFisher), following the manufacturer's instructions. The amplified DNA was purified, quantified with the Qubit™ (Qubit dsDNA HS Assay Kit ThermoFisher), and diluted to 80 pM before placing it in the Ion Chef™ equipment that automates preparation of the library and templates as well as chip loading, significantly reducing the hands-on time and interexperiment variability. The complete workflow from sample processing to reporting was completed in 12–14 h depending on the number of samples processed simultaneously.

For PGT-SR, the original protocol was modified by doubling the number of reads per sample, loading the 520 chips with half of the samples (12 instead of 24). Purification steps were improved to increase DNA integrity, yield, and purity, allowing enrichment of the final library for fragments with the optimum length for the sequencer to read and increasing the quality of the sequencing.

Quality parameters (QC) for both the entire run and individual samples were examined, with the most critical run parameters being loading percentage, live Ion Sphere Particles (ISPs) percentage, polyclonality and usable reads. The first factor impacting the average number of useful reads is the loading of the run, which indicates the number of chip wells containing ISP (with DNA (templated) or without (non-templated)). Templated ISPs, the ones that are sequenced, are termed 'live'. Polyclonality refers to ISPs with more than one library template population (different DNA fragments). Each ISP should have only one DNA population, hence reads from ISPs with polyclonality are removed from analysis. The combination of these factors determines the usable read number, that will be divided among all samples in the run. Acceptable values for a run were: ≥70% loading, >98%, Live ISPs, <50% polyclonality, and >30% usable reads. For individual samples, the most important QC parameters were: the number of reads (required to be >70,000 for PGT-A and >120,000 for PGT-SR), the dispersion/noise of the profile as measured by the mean absolute percent deviation (MAPD) (required to be <0.3), and the number of duplicates (required to be < 30%). A sample was considered informative if these parameters were met.

2.3. Bioinformatics Analysis and Interpretation of Results

Phase I: PGT-A for uniform whole chromosome and segmental aneuploidies ≥ 10 Mb and mosaicism

Sequencing data obtained by the S5 sequencer were processed and transferred to Ion Reporter software for data analysis. This software uses the bioinformatic tool ReproSeq w1.1 workflow to detect 24-chromosome aneuploidies from a single whole-genome sample with low coverage (minimum 0.01×). Normalization was done using the bioinformatics baseline ReproSeq Low-Coverage Whole-Genome Baseline generated from multiple normal samples.

For all full/partial chromosomal regions detected by the software, we computed the difference value (DV) parameter, defined as $DV = SNMC + CNMP \times EP$, where:

- Sample Normalized Mean Coverage (SMNC) is the observed ratio of reads in the sample;
- Control Normalized Mean Coverage for 1 copy (CNMP1) is the expected ratio of reads for one copy if the sample is normal;
- Expected Ploidy (EP) is the expected number of copies.

The DVs from all regions (positives for gains and negatives for losses) were used to establish the mosaicism and ploidy cutoffs according to the median values obtained in the different experiments that included uniform aneuploidy and different levels of mosaicism (0%, 30%, 50%, 70% or 100%). Different thresholds were defined to classify four levels of aneuploidy: euploid (<30% aneuploid), low-degree mosaicism (from 30 to <50% aneuploid), high-degree mosaicism (from 50 to <70% aneuploid) and aneuploid (≥70% aneuploid). In the pipeline for the diagnosis algorithm, all run and individual sample QC parameters were uploaded as well as the individual bam files, incorporating the aneuploidy classification described above.

After validation and development, the algorithm was verified by calculating the incidence of mosaicism retrospectively in 14, 108 TE biopsies from 10 diagnostic laboratories (January–June 2019). The difference among the laboratories was studied using ANOVA.

Phase II: PGT-SR for Del/Dup ≥ 6 Mb

The analysis of these of samples was subjected to small changes in the workflow of the bioinformatic analysis. The confidence filter was lowered to increase sensitivity for smaller chromosome segments.

2.4. Evaluation of Efficiency, Concordance, Sensitivity and Specificity

To determine the efficiency of the protocols, the percentage of informative samples was determined for each individual experiment. Sensitivity and specificity values were determined using only the informative samples (those meeting QC criteria). Concordance rates per sample were estimated as the percentage of samples showing the expected result according to the cell line karyotype. Sensitivity was defined as the percentage of samples showing the expected aneuploidy for each cell line and was calculated as True Positive ÷ (True Positive + False Negative). Specificity was defined as the probability of diagnosing a sample as euploid when there is no aneuploidy and it was defined as True Negative ÷ (True Negative + False Positive).

3. Results

3.1. Phase I: PGT-A for Uniform Whole Aneuploidies, Mosaicism, and Segmental Aneuploidies (≥10 Mb)

For uniform whole-chromosome aneuploidies, 96 samples from 11 cell lines with known karyotype (2 of them normal XX and XY) were analyzed in one 530 chip sequencing run. All uniform samples met QC criteria and had perfect informativity and concordance rates (Table 1). The average of reads per sample was 173,053 (87,767–374,809; SD = 67,485) and the MAPD (Median Absolute Pair-wise Difference) that gives information about the noise of the profile was remarkable (0.17 (0.111–0.288; SD = 0.038). Importantly, no false negatives or positives were identified; hence, both sensitivity and specificity were 100%.

Table 1. Number of samples; informativity, and media of the quality parameters for all sample categories used in the validations.

TEST	Type of Sample	Total Samples	Informativity	Concordance Rates	Reads *	MAPD *	Duplicates
PGT-A	Uniform whole aneuploidies	96	100% (96/96)	100% (96/96)	173,053	0.170	10.00%
	Segmentals (≥ 10 Mb)	48	98% (47/48)	100% (47/47)	126,780	0.194	9.60%
	Mosaicism (0%, 40%, 60%, 100%)	18	100% (18/18)	94.4% (17/18)	148,874	0.174	6.63%
PGT-SR	Small rearrangements (≥ 6 Mb)	48	100% (48/48)	100% (48/48)	305,287	0.145	7.00%

* Mean of all samples for that category; MAPD: Median Absolute Pair-wise Difference

For segmental aneuploidies (Del/Dup ≥ 10 Mb), 48 samples from four cell lines were analyzed in two 520 chip runs. Again, all samples passed QC, and informativity and concordance rates were high as summarized in Table 1. On average, there were 126,780 reads (78,606–264,095; SD = 47,676) per sample and an MAPD value of 0.194 (0.151–0.234; SD = 0.031). Sensitivity and specificity were 100%.

For determining thresholds for different degrees of mosaicism, 168 gDNA samples from 10 different cell lines were analyzed in one 530 chip and three 520 chips. Informativity was 99.4% (167/168), mean number of reads 154,934 (75,598–290,805; SD = 38,562), and MAPD 0.180 (0.127–0.285; SD = 0.033).

Four categories were established: euploidy (<30% aneuploid cells), low degree mosaicism (30–50%), high degree mosaicism (>50–70%), and aneuploidy (>70%). To classify samples in these categories, we defined the thresholds of different degrees of mosaicism. These thresholds were calculated using our cell line models to mimic different levels of mosaicism. The mean difference values for each category were 0.05 (SD = 0.04), 0.33 (SD = 0.08), 0.52 (SD = 0.09), 0.72 (SD = 0.12), 0.94 (SD = 0.08) for the 0%, 30%, 50%, 70%, and 100% categories, respectively. Figure 2A displays the distributions and confidence intervals of the different CNV thresholds when considering all chromosomes at different percentages of mosaicism (0%, 30%, 50%, 70% and 100%). The distribution obtained using all chromosomes is very similar to the distribution obtained when each chromosome was analyzed separately using the same method (Figure 2B).

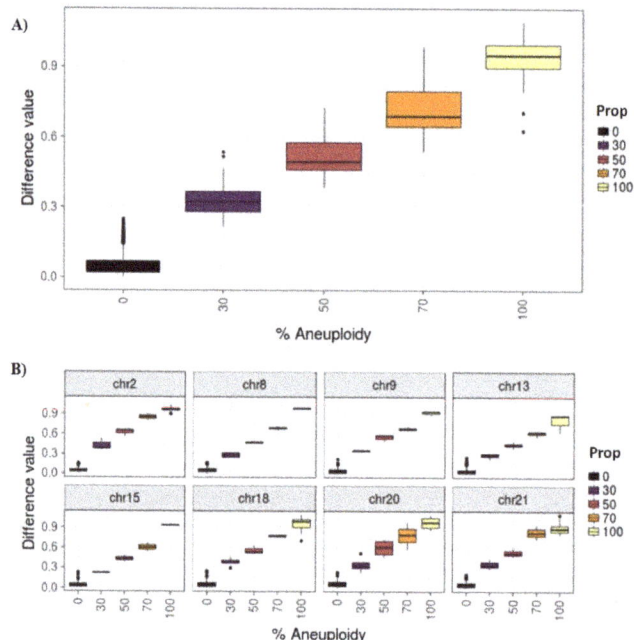

Figure 2. (**A**) Difference values for all chromosomes by known percentage of mosaicism. (**B**) All samples by selected chromosomes and proportion.

To check if our algorithm was correctly diagnosing percent mosaicism, 18 samples with different percentages of mosaicism (40%, 60% and 100%) generated using two cell lines with trisomy in chromosome 8 and 9 (GM00425 and NA09287, respectively) were analyzed. 100% of the samples amplified correctly (18/18), and 94.4% (17/18) were correctly categorized; only one 40% mosaic sample was mis-categorized as being high mosaic instead of low. All QC criteria were met (Table 1).

Finally, to estimate the percentage of mosaicism in TE biopsies, we applied the algorithm retrospectively to 14, 108 TE biopsies analyzed in 10 different diagnostic laboratories from our group. The overall percentage of mosaicism was 5%, with 3.66% (SD = 0.86) of samples classified as low-degree mosaicism and 1.34% (SD = 0.36) samples as high-degree mosaicism. The differences among laboratories were not significant ($p < 0.05$). These data are in concordance with previously reported percentages [21].

3.2. Phase II: PGT-SR

For these samples, the amplification rate was 100% (48/48). Samples were sequenced in four 520 chips, with only 12 samples per run. The average number of reads per sample was 305,287 (156,970–604,356; SD = 120,052) and the MAPD mean value was 0.145 (0.106–0.3; SD = 0.037).

All deletions were detected (48/48), including the smallest, setting the detection limit to 5.6 Mb and making the concordance rate and sensitivity/specificity 100% (48/48) (Table 1).

4. Discussion

In recent years, several sequencing platforms have been applied to PGT-A, and initial publications [10–15] have highlighted the need for a proper validation of each platform, mostly for mosaicism levels and resolution for de novo and inherited Del/Dup. Here, we describe an improved, mostly automatized, fast, and accurate protocol for detecting whole uniform aneuploidies, de novo Del/Dup (≥10 Mb), unbalanced Del/Dup up to 6 Mb in carriers of structural rearrangements, as well as mosaic aneuploidies. A key advantage of NGS is that portions of the protocols can be automated minimizing the contamination risk, mismatch of samples, time, and cost. In this study, introducing automated library preparation with the Ion Chef™ increased the robustness and reproducibility of the NGS protocol. To our knowledge, this is the first study to extensively validate a semiautomated NGS protocol with the Ion Chef + S5 sequencer for PGT-A, PGT-SR (≥ 6 Mb), and mosaicism detection using a proprietary algorithm.

To validate our PGT-A strategy for detecting whole uniform chromosome aneuploidies and large Del/Dup, we used cell lines of known karyotypes. These cell lines have been utilized previously by other groups to validate PGT-A with both aCGH and NGS techniques [1], but, to our knowledge, our study was the most comprehensive regarding the number of different cell lines and different chromosomes affected (14 chromosomes divided between nine cell lines for whole uniform chromosome aneuploidy and six cell lines for large segmentals ≥ 10 Mb). Other authors, e.g., Kung et al. (2015) [1] and Goodrich et al. (2017) [28], used six and four cell lines, respectively, and only for whole-chromosome aneuploidies and without the benefit of the automation steps used in this study.

Our PGT-A protocol was highly effective at detecting segmentals (≥ 10 Mb) in pools of 5-6 cells, mimicking TE biopsy. In 100% of samples, we not only correctly determined whole uniform chromosome aneuploidies, but also detected Del/Dup. These results are consistent with or improve upon those obtained in previous works, e.g., the Fiorentino et al. (2014) study [29], where authors set the size of de novo detectable segmentals to 14 Mb using the Illumina NGS platform.

Our protocol was also highly effective at predicting mosaicism. We established thresholds for this using multiple mixtures of gDNA from cell lines with known karyotype, mimicking different mosaic percentages. Other groups have used distinct strategies combining different numbers of euploid and aneuploid individual cells [28,30]. Our gDNA approach allowed us to test mosaicism for more chromosomes than commercial cell lines (eight in total) can test, covering potential variability among chromosomes, since it is known that amplification can be biased by GC content [31]. Using the sequencing information from our samples, we developed a proprietary algorithm allowing the automated assignation of mosaic embryos to different categories, avoiding the subjectivity of both the scientist performing the diagnosis and the laboratory where the analysis has taken place. For this, we divided mosaic embryos into two categories: low and high. Such categorization is clinically relevant since implantation and ongoing pregnancy rates after the transfer of mosaic embryos relates to the degree of mosaicism, with low mosaic embryos exhibiting better implantation rates [17,20,24,32,33]. Nevertheless, euploid embryos should be chosen first for transfer, and the transfer of mosaic embryos should be coupled with pre- and post-genetic counselling, including the option of a new IVF cycle if there are no euploid embryos in the current cycle, to yield a better prognosis [34]. Segmental aneuploidies which are not uniformly present in blastocysts and have low predictive value in IVF/PGT-A [35,36] were not considered when determining mosaicism in embryos.

Our algorithm to detect mosaicism is robust even when considering samples from different laboratories. We retrospectively analyzed the incidence of mosaicism in TE biopsies from 10 diagnostic Igenomix laboratories, finding an average incidence of 5% (3.6% low and 1.4% high), with no significant differences among laboratories, demonstrating the consistency of the algorithm. A wide range of mosaicism has been reported by different authors, suggesting that mosaicism may be over-diagnosed and highlighting the need to set thresholds for the degree of mosaicism that can be detected in a TE biopsy based upon the background signal that can interfere with the interpretation of results [37]. Interestingly, the different percentages of mosaic embryos reported in the bibliography are linked with the cutoffs used [38]. Some laboratories broadly defined mosaicism as being between 20% and 80% admixed aneuploid and euploid DNA and others, including us, used thresholds of 30% and 70%. Using the 20–80% range detected mosaicism in up to 17% of embryos, whereas the 30–70% threshold range decreased the mosaicism rate to 5%. Miscarriage rates are similar in both scenarios, indicating the 20–80% range may overdiagnoses mosaicism [38].

Finally, our protocol was successfully modified to create the PGT-SR protocol for detecting smaller Del/Dup (≥6 Mb). For this, we used four different cells lines with deletions in different chromosomes and with different breakpoints to assay the robustness of the technique in dealing with different chromosomal conditions. Other groups have reported the detection of deletions as small as 5 Mb in embryos using a similar platform [39]. However, these samples were amplified twice, first with Sureplex (Illumina, San Diego, CA, USA) and then during WGA, and therefore more DNA (100 g) than seen in regular protocols was used to prepare the libraries [39]. In an additional study, the authors reported automatic calling of deletions as small as 10 Mb but detected fragments around 5 Mb when data were examined manually, during which subjectivity could alter the diagnosis [40]. Additionally, the abovementioned studies all used TE biopsies not cell lines, likely contributing to the variation in the fragment sizes detected.

5. Conclusions

Our study indicates that the NGS platform Ion Chef plus S5 sequencer from ThermoFisher is a reliable tool for testing the chromosomal complement of preimplantation embryos, detecting whole uniform aneuploidies, segmentals (≥10 Mb), small rearrangements (Del/Dup ≥ 6 Mb), and degree of mosaicism. Part of the protocol is automated, remarkably reducing user error and the subjectivity often seen in manual PGT-A evaluation. Our automated algorithm allows for accurate, unbiased, and reproducible diagnoses for PGT-A and PGT-SR application. The next steps would be trying to enhance the detection of small rearrangements by improving the resolution to 6 Mb and moreover, to improve the accuracy of the diagnostic algorithm of mosaicism including data from the chromosomal analysis of the products of conception and livebirths.

Author Contributions: C.R., C.S., and C.M.G.-P. participated in conceptualizing the study; Methodology was developed by L.R., L.N.-S., and C.M.G.-P.; Most experiments were performed by L.M. and L.N.-S.; R.N., L.N.-S., and C.M.G.-P. curated and analyzed the data; Software application and visualization were carried out by R.N. and J.J., C.R. was involved in supervising and administering the project. The manuscript was written by C.M.G.-P. and L.N.-S. and reviewed by L.R., C.S. and C.R. All authors have read and agreed to the published version of the manuscript.

Funding: This study has been funded by Igenomix.

Acknowledgments: Authors would like to thank all Igenomix laboratory staff around the world for sharing valuable data.

Conflicts of Interest: The authors declare no conflict of interest.

References

1. Kung, A.; Munné, S.; Bankowski, B.; Coates, A.; Wells, D. Validation of next-generation sequencing for comprehensive chromosome screening of embryos. *Reprod. Biomed. Online* **2015**, *31*, 760–769. [CrossRef] [PubMed]
2. Franasiak, J.M.; Forman, E.J.; Hong, K.H.; Werner, M.D.; Upham, K.M.; Treff, N.R.; Scott, R.T., Jr. The nature of aneuploidy with increasing age of the female partner: A review of 15,169 consecutive trophectoderm biopsies evaluated with comprehensive chromosomal screening. *Fertil. Steril.* **2014**, *101*, 656–663.e1. [CrossRef] [PubMed]
3. Rubio, C.; Rodrigo, L.; Garcia-Pascual, C.; Peinado, V.; Campos-Galindo, I.; Garcia-Herrero, S.; Simón, C. Clinical application of embryo aneuploidy testing by NGS. *Biol. Reprod.* **2019**. [CrossRef] [PubMed]

4. Scott, R.T., Jr.; Ferry, K.; Su, J.; Tao, X.; Scott, K.; Treff, N.R. Comprehensive chromosome screening is highly predictive of the reproductive potential of human embryos: A prospective, blinded, nonselection study. *Fertil. Steril.* **2012**, *97*, 870–875. [CrossRef]
5. Rubio, C.; Bellver, J.; Rodrigo, L.; Castillón, G.; Guillén, A.; Vidal, C.; Giles, J.; Ferrando, M.; Cabanillas, S.; Remohí, J.; et al. In vitro fertilization with preimplantation genetic diagnosis for aneuploidies in advanced maternal age: A randomized, controlled study. *Fertil. Steril.* **2017**, *107*, 1122–1129. [CrossRef]
6. Lean, S.C.; Derricott, H.; Jones, R.L.; Heazell, A.E.P. Advanced maternal age and adverse pregnancy outcomes: A systematic review and meta-analysis. *PLoS ONE* **2017**, *12*, e0186287. [CrossRef]
7. Pinheiro, R.L.; Areia, A.L.; Mota Pinto, A.; Donato, H. Advanced maternal age: Adverse outcomes of pregnancy, a meta-analysis. *Acta Med. Port.* **2019**, *32*, 219–226. [CrossRef]
8. Neal, S.A.; Morin, S.J.; Franasiak, J.M.; Goodman, L.R.; Juneau, C.R.; Forman, E.J.; Werner, M.D.; Scott, R.T., Jr. Preimplantation genetic testing for aneuploidy is cost-effective, shortens treatment time, and reduces the risk of failed embryo transfer and clinical miscarriage. *Fertil. Steril.* **2018**, *110*, 896–904. [CrossRef]
9. Somigliana, E.; Busnelli, A.; Paffoni, A.; Vigano, P.; Riccaboni, A.; Rubio, C.; Capalbo, A. Cost-effectiveness of preimplantation genetic testing for aneuploidies. *Fertil. Steril.* **2019**, *111*, 1169–1176. [CrossRef]
10. Harper, J.C.; Harton, G. The use of arrays in preimplantation genetic diagnosis and screening. *Fertil. Steril.* **2010**, *94*, 1173–1177. [CrossRef]
11. Fiorentino, F.; Caiazzo, F.; Napolitano, S.; Spizzichino, L.; Bono, S.; Sessa, M.; Nuccitelli, A.; Biricik, A.; Gordon, A.; Rizzo, G.; et al. Introducing array comparative genomic hybridization into routine prenatal diagnosis practice: A prospective study on over 1000 consecutive clinical cases. *Prenat. Diagn.* **2011**, *31*, 1270–1282. [CrossRef] [PubMed]
12. Treff, N.R.; Tao, X.; Ferry, K.M.; Su, J.; Taylor, D.; Scott, R.T., Jr. Development and validation of an accurate quantitative real-time polymerase chain reaction-based assay for human blastocyst comprehensive chromosomal aneuploidy screening. *Fertil. Steril.* **2012**, *97*, 819–824. [CrossRef] [PubMed]
13. Rodrigo, L.; Mateu, E.; Mercader, A.; Cobo, A.C.; Peinado, V.; Milán, M.; Al-Asmar, N.; Campos-Galindo, I.; García-Herrero, S.; Mir, P.; et al. New tools for embryo selection: Comprehensive chromosome screening by array comparative genomic hybridization. *Biomed. Res. Int.* **2014**, *2014*, 517125. [CrossRef] [PubMed]
14. Vera-Rodríguez, M.; Michel, C.E.; Mercader, A.; Bladon, A.J.; Rodrigo, L.; Kokocinski, F.; Mateu, E.; Al-Asmar, N.; Blesa, D.; Simón, C.; et al. Distribution patterns of segmental aneuploidies in human blastocysts identified by next-generation sequencing. *Fertil. Steril.* **2016**, *105*, 1047–1055. [CrossRef] [PubMed]
15. Lai, H.H.; Chuang, T.H.; Wong, L.K.; Lee, M.J.; Hsieh, C.L.; Wang, H.L.; Chen, S.U. Identification of mosaic and segmental aneuploidies by next-generation sequencing in preimplantation genetic screening can improve clinical outcomes compared to array-comparative genomic hybridization. *Mol. Cytogenet.* **2017**, *10*, 14. [CrossRef] [PubMed]
16. Wells, D.; Kaur, K.; Grifo, J.; Glassner, M.; Taylor, J.C.; Fragouli, E.; Munne, S. Clinical utilisation of a rapid low-pass whole genome sequencing technique for the diagnosis of aneuploidy in human embryos prior to implantation. *J. Med. Genet.* **2014**, *51*, 553–562. [CrossRef]
17. Munné, S.; Blazek, J.; Large, M.; Martinez-Ortiz, P.A.; Nisson, H.; Liu, E.; Tarozzi, N.; Borini, A.; Becker, A.; Zhang, J.; et al. Detailed investigation into the cytogenetic constitution and pregnancy outcome of replacing mosaic blastocysts detected with the use of high-resolution next-generation sequencing. *Fertil. Steril.* **2017**, *108*, 62–71. [CrossRef]
18. Miroslav, H.; Jakub, H.; David, K.; Rostislav, N.; Gabriela, T.; Pavel, T.; Katerina, V. The incidence and origin of segmental chromosome abnormalities in human IVF embryos detected during PGD and PGS. *Rep. Biomed. Online* **2018**, *36*, e13–e14.
19. Popovic, M.; Dheedene, A.; Christodoulou, C.; Taelman, J.; Dhaenens, L.; Van Nieuwerburgh, F.; Deforce, D.; Van den Abbeel, E.; De Sutter, P.; Menten, B.; et al. Chromosomal mosaicism in human blastocysts: The ultimate challenge of preimplantation genetic testing? *Hum. Reprod.* **2018**, *33*, 1342–1354. [CrossRef]
20. Victor, A.R.; Tyndall, J.C.; Brake, A.J.; Lepkowsky, L.T.; Murphy, A.E.; Griffin, D.K.; McCoy, R.C.; Barnes, F.L.; Zouves, C.G.; Viotti, M. One hundred mosaic embryos transferred prospectively in a single clinic: Exploring when and why they result in healthy pregnancies. *Fertil. Steril.* **2019**, *111*, 280–293. [CrossRef]
21. Greco, E.; Minasi, M.G.; Fiorentino, F. Healthy babies after intrauterine transfer of mosaic Aneuploid blastocysts. *N. Engl. J. Med.* **2015**, *373*, 2089–2090. [CrossRef] [PubMed]

22. Fragouli, E.; Alfarawati, S.; Spath, K.; Babariya, D.; Tarozzi, N.; Borini, A.; Wells, D. Analysis of implantation and ongoing pregnancy rates following the transfer of mosaic diploid-aneuploid blastocysts. *Hum. Genet.* **2017**, *136*, 805–819. [CrossRef]
23. Chuang, T.-H.; Hsieh, J.-Y.; Lee, M.-J.; Lai, H.-L.; Hsieh, C.-L.; Wang, H.-L.; Chang, Y.-J.; Chen, S.-U. Concordance between different trophectoderm biopsy sites and the inner cell mass of chromosomal composition measured with a next-generation sequencing platform. *Mol. Hum. Rep.* **2018**, *21*, 593–601. [CrossRef] [PubMed]
24. Spinella, F.; Fiorentino, F.; Biricik, A.; Bono, S.; Ruberti, A.; Cotroneo, E.; Baldi, M.; Cursio, E.; Minasi, M.G.; Greco, E. Extent of chromosomal mosaicism influences the clinical outcome of in vitro fertilization treatments. *Fertil. Steril.* **2018**, *109*, 77–83. [CrossRef] [PubMed]
25. Grati, F.R.; Gallazzi, G.; Branca, L.; Maggi, F.; Simoni, G.; Yaron, Y. An evidence-based scoring system for prioritizing mosaic aneuploid embryos following preimplantation genetic screening. *Reprod. Biomed. Online* **2018**, *36*, 442–449. [CrossRef]
26. Maxwell, S.M.; Colls, P.; Hodes-Wertz, B.; McCulloh, D.H.; McCaffrey, C.; Wells, D.; Munné, S.; Grifo, J.A. Why do euploid embryos miscarry? A case-control study comparing the rate of aneuploidy within presumed euploid embryos that resulted in miscarriage or live birth using next-generation sequencing. *Fertil. Steril.* **2016**, *106*, 1414–1419.e5. [CrossRef]
27. Tsuji, K.; Ojima, M.; Otabe, K.; Horie, M.; Koga, H.; Sekiya, I.; Muneta, T. Effects of different cell-detaching methods on the viability and cell surface antigen expression of synovial mesenchymal stem cells. *Cell Transpl.* **2017**, *26*, 1089–1102. [CrossRef]
28. Goodrich, D.; Xing, T.; Tao, X.; Lonczak, A.; Zhan, Y.; Landis, J.; Zimmerman, R.; Scott, R.T., Jr.; Treff, N.R. Evaluation of comprehensive chromosome screening platforms for the detection of mosaic segmental aneuploidy. *J. Assist. Reprod. Genet.* **2017**, *34*, 975–981. [CrossRef] [PubMed]
29. Fiorentino, F.; Biricik, A.; Bono, S.; Spizzichino, L.; Cotroneo, E.; Cottone, G.; Kokocinski, F.; Michel, C.E. Development and validation of a next-generation sequencing-based protocol for 24-chromosome aneuploidy screening of embryos. *Fertil. Steril.* **2014**, *101*, 1375–1382. [CrossRef] [PubMed]
30. Goodrich, D.; Tao, X.; Bohrer, C.; Lonczak, A.; Xing, T.; Zimmerman, R.; Zhan, Y.; Scott, R.T., Jr.; Treff, N.R. A randomized and blinded comparison of qPCR and NGS based detection of aneuploidy in a cell line mixture model of blastocyst biopsy mosaicism. *J. Assist. Reprod. Genet.* **2016**, *33*, 1473–1480. [CrossRef] [PubMed]
31. Kebschull, J.M.; Zador, A.M. Sources of PCR-induced distortions in high-throughput sequencing data sets. *Nucleic Acids Res.* **2012**, *43*, e143. [CrossRef] [PubMed]
32. Munné, S. Origins of mosaicism and criteria for the transfer of mosaic embryos. *Reprod. Biomed. Online* **2018**, *36*, 369–370. [CrossRef] [PubMed]
33. Cram, D.S.; Leigh, D.; Handyside, A.; Rechitsky, L.; Xu, K.; Harton, G.; Grifo, J.; Rubio, C.; Fragouli, E.; Kahraman, S.; et al. PGDIS newsletter, 27 May 2019. In Proceedings of the Pgdis Position Statement On The Transfer Of Mosaic Embryos In Preimplantation Ganetic Testing For Aneuploidy (PGT-A) * Based On Materials Of 18th International Conference On Preimplantation Genetics, Geneva, Switzerland, 15–18 April 2019.
34. Kushnir, V.A.; Darmon, S.K.; Barad, D.H.; Gleicher, N. Degree of mosaicism in trophectoderm does not predict pregnancy potential: A corrected analysis of pregnancy outcomes following transfer of mosaic embryos. *Reprod. Biol. Endocrinol.* **2018**, *16*, 6. [CrossRef]
35. Girardi, L.; Romanelli, V.; Fabiani, M.; Cimadomo, D.; Rienzi, L.; Ubaldi, F.M.; Serdarogulları, M.; Coban, O.; Findikli, N.; Boynukalin, K.; et al. Segmental aneuploidies show mosaic pattern reducing predictive value compared to high whole chromosome aneuploidies representativeness. *Reprod. Biomed. Online* **2019**, *39*, 18–19. [CrossRef]
36. Zhou, S.; Cheng, D.; Ouyang, Q.; Xie, P.; Lu, C.; Gong, F.; Hu, L.; Tan, Y.; Lu, G.; Lin, G. Prevalence and authenticity of de-novo segmental aneuploidy (>16 Mb) in human blastocysts as detected by next-generation sequencing. *Reprod. Biomed. Online* **2018**, *37*, 511–520. [CrossRef] [PubMed]
37. Capalbo, A.; Ubaldi, F.; Rienzi, L.; Scott, R.; Treff, N. Detecting mosaicism in trophectoderm biopsies: Current challenges and future possibilities. *Hum. Reprod.* **2017**, *32*, 492–498. [CrossRef]
38. Monahan, D.; Harton, G.; Griffin, D.; Angle, D.; Smikle, C. Clinical comparison of two PGT-A platforms utilizing different thresholds to determine ploidy status. *Reprod. Biomed. Online* **2019**, *39*, 27–28. [CrossRef]

39. Bono, S.; Biricik, A.; Spizzichino, L.; Nuccitelli, A.; Minasi, M.; Greco, E.; Spinella, F.; Fiorentino, F. Validation of a semiconductor next-generation sequencing-based protocol for preimplantation genetic diagnosis of reciprocal translocations. *Prenat. Diagn.* **2015**, *35*, 938–944. [CrossRef]
40. Blanca, H.; González-Reig, S.; Penacho, V.; Castejón-Fernández, N.; Amoros, D.; Galán, F.; Alcaraz, L.A. Detection limit of partial insertions and deletions for PGS in terms of NGS by analyzing 242 embryos of couples with balanced translocations. *Reprod. Biomed. Online* **2018**, *36* (Suppl. 1), e17. [CrossRef]

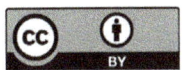

© 2020 by the authors. Licensee MDPI, Basel, Switzerland. This article is an open access article distributed under the terms and conditions of the Creative Commons Attribution (CC BY) license (http://creativecommons.org/licenses/by/4.0/).

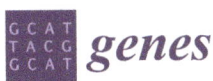

Review

Preimplantation Genetic Testing for Monogenic Disorders

Martine De Rycke * and Veerle Berckmoes

Center for Medical Genetics, Universitair Ziekenhuis Brussel, Laarbeeklaan 101, 1090 Brussels, Belgium; veerle.berckmoes@uzbrussel.be
* Correspondence: martine.derycke@uzbrussel.be

Received: 4 July 2020; Accepted: 29 July 2020; Published: 31 July 2020

Abstract: Preimplantation genetic testing (PGT) has evolved into a well-established alternative to invasive prenatal diagnosis, even though genetic testing of single or few cells is quite challenging. PGT-M is in theory available for any monogenic disorder for which the disease-causing locus has been unequivocally identified. In practice, the list of indications for which PGT is allowed may vary substantially from country to country, depending on PGT regulation. Technically, the switch from multiplex PCR to robust generic workflows with whole genome amplification followed by SNP array or NGS represents a major improvement of the last decade: the waiting time for the couples has been substantially reduced since the customized preclinical workup can be omitted and the workload for the laboratories has decreased. Another evolution is that the generic methods now allow for concurrent analysis of PGT-M and PGT-A. As innovative algorithms are being developed and the cost of sequencing continues to decline, the field of PGT moves forward to a sequencing-based, all-in-one solution for PGT-M, PGT-SR, and PGT-A. This will generate a vast amount of complex genetic data entailing new challenges for genetic counseling. In this review, we summarize the state-of-the-art for PGT-M and reflect on its future.

Keywords: preimplantation genetic testing; monogenic disease; multiplex PCR; SNP array; NGS

---

1. Introduction

Preimplantation genetic testing (PGT) can be performed for monogenic disorders or single gene defects (PGT-M), for chromosomal structural rearrangements (PGT-SR), and for aneuploidy detection (PGT-A) [1]. PGT involves the biopsy of a single or few cells from in vitro fertilized embryos and testing of the biopsied samples for genetic aberrations followed by the selective transfer of embryos unaffected for the condition under study. Although genetic testing of single or few cells is challenging and the overall procedure is quite complex, PGT has evolved from an experimental procedure in the early 1990s to a well-established alternative to invasive prenatal diagnosis and possible therapeutic termination of pregnancy. The first report on children born after PGT was published by Handyside and colleagues in 1990, describing the use of PCR amplification for the detection of repetitive Y-sequences for gender determination in families with X-linked diseases [2]. The single cell simplex PCR applied in this earliest PGT-M approach was soon replaced by multiplex PCR testing, in which closely linked informative short tandem repeat (STR) markers are co-amplified, with or without the pathogenic variant amplicon. Single cell biopsy at day 3 followed by multiplex PCR became the method of choice for the detection of monogenic disorders [3]. Biopsy at the blastocyst stage followed by genome-wide technologies began to replace this gold-standard method over the last decade. The genome-wide methods yield data on genotyping as well as on chromosome copy number, allowing for concurrent analysis of PGT-M and PGT-A [4–8].

As PGT and especially PGT-M is technically complex, transport PGT was implemented, a procedure in which embryo samples biopsied in a satellite IVF laboratory are transported to a genetics unit for testing. Transport PGT has the advantage that testing can be performed by experienced teams in genetic laboratories specialized in single cell molecular diagnostics. Transport PGT is a service that has expanded substantially, despite the challenges related to transport and collaborations over (long) distances [9].

PGT guidelines and recommendations for good practice have been designed by several international societies such as the PGD International Society (PGDIS), the American Society for Reproductive Medicine (ASRM), and the European Society for Human Reproduction and Embryology (ESHRE) PGT Consortium. The latter society has recently updated and extended four sets of recommendations, covering guidance on the organization of PGT service as well as technical guidance on embryo biopsy and genetic testing [9–12].

In this review, we present an overview of current PGT-M practice from patient inclusion to baby follow-up and reflect on future developments.

2. Indications for PGT-M

The provision of PGT is legally restricted in many countries, yet, policies and regulations differ [13]. Some countries have quite restrictive laws with a clear line between acceptable and unacceptable indications with specific mechanisms in place for delineating which indications are eligible for PGT. For instance, the Human Fertilization and Embryology Authority oversees the acceptable use of PGT in the UK. In France, l'Agence de la Biomédecine is charged with the regulation of PGT. In other countries, the law is more liberal. A minority of countries have no government regulation. The USA, for example, has no established restrictions on PGT practice and as such, PGT is also used for nonmedical reasons such as social sexing [14]. A recent overview of regulatory frameworks in 43 European countries shows only two countries where PGT is not allowed (Malta and Bosnia & Herzegovina) [15]. The main concern raised from the dawn of PGT has been the fear for eugenics. Many countries have a legislation banning any form of eugenic selection, allowing to select against high risk and serious disorders in PGT-M and PGT-SR but excluding the selection or enhancement of non-pathological characteristics in humans. PGT-A fails to meet the standard of a 'high risk and serious disorder' and is therefore not permitted in 11 out of 43 European countries [15]. As the field is rapidly progressing, it is essential to continue the scientific, ethical, and legal debate about embryo selection and to make amendments when necessary. For instance, the implementation of preconception carrier screening is likely to bring more requests for double or triple conditions, which may not all meet the 'high risk and serious disorder' standard. It is clear that this should be balanced with thorough discussions and ethical reflections [16]. PGT-M can in theory be offered for all (combinations of) monogenic disorders for which the disease-causing loci have been unequivocally identified. These loci are nuclear (X-linked, autosomal, dominantly or recessively inherited) or mitochondrial (maternally inherited) and involve (likely) pathogenic genetic variant(s) (class 4–5) [17].

The requests can be for rare or for more common diseases. The more frequent indications for which PGT-M are currently applied are cystic fibrosis and hereditary hemoglobinopathies for the autosomal recessive disorders, and myotonic dystrophy type 1, neurofibromatosis, Huntington's disease, and hereditary cancer syndromes for the autosomal dominant disorders. For the X-linked disorders, PGT is mainly carried out for Duchenne's muscular dystrophy, hemophilia, and fragile X syndrome (unpublished data from the ESHRE PGT consortium). The advantages of specific DNA diagnosis over sexing for recessive X-linked disorders are twofold: healthy male embryos are not discarded and female carrier embryos can be identified and possibly used for transfer, according to the patient's wishes and the center's policy. PGT with sex selection for non-medical reasons such as family balancing is prohibited in most countries.

Some special indications have raised further ethical concerns. For instance, Human Leucocyte Antigen (HLA) matching of preimplantation embryos is an exceptional indication as it is not a pathological condition. PGT is applied to select an embryo that is HLA compatible with an affected sibling who will need a bone marrow transplantation in the future. Hematopoietic stem cells from the cord blood at birth or later from bone marrow of the PGT baby are used to transplant and cure the affected sibling. HLA typing alone is carried out for couples having a child with an acquired hematological malignancy, but mostly, HLA typing is combined with PGT for a monogenic disorder, commonly immunodeficiencies and hemoglobinopathies [18]. The selection of HLA-matched embryos has evoked many ethical debates. The possible instrumentalization of the child to be born is the main issue raised in these discussions. As a result, the regulation of PGT and HLA matching varies in different countries around the world. Local and national legislation usually allow the use of PGT to avoid the transmission of diseases for which no treatment exists, but only a subset of frameworks is permissive for PGT and HLA typing.

In families with a history of late-onset neurodegenerative disorders such as Huntington's disease, individuals at risk who want to avoid pre-symptomatic testing but wish for their own biological unaffected children may opt for PGT with exclusion testing [19]. Exclusion testing recognizes the right of the parent not to know whether they are themselves affected while enabling them to have children not affected by the disease. Genetic implication counseling is a necessary part of the procedure [11]. Exclusion testing is indirect, based only on genetic markers, and involves the transfer of embryos carrying the haplotype derived from the non-affected grandparent. Embryos which have inherited the haplotype of the affected grandparent will be discarded as they have a 50% chance of being affected. These embryos have as well a 50% chance of being healthy for the disease under study. This fact together with the fact that about half of the couples will have an unnecessary IVF/PGT treatment with exposure to side effects and risks for the female and embryo, may be considered unethical. PGT with exclusion testing is therefore prohibited in some countries. The alternative with direct testing and non-disclosure of the results is not recommended as it obligates extreme confidentiality and may impose unethical behavior on the practitioners (for instance, fake embryo transfers) [20].

PGT for mitochondrial (mt) DNA pathogenic variants is offered in only few centers worldwide. The majority of mitochondrial DNA (mtDNA) pathogenic variants implicated in diseases show heteroplasmy, which is the co-existence of wildtype and pathogenic variant mtDNA in a single cell. The mtDNA pathogenic variant load (proportion of pathogenic variant mtDNA) may vary over time and differ from one cell type to another. Clinical symptoms manifest once a particular pathogenic variant load threshold has been exceeded. Because of a genetic bottleneck during oogenesis, the proportion of pathogenic variant mtDNA inherited from one generation to the next varies widely. PGT can be applied to select for embryos with a mtDNA pathogenic variant load below the threshold of clinical expression. It is an ethically difficult indication group as the approach reduces the risk for an affected child rather than eliminating it and this requires case-by-case counseling [21].

3. Genetic and Reproductive Counseling—Preclinical Workup

Before starting a clinical cycle, extensive genetic and reproductive counseling is provided to the prospective parent(s). Psychological support may be offered as well. Parents are asked to sign informed consent and blood samples are collected for preclinical workup. For PGT-M this usually includes blood samples and genetic reports from relevant first-degree family members. The preclinical reproductive workup and ovarian stimulation is similar as for patients undergoing conventional IVF. The preclinical genetic workup requires a conventional karyotype of both partners. This can be complemented by screening tests for carriership of common genetic variants for cystic fibrosis, spinomuscular atrophy, or hemoglobinopathies. In the near future, these individual screening tests will be most likely replaced by extended carrier screening. Genetic reports should be available at the intake of a PGT request. The preclinical genetic workup for the monogenic disorder depends on the test methodology (targeted versus genome-wide testing) and the strategy (an indirect test based on genetic markers versus a direct test including the detection of the pathogenic variant).

4. IVF, Embryo Biopsy, Transfer, and Cryopreservation

4.1. IVF and Current Embryo Biopsy Methods

Fertilization by ICSI rather than regular IVF is recommended for PGT treatment, in order to avoid contamination from remaining cumulus cells or residual sperm cells attached to the zona pellucida. Certain PGT indications may be associated with reduced spermatogenesis, and present with lowered fertilization rates. For instance, it has been known that the *PKD1* and *PKD2* genes underlying autosomal dominant polycystic kidney disease (ADPKD) play a role in the male reproductive system. Males affected with ADPKD may present with lower sperm motility and lower sperm concentration. A recent study showed that fertilization rates and live birth delivery rates tended to be lower for couples with the male partner affected with ADPKD, compared to couples with the female partner affected with ADPKD, although the higher female age in the former group was a confounding factor [22]. In some centers, oocyte or embryo vitrification before biopsy is applied as a systematic approach to accumulate a larger number of embryos for testing while in other cases it is applied as a rescue strategy in a minority of cycles, when in need for rapid interventions to preserve fertility such as in cases of cancer treatment [23–25].

Biopsy can be performed at different developmental stages. All present methods are invasive. Biopsy of the first and second polar body (both are required for an accurate diagnosis) is currently applied in only a minority of centers (unpublished data from the ESHRE PGT consortium of 2016 and 2017). An advantage is that the removal of polar bodies has no detrimental effect on embryonic development, however the most important limitation is that only the maternal genetic contribution can be evaluated.

Cleavage-stage embryo biopsy has been the gold-standard for many years. It implies zona opening (mechanically, chemically, or by using laser energy) and blastomere removal, mainly by aspiration, on day 3 of preimplantation development. Major disadvantages of day 3 biopsy are the limited amount of DNA available for testing and the negative impact of the removal of embryonic cells. It was shown that a two-cell removal at the cleavage stage harms embryonic development and implantation potential more than the removal of one cell [26]. Therefore, the removal of a single cell at the cleavage stage has been recommended. Cleavage-stage biopsy leaves sufficient time for genetic analysis before fresh embryo transfer on day 5. If available, supernumerary genetically transferable embryos can be cryopreserved for later use.

Blastocyst or trophectoderm (TE) biopsy is at present the most widely used technique [27]. Laser energy is used to open the zona pellucida, either on day 3/4 or on day 5. TE cells are aspirated and excised with a laser from herniating blastocysts, or aspirated in combination with mechanical dissection from blastocysts, usually on day 5/6. TE biopsy provides more cells (ideally five to eight cells) for genetic analysis providing a better accuracy [28]. This embryonic stage is also considered less sensitive to possible embryo damage as the inner cell mass from which the fetus originates is left intact. A paired clinical trial showed that implantation rates of 50% in the nonbiopsied group were diminished to 30% in the cleavage-stage biopsy group, while similar implantation rates were obtained for the blastocyst-biopsy group versus the nonbiopsied group [29]. Another benefit of TE biopsy is the lower level of chromosomal mosaicism at this stage as compared to the cleavage stage. The problem of limited time for analysis in the case of a fresh embryo transfer at day 5/6 is overcome by vitrification and embryo transfer in a deferred cycle.

4.2. Current Developments and Future Sampling Methods

An alternative method is morula-stage biopsy, performed on day 4, after artificial decompaction using Ca/Mg-free medium [30]. This option is attractive as more cells are obtained compared with cleavage-stage biopsy, cells are intact in contrast to TE biopsy where cells may be damaged and fresh embryo transfer is still possible. A drawback is the inability to distinguish between inner cell mass and TE cells. Whether or not the removal of several cells at day 4 has a negative impact on embryo development and implantation remains largely unknown. Irani and colleagues relied on morula biopsy at day 6 for slowly developing embryos in order to enlarge the cohort of available embryos for testing. Of note were findings of lower implantation and live birth rates as well as higher rates of complex aneuploidy [31].

Another option is blastocentesis, which is the aspiration of blastocoel fluid (BF) containing cell-free DNA (cfDNA) from the blastocoel cavity with a fine needle [32]. This procedure is considered less invasive than TE biopsy and results in embryo collapse which is a manipulation applied in routine vitrification practice to maximize embryo survival post-vitrification [33]. A true non-invasive alternative is to rely on cfDNA present in the spent blastocyst medium (SBM) [34]. Several studies showed that the karyotype concordance between blastocoel fluid samples and inner cell mass and/or TE cells varied widely, indicating that genetic analysis following blastocentesis is insufficiently accurate for clinical PGT-A/PGT-SR [35]. Moreover, the diagnostic efficiency was low with high amplification failure rates, making blastocentesis also unsuitable for PGT-M.

Analysis of cfDNA of spent embryo culture medium collected at the blastocyst stage seems a more promising sampling method. A recent study of Capalbo and colleagues compared blastocoel fluid and spent culture medium samples with TE cells as template for PGT-M [35]. TE samples showed 100% amplification and a high genotype concordance rate (99.8%). Blastocoel fluid samples gave high amplification failure (72.6%) with low genotype concordance (13.3%). SBM samples performed better with low amplification failure (10.3%) and an intermediate accordance rate of 59.5%. The lower diagnostic accuracy rate was due to contamination derived from maternal DNA due to incomplete oocyte denudation and from exogenous DNA present in supplements of culture media. As contamination is a major risk factor for genetic misdiagnosis, it is necessary to further optimize current protocols to favor embryo-specific analysis and allow discrimination between embryonic and non-embryonic DNA. This will provide more reliable and accurate testing for PGT-M in the short-term. Future research should also focus on the origin of the cell-free DNA to determine whether collected samples reflect the real genetic status of the embryo [36]. Substituting the laser-based biopsy methods by non-invasive sampling would definitely transform the field of PGT as it represents a safer option for the embryo and it would make the overall treatment less expensive.

4.3. Embryo Transfer and Cryopreservation

More and more PGT centers carry out a single embryo transfer (SET), a policy that can be linked with mechanisms of reimbursement and legislation, but also with the acknowledgement that SET is associated with a safer clinical outcome for any ensuing pregnancy. The substitution of slow-freezing by vitrification greatly contributed to the widespread use of SET. Vitrification has been shown to be superior to slow-freezing in terms of survival rate for both cleavage-stage embryos and blastocysts [37]. The evidence overall indicates that clinical outcomes after elective frozen embryo transfer are equivalent with the outcome after fresh embryo transfer for the general population (normo-ovulatory patients) and prove even better for specific subgroups such as patients at high risk of ovarian hyperstimulation syndrome (OHSS) [38].

The implementation of vitrification also changed the overall timeline of a PGT cycle. For many years, embryo biopsy on day 3, and testing and embryo transfer on day 5/6 were carried out within the timeframe of one cycle; the transfer was a 'fresh embryo transfer' and any surplus embryo from that cycle was cryopreserved. An alternative timeline emerged for cases for which no fresh embryo transfer was possible (high risk of OHSS or endometrium problems). During this freeze-all strategy, all genetically suitable embryos are vitrified and transfer was scheduled in a later cycle. Current comprehensive genetic testing is mostly linked with TE biopsy and a freeze-all strategy. This enables a more efficient and cost-effective laboratory organization as the larger time windows make it possible to pool and co-process samples of multiple patients. Once the genetic testing results have been disclosed, only genetically suitable embryos remain cryopreserved.

5. Diagnostic Methods

5.1. Early Methods of PGT-M

An overview of past, present, and future methods for PGT-M is summarized in Figure 1. At the start of PGT-M in the early 1990s, single cell simplex PCR amplification was applied. From these earliest approaches, contamination and allele drop out (ADO) surfaced as important issues that could lead to misdiagnosis [39]. Contamination with extraneous DNA or carry-over from previous amplification reactions was and still is a major problem, given the high number of amplification cycles that is required to increase the minute amount of DNA. It can be minimized by taking rigorous prevention measures. ADO originates from the unequal amplification of alleles present in a heterozygous sample (called preferential amplification) to the point where an allele remains undetected. Control for ADO relies on optimized methods for cell lysis and amplification and on sensitive methods for allele detection. By far, the most important measure to control and detect ADO as well as contamination was the inclusion of closely linked informative short tandem repeat (STR) markers in the PCR reaction. The co-amplification of STR markers with or without the pathogenic variant amplicon(s) at the level of a single or few cells yields a more accurate test and this so-called haplotyping approach has been the gold-standard for over two decades [27,40]. A major limitation of this approach is that the development and validation of a single cell multiplex PCR is labor intensive for the laboratory and couples face a long waiting time.

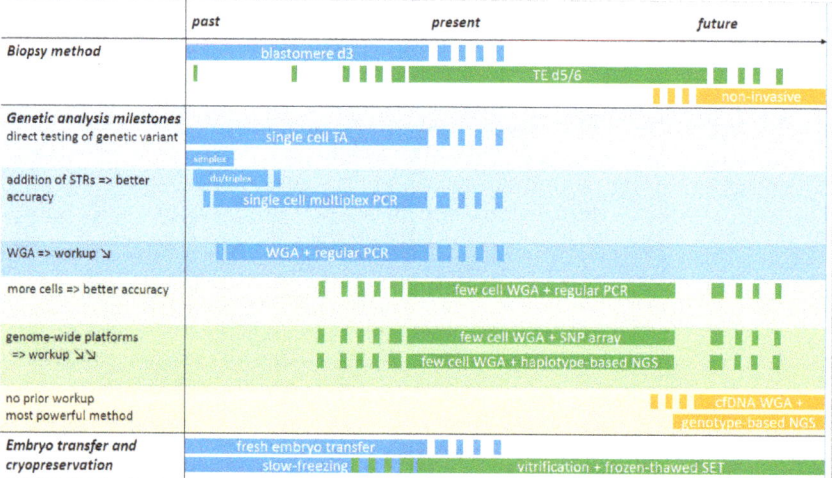

Figure 1. Overview of past, present, and future methods for PGT-M. The timeline is divided over past, present, and future sections without precise timepoints and starts in the early 1990s with blastomere biopsy and simplex PCR amplification for detection of the genetic variant in PGT-M. If the amplicon did not generate a difference in fragment length, post-PCR reactions were applied to allow low- and high-risk allele discrimination. These methods are currently still employed, for instance for detection of (de novo) genetic variants following WGA and SNP array. The addition of STR markers flanking the region of interest increased the accuracy of the PCR test: with every informative marker added, the diagnosis is confirmed and contamination and ADO pitfalls can be detected. The use of commercial PCR multiplex kits facilitated the development of single cell PCR reactions and duplex or triplex PCRs became multiplexes of 10 or more amplicons. Single cell multiplex PCR has been the gold standard for over two decades, alongside blastomere biopsy at day 3 and fresh embryo transfer on day 5/6. TE biopsy is currently the norm for embryo biopsy and is linked with the freeze-all strategy. The substitution of slow-freezing by vitrification greatly contributed to the widespread use of SET. WGA represents a technical milestone. The method of single or few cell WGA followed by regular PCR of multiple STRs with or without the genetic variant amplicon is a more universal method with a reduced

workup as the adaptation/validation of PCR reactions to the level of single or few cells can be omitted. The implementation of WGA followed by genome-wide SNP array or NGS represents a truly generic method, making it possible to combine haplotyping results for PGT-M with genome-wide chromosome copy number PGT-A data. Both platforms require a sample of a valid reference family member for haplotyping. Genotype-based NGS is regarded as the most powerful platform for future PGT as it will allow an all-in-one solution for direct genotyping and chromosome aberration assessment. Whether TE biopsy will be replaced by non-invasive sampling methods for PGT in the future requires further investigations. TA: targeted amplification: i.e., PCR-based amplification of the region of interest, either the genetic variant and/or a genetic marker(s); WGA: whole genome amplification: WGA products are used in downstream amplification reactions, either TA (regular PCR) or via genome-wide platforms (SNP array or NGS); STR: short tandem repeat marker; SNP: single nucleotide polymorphism marker; TE: trophectoderm; cfDNA: cell-free DNA; SET: single embryo transfer.

5.2. Whole Genome Amplification Approaches

The implementation of single or few cell whole genome amplification (WGA) was a technical improvement which stimulated the development of more generic approaches. The first WGA methods were PCR-based and suffered from incomplete genome coverage and amplification bias. The use of *Taq* DNA polymerase yielded an average fragment length of 400–500 bp (with a maximum size of 3 kb) and introduced many DNA sequence errors [41]. A multiple displacement amplification (MDA) method relying on isothermal strand displacement amplification was developed at the single cell level more than a decade ago [41]. In a MDA reaction, random exonuclease-resistant primers anneal to the denatured target DNA and a DNA polymerase with strand-displacement activity such as *Phi29* elongating the primers in an isothermal reaction at 30 °C. Additional priming events can occur on each displaced strand leading to a network of branched DNA strands over 10 kb. Because of the proofreading activity of the *Phi29* polymerase, the error rate of MDA-based WGA is much lower compared with *Taq* DNA polymerase-based methods, but the non-linear amplification yields over- or under-representation of genomic regions [42]. Afterwards, WGA methods combining MDA and PCR amplification were introduced. Both the Rubicon PicoPLEX and the MALBAC (Multiple Annealing and Looping Based Amplification Cycles) protocol initiate with DNA fragmentation and a pre-amplification MDA reaction using hybrid primers, followed by PCR [43,44].

None of the WGA methods are producing a true linear representation of the single or few cell genome and the results vary in ADO, preferential amplification rate, coverage, and nucleotide copy errors. As a consequence, a specific WGA method is chosen in function of the downstream application: the Rubicon PicoPLEX protocol is currently the method of choice for the detection of chromosomal copy number because of the reduced amplification bias while MDA is preferred for haplotyping applications in case of monogenic disorders because of the better genome coverage and low error rates [45–47]. Final data interpretation has to take into account bias and artefacts introduced from WGA. Also artefacts from the cell cycle phase should be considered. Analysis of TE samples containing cells in different cell cycle stages may overcome this problem while the WGA representation bias may be partially filtered out by computational algorithms but can not be completely eliminated.

WGA followed by standard PCR reactions of a multitude of STR markers flanking the region(s) of interest is simpler and requires a shorter validation, compared to single or few cell multiplex PCR [48]. WGA followed by genome-wide methods based on single nucleotide polymorphism (SNP) array or next-generation sequencing (NGS), represents a truly comprehensive approach.

5.3. SNP Array for PGT-M

SNP arrays are high density oligo arrays containing up to several million probes, which allow genotyping of hundreds of thousands of selected SNPs across all chromosomes in a single reaction. SNPs are mostly biallelic, alleles are indicated as A and B and genotypes are homozygous AA or

BB, or heterozygous AB. The commercially available SNP arrays use different methods for SNP genotyping: hybridization to SNP allele-specific probes or single base extension reactions are often applied [49]. The arrays are scanned and SNP genotypes are called based on the total fluorescence and the ratio of hybridization intensities for A and B (allele frequencies) (for example AB is called in case of similar intensities of an intermediate level). Targeted multiplex PCR and SNP array share the same principle of linkage-based testing for PGT-M, but the SNP array workflow is much more standardized and uniform, without the need for a locus-specific preclinical workup. This reduces the laboratory workload and the waiting time for the couples substantially. A drawback of SNP arrays is the high cost of equipment and consumables which seems to hamper their widespread clinical use. The SNP array platform is especially powerful for double indications (for instance two monogenic disorders or a monogenic disorder plus HLA matching) as whole genome haplotyping is accomplished from a single data set. Haplotyping via SNP array can also be applied for balanced translocations or inversions. Analysis reaches a high resolution and can distinguish normal from balanced translocation carriers. The major requirements for SNP array application are that the chromosomal or monogenic aberration(s) is/are inherited and relevant family samples are available for haplotyping.

Different SNP genotyping algorithms are available. Handyside and coworkers developed karyomapping, a family-based computational phasing approach for reconstruction of SNP haplotypes which flank the pathogenic variant(s) [5,50]. It is applicable for both SNP arrays and NGS. The commercially available karyomapping algorithm uses discrete diploid SNP calls (assuming AA, BB, AB, or No call as possible states for each SNP) together with basic Mendelian laws and requires a close relative for phasing.

5.4. PGT-M for De Novo Pathogenic Variants

In case of a de novo pathogenic variant(s) or when relevant DNA samples of family members cannot be obtained, it is necessary to include the genetic variant detection in the test strategy. This is feasible in targeted—as well as in genome-wide—methods, but the validation step of the latter methods is much easier. Many types of genetic variants can be detected by PCR supplemented with a post-PCR reaction if necessary. Deletion or duplication variants of a few nucleotides can be detected directly via fragment length difference. For single nucleotide substitutions, different strategies of allele discrimination have been developed, e.g., minisequencing [51]. The direct detection of complex and/or larger gene rearrangements has so far been difficult since the exact breakpoints of the rearrangement are frequently unknown. High-resolution characterization of breakpoints located outside highly repetitive regions is now achievable with long-read nanopore sequencing [52].

Since high-risk and low-risk haplotypes cannot be established during workup, segregation must be determined and diagnosis can be obtained during the first PGT cycle(s), provided that sufficient embryos are available with at least one embryo diagnosed as affected and with the pathogenic variant consistently detected in the presence of the same parental haplotype.

5.5. SNP Array for Concurrent PGT-M and PGT-A

SNP array can allow for simultaneous analysis of PGT-M and PGT-A as both SNP genotype and chromosome copy number info are obtained from the raw data set. As such, SNP arrays can reveal the presence of aneuploidies, polyploidies, and uniparental disomy [53]. Two measures provide evidence about the copy number state: the log R ratio (the log2 transformed value of the normalized intensity of the SNP) and the B allele frequency (BAF, which is the signal intensity of the B allele over the total signal intensity for a SNP). BAF values of 0, 0.5, and 1 represent a normal copy number ($n = 2$) but aberrations will cause a decrease or increase of the total intensity and allele frequencies. SNP arrays at the level of a single or few cells yield a lot of noise because of WGA pitfalls and therefore demand particularly well-developed algorithms for data interpretation. Genotyping algorithms using discrete diploid SNP calls such as karyomapping will yield errors across regions with copy number variations (true or WGA-induced) and therefore have restrictions in the detection of copy number aberrations. So far, few well-developed algorithms providing an all-in-one solution for data interpretation have been published. Some PGT centers rely on in-house developed extended or novel algorithms, to overcome this limitation. For instance, haplarithmisis is a computational pipeline that primarily relies on continuous BAFs and allows haplotype and copy number detection as well as determination of the parental origin of the chromosomal anomaly [6].

The true clinical benefit of PGT-A remains a topic of discussion, neither is there a consensus about adding PGT-A routinely to PGT-M cases, yet, concurrent PGT-A and PGT-M is increasingly regarded as an acceptable option, since it does not entail additional procedures or higher risks for the couple or future child.

5.6. NGS for Concurrent PGT-M and PGT-A

NGS involves DNA fragmentation and preparation of a library of templates using adapters containing barcodes for a more affordable analysis with multiple samples in a single run. The single molecule templates are then sequenced in parallel from one end or from both ends, either directly (third-generation) or after prior clonal amplification (second-generation) and the sequence reads are mapped to a reference genome. A crucial parameter is the genome coverage or read depth referring to the number of reads that is found at a given genomic position. A relatively low average coverage has been demonstrated as sufficient for accurate numerical chromosome analysis [54]. For monogenic disorders, sequencing at high coverage is required, which at this time is still too expensive for routine clinical applications at a whole-genome scale, and therefore, various strategies, aiming at affordable and rapid protocols are being developed. These protocols often provide a tandem solution, combining PGT-A with PGT-M, and can be classified in two groups, depending on whether sequencing data for the monogenic locus are derived with a targeted or a genome-wide method.

The three approaches of targeted sequencing presented here are merely an illustration of the wide range of possibilities. A more affordable solution is to increase the read depth across the site of the pathogenic variant (minimum 100×) only. In one report, the pathogenic variant loci were captured in a preamplification reaction with pathogenic variant specific primers while the concurrent inclusion of a specially designed primer pool allowed for parallel aneuploidy screening via real-time quantitative PCR [4]. The MARSALA method (mutated allele revealed by sequencing with aneuploidy and linkage analyses) works in a similar way: an aliquot of MALBAC-based WGA products undergoes targeted amplification and the mixture of WGA and targeted enriched templates is subsequently sequenced at low depth (0.1–2×), yielding targeted SNP haplotyping results for PGT-M together with genome-wide PGT-A data [55]. Chamayou and colleagues developed a universal strategy for concurrent PGT-M for cystic fibrosis and PGT-A [56]. Part of the MDA-based WGA products undergo multiplex PCR for coverage of the *CFTR* gene (pathogenic variants and SNPs), generating a targeted DNA library. Another aliquot of the WGA products is processed for comprehensive chromosome analysis, generating a genome-wide DNA library. Both DNA libraries are subsequently sequenced. In these three examples, the targeted amplification is coupled with the need for a locus-specific preclinical workup.

Genome-wide NGS is regarded as the most powerful platform for future PGT, as it will offer simultaneously genotype and chromosome copy number data with increased accuracy, reliability, and resolution, allowing a generic protocol for monogenic disorders (including the detection of de novo pathogenic variants and repeat expansions) and numerical and structural chromosomal aberrations (including balanced rearrangements). As the current cost is too high, the main approach has been to decrease the number of reads by reducing the complexity of the libraries. Some of these strategies are listed below (non-exhaustive).

The OnePGT solution, commercialized by Agilent, is a NGS-based generic application for PGT-M, PGT-SR, and PGT-A [8]. The method takes advantage of reduced-representation genome sequencing in offering a single workflow, starting from MDA-based WGA and followed by library preparation with double restriction enzyme digestion and enrichment for fragments in a specific range of length; sequencing data interpretation relies on the haplarithmisis algorithm with concurrent chromosome copy number detection and SNP linkage-based haplotyping. The PGT-M module requires a minimum of 1.6× coverage and cosequencing of samples from the parents and a valid reference family member.

Haploseek is another universal workflow offering an economical analysis of PGT-M and PGT-A within a 24-hour protocol, starting from PicoPLEX-based WGA and genome-wide low coverage sequencing (0.3–1.4×) [7]. The information of high quality whole genome haplotypes of the couple and a reference obtained through SNP array is then integrated with the sample sequencing data and a hidden Markov model is used to predict whether haplotypes of the samples are shared with the reference or not.

In another NGS approach, a target enrichment gene panel with nearly 5000 Mendelian disease-associated genes (TruSight One sequencing panel) was applied on MDA-based WGA products, thereby offering direct testing of family pathogenic variant(s) plus indirect pathogenic variant detection through haplotyping of SNPs together with chromosome copy number detection through the log ratio of signal intensities, i.e., PGT-M and PGT-A together in a single workflow [57].

It is clear that the implementation of concurrent PGT-M and PGT-A offers further possibilities but may also generate incidental findings and more complex genetic information which we currently do not fully understand. This entails many ethical discussions and challenges for genetic counseling, because we lack knowledge to support data interpretation.

6. Clinical Outcome

It is difficult to compare clinical outcomes between individual centers because of varying factors such as maternal age, indication type, or differences in genetic testing and IVF procedures. Proper benchmarking against consortia data is neither straightforward, since reports of large data collections have been lagging. The most recent publication is about summary PGT data for 2015 from the ESHRE European IVF-Monitoring Consortium. This data set, which had been collected from 23 countries, showed a pregnancy rate of 39.7% per fresh embryo transfer cycle and a rate of 41.0% per frozen embryo transfer, over all PGT indications [58].

A high diagnostic efficiency is a prerequisite for any laboratory wishing to perform PGT as this potentially increases the clinical outcome. This is particularly true for indications with limited success rate a priori, such as for PGT-M with HLA typing where the chance of finding a genetically compatible embryo was shown to be only 16% [59]. This yielded a live birth delivery rate of 30.3% per transfer, showing that PGT with HLA typing is a valuable procedure where the high complexity and limited delivery rate are balanced by the successful transplantation outcome and the positive impact on families.

Apart from technical errors due to ADO and contamination, possible causes of misdiagnosis involve human errors such as mislabeling or incorrect embryo transfer. The misdiagnosis rate as published by the ESHRE PGT consortium is generally very low (<0.1%) [27]. The true misdiagnosis rate is difficult to assess as many embryo transfers yield no pregnancy or birth and only a minority of children have pre- or postnatal testing. PGT centers are encouraged to re-analyse part of the non-transferred embryos to provide an in-house estimate of the misdiagnosis rate.

7. Children Follow-Up

It was hypothesized that assisted reproductive technologies, especially the more invasive techniques like ICSI, would increase the risk for birth defects. Studies showed that IVF and ICSI are associated with a small but statistically significant increase in congenital anomalies at birth, compared with the general population [60,61]. No difference was observed between ICSI and IVF [62].

Follow-up data on children conceived after PGT with ICSI and embryo biopsy procedures are still limited. Neonatal follow-up studies did not report a higher rate of major congenital malformations after PGT when compared to IVF/ICSI [63–65]. The study from our center compared neonatal data of 995 live born children after PGT with the outcome data of 1507 live born children after ICSI and showed that embryo biopsy at cleavage stage did not add a significant risk to the overall medical condition of newborn children nor did it change the risk for major malformations [63]. These results were in line with studies carried out in other centers using embryo biopsy at cleavage stage [64,65]. The recent retrospective study in which a cohort of 1,721 children born after PGT with blastocyst biopsy and cryopreservation was compared with an IVF/ICSI control group showed no significant difference in neonatal outcome, indicating that neither embryo biopsy at blastocyst stage nor cryopreservation added further risk to the health of PGT children [66].

The follow-up of PGT children at a young age has been studied in smaller cohorts. Developmental neurological and cognitive assessment and follow-up on psychomotor and social functioning showed that PGT pre-schoolers were comparable with controls born after ICSI or after spontaneous conception [67–70]. Another study on body composition and blood pressure showed no adverse outcomes for 6-year-old children born after PGT (with day 3 embryo biopsy followed by blastocyst transfer) compared to children born after ICSI without embryo biopsy [71]. In summary, the follow-up results have so far been reassuring but further monitoring of the safety of PGT and the long-term health of the children remains necessary.

8. Conclusions and Future Perspectives

Major advancements have been introduced in the area of PGT and assisted reproduction over the years, making PGT a well-established, accurate, and safe clinical procedure. The implementation of genome-wide methods has allowed more standardization and uniformity for the genetic laboratories. However, additional genetic findings other than the requested genetic condition—such as chromosomal mosaicism in embryos tested for a monogenic disorder— have posed new dilemmas for genetic counseling and embryo transfer policy making. As the cost of sequencing continues to decline, PGT moves technically towards a sequencing-based, all-in-one solution for PGT-M, PGT-SR, and PGT-A. As there is more awareness among patients about the risks of transmitting genetic disorders and since the number of diseases with identifiable genetic cause(s) continues to rise, the total number of treatments as well as the list of indications for PGT is likely to expand. Whether the scope of PGT indications will broaden in the future from diagnosis of monogenic disorders to also predicting the risk of polygenic disorders (PGT-P) represents an emerging ethical challenge for PGT practice. It is clear that the rapid technological advances should be balanced with ethical reflection and thorough discussions.

Author Contributions: M.D.R. wrote the review. Both authors participated in critical reading and editing of the review. Both authors have read and agreed to the published version of the manuscript.

Funding: This research received no external funding.

Conflicts of Interest: The authors declare no conflict of interest.

References

1. Zegers-Hochschild, F.; Adamson, G.D.; Dyer, S.; Racowsky, C.; de Mouzon, J.; Sokol, R.; Rienzi, L.; Sunde, A.; Schmidt, L.; Cooke, I.D.; et al. The International Glossary on Infertility and Fertility Care, 2017. *Hum. Reprod.* **2017**, *32*, 1786–1801. [CrossRef] [PubMed]
2. Handyside, A.H.; Kontogianni, E.H.; Hardy, K.; Winston, R.M. Pregnancies from biopsied human preimplantation embryos sexed by Y-specific DNA amplification. *Nature* **1990**, *344*, 768–770. [CrossRef] [PubMed]
3. Laurie, A.D.; Hill, A.M.; Harraway, J.R.; Fellowes, A.P.; Phillipson, G.T.; Benny, P.S.; Smith, M.P.; George, P.M. Preimplantation genetic diagnosis for hemophilia A using indirect linkage analysis and direct genotyping approaches. *J. Thromb. Haemost.* **2010**, *8*, 783–789. [CrossRef] [PubMed]
4. Treff, N.R.; Fedick, A.M.; Tao, X.; Devkota, B.; Taylor, D.; Scott, R.T., Jr. Evaluation of targeted next-generation sequencing–based preimplantation genetic diagnosis of monogenic disease. *Fertil. Steril.* **2013**, *99*, 1377–1384. [CrossRef] [PubMed]
5. Natesan, S.A.; Bladon, A.J.; Coskun, S.; Qubbaj, W.; Prates, R.; Munné, S.; Coonen, E.; Dreesen, J.C.; Stevens, S.J.; Paulussen, A.D.; et al. Genome-wide karyomapping accurately identifies the inheritance of single-gene defects in human preimplantation embryos in vitro. *Genet. Med.* **2014**, *16*, 838–845. [CrossRef]

6. Esteki, M.Z.; Dimitriadou, E.; Mateiu, L.; Melotte, C.; Van Der Aa, N.; Kumar, P.; Das, R.; Theunis, K.; Cheng, J.; Legius, E.; et al. Concurrent Whole-Genome Haplotyping and Copy-Number Profiling of Single Cells. *Am. J. Hum. Genet.* **2015**, *96*, 894–912. [CrossRef]
7. Backenroth, D.; Zahdeh, F.; Kling, Y.; Peretz, A.; Rosen, T.; Kort, D.; Zeligson, S.; Dror, T.; Kirshberg, S.; Burak, E.; et al. Haploseek: A 24-hour all-in-one method for preimplantation genetic diagnosis (PGD) of monogenic disease and aneuploidy. *Genet. Med.* **2018**, *21*, 1390–1399. [CrossRef]
8. Masset, H.; Esteki, M.Z.; Dimitriadou, E.; Dreesen, J.; Debrock, S.; Derhaag, J.; Derks, K.; Destouni, A.; Drüsedau, M.; Meekels, J.; et al. Multi-centre evaluation of a comprehensive preimplantation genetic test through haplotyping-by-sequencing. *Hum. Reprod.* **2019**, *34*, 1608–1619. [CrossRef]
9. Carvalho, F.; Coonen, E.; Goossens, V.; Kokkali, G.; Rubio, C.; Meijer-Hoogeveen, M.; Moutou, C.; Vermeulen, N.; De Rycke, M. ESHRE PGT Consortium good practice recommendations for the organisation of PGT. *Hum. Reprod. Open* **2020**, *2020*. [CrossRef]
10. Kokkali, G.; Coticchio, G.; Bronet, F.; Celebi, C.; Cimadomo, D.; Goossens, V.; Liss, J.; Nunes, S.; Sfontouris, I.; Vermeulen, N.; et al. ESHRE PGT Consortium and SIG Embryology good practice recommendations for polar body and embryo biopsy for PGT. *Hum. Reprod. Open* **2020**, *2020*. [CrossRef]
11. Carvalho, F.; Moutou, C.; Dimitriadou, E.; Dreesen, J.; Giménez, C.; Goossens, V.; Kakourou, G.; Vermeulen, N.; Zuccarello, D.; De Rycke, M. ESHRE PGT Consortium good practice recommendations for the detection of monogenic disorders. *Hum. Reprod. Open* **2020**, *2020*. [CrossRef] [PubMed]
12. Coonen, E.; Rubio, C.; Christopikou, D.; Dimitriadou, E.; Gontar, J.; Goossens, V.; Maurer, M.; Spinella, F.; Vermeulen, N.; De Rycke, M. ESHRE PGT Consortium good practice recommendations for the detection of structural and numerical chromosomal aberrations. *Hum. Reprod. Open* **2020**, *2020*. [CrossRef] [PubMed]
13. Ginoza, M.E.C.; Isasi, R. Regulating Preimplantation Genetic Testing across the World: A Comparison of International Policy and Ethical Perspectives. *Cold Spring Harb. Perspect. Med.* **2019**, *10*. [CrossRef] [PubMed]
14. Bayefsky, M.J. Comparative preimplantation genetic diagnosis policy in Europe and the USA and its implications for reproductive tourism. *Reprod. Biomed. Soc. Online* **2016**, *3*, 41–47. [CrossRef]
15. Calhaz-Jorge, C.; De Geyter, C.H.; Kupka, M.S.; Wyns, C.; Mocanu, E.; Motrenko, T.; Scaravelli, G.; Smeenk, J.; Vidakovic, S.; Goossens, V. Survey on ART and IUI: Legislation, regulation, funding and registries in European countries: The European IVF-monitoring Consortium (EIM) for the European Society of Human Reproduction and Embryology (ESHRE). *Hum. Reprod. Open* **2020**, *2020*. [CrossRef]
16. Dondorp, W.; De Wert, G. Refining the ethics of preimplantation genetic diagnosis: A plea for contextualized proportionality. *Bioethics* **2019**, *33*, 294–301. [CrossRef]
17. Richards, S.; Aziz, N.; Bale, S.; Bick, D.; Das, S.; Gastier-Foster, J.; Grody, W.W.; Hegde, M.; Lyon, E.; Spector, E.; et al. Standards and Guidelines for the Interpretation of Sequence Variants: A Joint Consensus Recommendation of the American College of Medical Genetics and Genomics and the Association for Molecular Pathology. *Genet. Med.* **2015**, *17*, 405–424. [CrossRef]
18. Kakourou, G.; Kahraman, S.; Ekmekci, G.C.; Tac, H.A.; Kourlaba, G.; Kourkouni, E.; Sanz, A.C.; Martin, J.; Malmgren, H.; Giménez, C.; et al. The clinical utility of PGD with HLA matching: A collaborative multi-centre ESHRE study. *Hum. Reprod.* **2018**, *33*, 520–530. [CrossRef]
19. Van Rij, M.C.; De Rademaeker, M.; Moutou, C.; Dreesen, J.C.; De Rycke, M.; Liebaers, I.; Geraedts, J.P.; De Die-Smulders, C.E.; Viville, S. Preimplantation genetic diagnosis (PGD) for Huntington's disease: The experience of three European centres. *Eur. J. Hum. Genet.* **2012**, *20*, 368–375. [CrossRef]
20. Shenfield, F.; Pennings, G.; Devroey, P.; Sureau, C.; Tarlatzis, B.; Cohen, J. Taskforce 5: Preimplantation genetic diagnosis. *Hum. Reprod.* **2003**, *18*, 649–651. [CrossRef]
21. Smeets, B.; Sallevelt, S.C.E.H.; Dreesen, J.C.; De Die-Smulders, C.E.; De Coo, I.; Die-Smulders, C.E. Preventing the transmission of mitochondrial DNA disorders using prenatal or preimplantation genetic diagnosis. *Ann. N. Y. Acad. Sci.* **2015**, *1350*, 29–36. [CrossRef]
22. Berckmoes, V.; Verdyck, P.; De Becker, P.; De Vos, A.; Verheyen, G.; Van Der Niepen, P.; Verpoest, W.; Liebaers, I.; Bonduelle, M.; Keymolen, K.; et al. Factors influencing the clinical outcome of preimplantation genetic testing for polycystic kidney disease. *Hum. Reprod.* **2019**, *34*, 949–958. [CrossRef] [PubMed]
23. Ubaldi, F.M.; Capalbo, A.; Vaiarelli, A.; Cimadomo, D.; Colamaria, S.; Alviggi, C.; Trabucco, E.; Venturella, R.; Vajta, G.; Rienzi, L. Follicular versus luteal phase ovarian stimulation during the same menstrual cycle (DuoStim) in a reduced ovarian reserve population results in a similar euploid blastocyst formation rate: New insight in ovarian reserve exploitation. *Fertil. Steril.* **2016**, *105*, 1488–1495. [CrossRef] [PubMed]

24. Chamayou, S.; Sicali, M.; Alecci, C.; Ragolia, C.; Liprino, A.; Nibali, D.; Storaci, G.; Cardea, A.; Guglielmino, A. The accumulation of vitrified oocytes is a strategy to increase the number of euploid available blastocysts for transfer after preimplantation genetic testing. *J. Assist. Reprod. Genet.* **2017**, *34*, 479–486. [CrossRef] [PubMed]
25. Hu, X.; Ding, C.; Zhang, D.; Zhou, W.; Wang, J.; Zeng, Y.; Lv, J.; Xu, Y.; Zhou, C.-Q. Embryo pooling: A promising strategy for managing insufficient number of embryos in preimplantation genetic diagnosis. *Gynecol. Endocrinol.* **2017**, *33*, 867–871. [CrossRef]
26. De Vos, A.; Staessen, C.; De Rycke, M.; Verpoest, W.; Haentjens, P.; Devroey, P.; Liebaers, I.; Van de Velde, H. Impact of cleavage-stage embryo biopsy in view of PGD on human blastocyst implantation: A prospective cohort of single embryo transfers. *Hum. Reprod.* **2009**, *24*, 2988–2996. [CrossRef] [PubMed]
27. De Rycke, M.; Goossens, V.; Kokkali, G.; Meijer-Hoogeveen, M.; Coonen, E.; Moutou, C. ESHRE PGD Consortium data collection XIV-XV: Cycles from January 2011 to December 2012 with pregnancy follow-up to October 2013. *Hum. Reprod.* **2017**, *32*, 1974–1994. [CrossRef] [PubMed]
28. Cimadomo, D.; Rienzi, L.; Capalbo, A.; Rubio, C.; Innocenti, F.; García-Pascual, C.M.; Ubaldi, F.M.; Handyside, A. The dawn of the future: 30 years from the first biopsy of a human embryo. The detailed history of an ongoing revolution. *Hum. Reprod. Update* **2020**, *26*, 453–473. [CrossRef] [PubMed]
29. Scott, R.T.; Upham, K.M.; Forman, E.J.; Zhao, T.; Treff, N.R. Cleavage-stage biopsy significantly impairs human embryonic implantation potential while blastocyst biopsy does not: A randomized and paired clinical trial. *Fertil. Steril.* **2013**, *100*, 624–630. [CrossRef]
30. Zakharova, E.E.; Zaletova, V.V.; Krivokharchenko, A.S. Biopsy of Human Morula-Stage Embryos: Outcome of 215 IVF/ICSI Cycles with PGS. *PLoS ONE* **2014**, *9*. [CrossRef]
31. Irani, M.; Zaninovic, N.; Canon, C.; O'Neill, C.; Gunnala, V.; Zhan, Q.; Palermo, G.; Reichman, D.; Rosenwaks, Z. A rationale for biopsying embryos reaching the morula stage on Day 6 in women undergoing preimplantation genetic testing for aneuploidy. *Hum. Reprod.* **2018**, *33*, 935–941. [CrossRef] [PubMed]
32. Magli, M.C.; Albanese, C.; Crippa, A.; Tabanelli, C.; Ferraretti, A.P.; Gianaroli, L. Deoxyribonucleic acid detection in blastocoelic fluid: A new predictor of embryo ploidy and viable pregnancy. *Fertil. Steril.* **2019**, *111*, 77–85. [CrossRef] [PubMed]
33. Van Landuyt, L.; Polyzos, N.P.; De Munck, N.; Blockeel, C.; Van de Velde, H.; Verheyen, G. A prospective randomized controlled trial investigating the effect of artificial shrinkage (collapse) on the implantation potential of vitrified blastocysts. *Hum. Reprod.* **2015**, *30*, 2509–2518. [CrossRef] [PubMed]
34. Brouillet, S.; Martinez, G.; Coutton, C.; Hamamah, S.; Sophie, B.; Guillaume, M.; Charles, C.; Samir, H. Is cell-free DNA in spent embryo culture medium an alternative to embryo biopsy for preimplantation genetic testing? A systematic review. *Reprod. Biomed. Online* **2020**, *40*, 779–796. [CrossRef]
35. Capalbo, A.; Romanelli, V.; Patassini, C.; Poli, M.; Girardi, L.; Giancani, A.; Stoppa, M.; Cimadomo, D.; Ubaldi, F.M.; Rienzi, L. Diagnostic efficacy of blastocoel fluid and spent media as sources of DNA for preimplantation genetic testing in standard clinical conditions. *Fertil. Steril.* **2018**, *110*, 870–879. [CrossRef]
36. Leaver, M.; Wells, D. Non-invasive preimplantation genetic testing (niPGT): The next revolution in reproductive genetics? *Hum. Reprod. Update* **2019**, *26*, 16–42. [CrossRef]
37. Loutradi, K.E.; Kolibianakis, E.; Venetis, C.A.; Papanikolaou, E.G.; Pados, G.; Bontis, I.; Tarlatzis, B.C. Cryopreservation of human embryos by vitrification or slow freezing: A systematic review and meta-analysis. *Fertil. Steril.* **2008**, *90*, 186–193. [CrossRef]
38. Bosch, E.; De Vos, M.; Humaidan, P. The Future of Cryopreservation in Assisted Reproductive Technologies. *Front. Endocrinol.* **2020**, *11*. [CrossRef]
39. Rechitsky, S.; Ström, C.; Verlinsky, O.; Amet, T.; Ivakhnenko, V.; Kukharenko, V.; Kuliev, A.; Verlinsky, Y. Accuracy of Preimplantation Diagnosis of Single-Gene Disorders by Polar Body Analysis of Oocytes. *J. Assist. Reprod. Genet.* **1999**, *16*, 192–198. [CrossRef]
40. Spits, C.; De Rycke, M.; Verpoest, W.; Lissens, W.; Van Steirteghem, A.; Liebaers, I.; Sermon, K. Preimplantation genetic diagnosis for Marfan syndrome. *Fertil. Steril.* **2006**, *86*, 310–320. [CrossRef]
41. Coskun, S.; Alsmadi, O. Whole genome amplification from a single cell: A new era for preimplantation genetic diagnosis. *Prenat. Diagn.* **2007**, *27*, 297–302. [CrossRef] [PubMed]
42. Spits, C.; Le Caignec, C.; De Rycke, M.; Van Haute, L.; Van Steirteghem, A.; Liebaers, I.; Sermon, K. Whole-genome multiple displacement amplification from single cells. *Nat. Protoc.* **2006**, *1*, 1965–1970. [CrossRef] [PubMed]

43. Langmore, J.P. Rubicon Genomics, Inc. *Pharmacogenomics* **2002**, *3*, 557–560. [CrossRef] [PubMed]
44. Zong, C.; Lu, S.; Chapman, A.R.; Xie, X.S. Genome-Wide Detection of Single-Nucleotide and Copy-Number Variations of a Single Human Cell. *Science* **2012**, *338*, 1622–1626. [CrossRef] [PubMed]
45. Deleye, L.; Coninck, D.D.; Christodoulou, C.; Sante, T.; Dheedene, A.; Heindryckx, B.; Abbeel, E.V.D.; Sutter, P.D.; Menten, B.; Deforce, D.; et al. Whole genome amplification with SurePlex results in better copy number alteration detection using sequencing data compared to the MALBAC method. *Sci. Rep.* **2015**, *5*, 11711. [CrossRef]
46. De Bourcy, C.F.A.; Vlaminck, I.D.; Kanbar, J.N.; Wang, J.; Gawad, C.; Quake, S.R. A Quantitative Comparison of Single-Cell Whole Genome Amplification Methods. *PLoS ONE* **2014**, *9*, e105585. [CrossRef]
47. Deleye, L.; Gansemans, Y.; De Coninck, D.; Van Nieuwerburgh, F.; Deforce, D. Massively parallel sequencing of micro-manipulated cells targeting a comprehensive panel of disease-causing genes: A comparative evaluation of upstream whole-genome amplification methods. *PLoS ONE* **2018**, *13*, e0196334. [CrossRef]
48. Renwick, P.; Trussler, J.; Lashwood, A.; Braude, P.; Ogilvie, C.M. Preimplantation genetic haplotyping: 127 diagnostic cycles demonstrating a robust, efficient alternative to direct mutation testing on single cells. *Reprod. Biomed. Online* **2010**, *20*, 470–476. [CrossRef]
49. LaFramboise, T. Single nucleotide polymorphism arrays: A decade of biological, computational and technological advances. *Nucleic Acids Res.* **2009**, *37*, 4181–4193. [CrossRef]
50. Handyside, A.H.; Harton, G.L.; Mariani, B.; Thornhill, A.R.; Affara, N.; Shaw, M.-A.; Griffin, D.K. Karyomapping: A universal method for genome wide analysis of genetic disease based on mapping crossovers between parental haplotypes. *J. Med. Genet.* **2009**, *47*, 651–658. [CrossRef]
51. García-Bermúdez, M.; Piyamongkol, W.; Tomaz, S.; Dudman, E.; Sherlock, J.K.; Wells, D. Single-cell sequencing and mini-sequencing for preimplantation genetic diagnosis. *Prenat. Diagn.* **2003**, *23*, 669–677. [CrossRef] [PubMed]
52. Chow, J.F.C.; Cheng, H.H.Y.; Lau, E.Y.L.; Yeung, W.S.B.; Ng, E.H.Y. Distinguishing between carrier and noncarrier embryos with the use of long-read sequencing in preimplantation genetic testing for reciprocal translocations. *Genomics* **2020**, *112*, 494–500. [CrossRef] [PubMed]
53. Kubicek, D.; Hornak, M.; Horak, J.; Navratil, R.; Tauwinklova, G.; Rubes, J.; Vesela, K. Incidence and origin of meiotic whole and segmental chromosomal aneuploidies detected by karyomapping. *Reprod. Biomed. Online* **2019**, *38*, 330–339. [CrossRef] [PubMed]
54. Yin, X.; Tan, K.; Vajta, G.; Jiang, H.; Tan, Y.; Zhang, C.; Chen, F.; Chen, S.; Zhang, C.; Pan, X.; et al. Massively Parallel Sequencing for Chromosomal Abnormality Testing in Trophectoderm Cells of Human Blastocysts1. *Boil. Reprod.* **2013**, *88*, 69. [CrossRef] [PubMed]
55. Yan, L.; Huang, L.; Xu, L.; Huang, J.; Ma, F.; Zhu, X.; Tang, Y.; Liu, M.; Lian, Y.; Liu, P.; et al. Live births after simultaneous avoidance of monogenic diseases and chromosome abnormality by next-generation sequencing with linkage analyses. *Proc. Natl. Acad. Sci. USA* **2015**, *112*, 15964–15969. [CrossRef] [PubMed]
56. Chamayou, S.; Sicali, M.; Lombardo, D.; Alecci, C.; Ragolia, C.; Maglia, E.; Liprino, A.; Cardea, C.; Storaci, G.; Romano, S.; et al. Universal strategy for preimplantation genetic testing for cystic fibrosis based on next generation sequencing. *J. Assist. Reprod. Genet.* **2019**, *37*, 213–222. [CrossRef]
57. Del Rey, J.; Vidal, F.; Ramírez, L.; Borràs, N.; Corrales, I.; Garcia, I.; Garcia-Martínez, I.; Fernandez, S.F.; Garcia-Cruz, R.; Pujol, A.; et al. Novel Double Factor PGT strategy analyzing blastocyst stage embryos in a single NGS procedure. *PLoS ONE* **2018**, *13*, e0205692. [CrossRef]
58. De Geyter, C.; Calhaz-Jorge, C.; Kupka, M.S.; Wyns, C.; Mocanu, E.; Motrenko, T.; Scaravelli, G.; Smeenk, J.; Vidakovic, S.; Goossens, V.; et al. ART in Europe, 2015: Results generated from European registries by ESHRE. *Hum. Reprod. Open* **2020**, *2020*. [CrossRef]
59. De Rycke, M.; De Vos, A.; Belva, F.; Berckmoes, V.; Bonduelle, M.; Buysse, A.; Keymolen, K.; Liebaers, I.; Nekkebroeck, J.; Verdyck, P.; et al. Preimplantation genetic testing with HLA matching: From counseling to birth and beyond. *J. Hum. Genet.* **2020**, *65*, 445–454. [CrossRef]
60. Davies, M.J.; Moore, V.M.; Willson, K.J.; Van Essen, P.; Priest, K.; Scott, H.; Haan, E.A.; Chan, A. Reproductive Technologies and the Risk of Birth Defects. *Obstet. Gynecol. Surv.* **2012**, *67*, 527–528. [CrossRef]
61. Pandey, S.; Shetty, A.; Hamilton, M.; Bhattacharya, S.; Maheshwari, A. Obstetric and perinatal outcomes in singleton pregnancies resulting from IVF/ICSI: A systematic review and meta-analysis. *Hum. Reprod. Update* **2012**, *18*, 485–503. [CrossRef] [PubMed]

62. Zhu, J.; Zhu, Q.; Wang, Y.; Wang, B.; Lyu, Q.; Kuang, Y. Comparative study on risk for birth defects among infants after in vitro fertilization and intracytoplasmic sperm injection. *Syst. Boil. Reprod. Med.* **2018**, *65*, 54–60. [CrossRef] [PubMed]
63. Desmyttere, S.; De Rycke, M.; De Schrijver, F.; Verpoest, W.; Haentjens, P.; Staessen, C.; Liebaers, I.; Bonduelle, M. Neonatal follow-up of 995 consecutively born children after embryo biopsy for PGD. *Hum. Reprod.* **2011**, *27*, 288–293. [CrossRef] [PubMed]
64. Bay, B.; Ingerslev, H.J.; Lemmen, J.G.; Degn, B.; Rasmussen, I.A.; Kesmodel, U.S. Preimplantation genetic diagnosis: A national multicenter obstetric and neonatal follow-up study. *Fertil. Steril.* **2016**, *106*, 1363–1369. [CrossRef] [PubMed]
65. Heijligers, M.; Van Montfoort, A.; Meijer-Hoogeveen, M.; Broekmans, F.; Bouman, K.; Homminga, I.; Dreesen, J.; Paulussen, A.; Engelen, J.; Coonen, E.; et al. Perinatal follow-up of children born after preimplantation genetic diagnosis between 1995 and 2014. *J. Assist. Reprod. Genet.* **2018**, *35*, 1995–2002. [CrossRef]
66. He, H.; Jing, S.; Lu, C.F.; Tan, Y.Q.; Luo, K.L.; Zhang, S.P.; Gong, F.; Lu, G.X.; Lin, G. Neonatal outcomes of live births after blastocyst biopsy in preimplantation genetic testing cycles: A follow-up of 1721 children. *Fertil. Steril.* **2019**, *112*, 82–88. [CrossRef]
67. Winter, C.; Van Acker, F.; Bonduelle, M.; Desmyttere, S.; De Schrijver, F.; Nekkebroeck, J. Cognitive and psychomotor development of 5- to 6-year-old singletons born after PGD: A prospective case-controlled matched study. *Hum. Reprod.* **2014**, *29*, 1968–1977. [CrossRef]
68. Winter, C.; Van Acker, F.; Bonduelle, M.; Desmyttere, S.; Nekkebroeck, J. Psychosocial development of full term singletons, born after preimplantation genetic diagnosis (PGD) at preschool age and family functioning: A prospective case-controlled study and multi-informant approach. *Hum. Reprod.* **2015**, *30*, 1122–1136. [CrossRef]
69. Sacks, G.C.; Altarescu, G.; Guedalia, J.; Varshaver, I.; Gilboa, T.; Levy-Lahad, E.; Eldar-Geva, T. Developmental neuropsychological assessment of 4- to 5-year-old children born following Preimplantation Genetic Diagnosis (PGD): A pilot study. *Child Neuropsychol.* **2016**, *22*, 458–471. [CrossRef]
70. Heijligers, M.; Peeters, A.; Van Montfoort, A.; Nijsten, J.; Janssen, E.; Gunnewiek, F.K.; De Rooy, R.; Van Golde, R.; Coonen, E.; Meijer-Hoogeveen, M.; et al. Growth, health, and motor development of 5-year-old children born after preimplantation genetic diagnosis. *Fertil. Steril.* **2019**, *111*, 1151–1158. [CrossRef]
71. Belva, F.; Roelants, M.; Kluijfhout, S.; Winter, C.; De Schrijver, F.; Desmyttere, S.; De Rycke, M.; Tournaye, H.; Liebaers, I.; Bonduelle, M. Body composition and blood pressure in 6-year-old singletons born after pre-implantation genetic testing for monogenic and structural chromosomal aberrations: A matched cohort study. *Hum. Reprod. Open* **2018**, *2018*. [CrossRef] [PubMed]

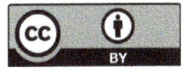

© 2020 by the authors. Licensee MDPI, Basel, Switzerland. This article is an open access article distributed under the terms and conditions of the Creative Commons Attribution (CC BY) license (http://creativecommons.org/licenses/by/4.0/).

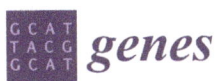

Review

Use of Customizable Nucleases for Gene Editing and Other Novel Applications

Pradeep Reddy [1,*], Felipe Vilella [2,3], Juan Carlos Izpisua Belmonte [1] and Carlos Simón [2,3,4,5]

1. Gene Expression Laboratory, Salk Institute for Biological Studies, La Jolla, CA 92037, USA; belmonte@salk.edu
2. Igenomix Foundation, Instituto de Investigación Sanitaria Hospital Clínico (INCLIVA), 46010 Valencia, Spain; felipe.vilella@igenomix.com (F.V.); carlos.simon@igenomix.com (C.S.)
3. Department of Obstetrics and Gynecology, BIDMC, Harvard University, Boston, MA 02215, USA
4. Department of Pediatrics, Obstetrics and Gynecology, School of Medicine, University of Valencia, 46010 Valencia, Spain
5. Department of Obstetrics and Gynecology, Baylor College of Medicine, Houston, TX 77030, USA
* Correspondence: preddy@salk.edu

Received: 25 July 2020; Accepted: 20 August 2020; Published: 22 August 2020

Abstract: The development of novel genome editing tools has unlocked new opportunities that were not previously possible in basic and biomedical research. During the last two decades, several new genome editing methods have been developed that can be customized to modify specific regions of the genome. However, in the past couple of years, many newer and more exciting genome editing techniques have been developed that are more efficient, precise, and easier to use. These genome editing tools have helped to improve our understanding of genetic disorders by modeling them in cells and animal models, in addition to correcting the disease-causing mutations. Among the genome editing tools, the clustered regularly interspaced short palindromic repeats (CRISPR)/CRISPR-associated (Cas) system has proven to be the most popular one due to its versatility and has been successfully used in a wide variety of laboratory animal models and plants. In this review, we summarize the customizable nucleases currently used for genome editing and their uses beyond the modification of genome. We also discuss the potential future applications of gene editing tools for both basic research and clinical purposes.

Keywords: genome editing; genetic diseases; embryos

1. Introduction

The ability to precisely manipulate the genome revolutionized not only molecular biology, but also opened several areas of biotechnology that are useful for research, agriculture, and medicine. Initial gene targeting primarily depended on homologous recombination to insert exogenous DNA sequences in the human cells [1]. The establishment of mouse embryonic stem (ES) cells led to the application of homologous recombination in pluripotent cells to modify the genome and generation of genetically engineered mice [2–4]. Initially, the efficiency of gene targeting using homologous recombination was extremely low, which was solved to an extent by enriching the edited cells using the antibiotic selection cassette. Interestingly, Russell and Hirata observed that recombinant adeno-associated virus (rAAV) vectors with homology arms proved efficient in modifying the chromosomal target sequences [5]. The mechanism behind this observation is not entirely clear. However, the single-stranded DNA of the AAV genome and higher transduction rates might be the reason for higher homology recombination.

Double-strand breaks (DSBs) on DNA are repaired using three different mechanisms, namely non-homology end joining (NHEJ), microhomology-mediated end joining (MMEJ), and homologous recombination (HR). Due to the nature of the repairs, NHEJ and HR are referred to as error-prone and error-free, respectively. NHEJ is active during all the cell cycle phases, whereas HR occurs only during the S-G2 phase of the cell cycle. For this reason, NHEJ is active in all the cell types, both dividing and non-dividing. During the repair of DSBs, the donor template with homology arms can get inserted at the site of repair using homology-directed repair (HDR) and dramatically increases the gene targeting efficiency [6]. Based on this method, rare cutting endonucleases such as the 18-bp cutter I-SceI have been used to introduce DSBs to increase the gene targeting efficiency [7]. Despite the presence of several natural meganucleases with unique recognition sites, the chances of finding a cutting site at the desired location are low. Nevertheless, modifications to meganucleases allowed some of the challenges to be overcome [8].

The discovery of customizable nucleases that can be programmed to induce DSBs at desired loci on the genome dramatically increased the efficiency of homologous recombination, leading to another revolution in gene editing with much broader implications in several different fields. This review aims to provide an overview of the recent developments in and applications of engineered nucleases that have helped lay the groundwork for their use not only for genome editing in various animal models, but also to correct the genetic mutations in human cells for clinical use. We also discuss the additional applications of genome editing tools in addition to modifying the genome, such as modulating the expression of genes and live-cell imaging. Finally, we review the use of genome editing tools in human embryos.

2. Customizable Nuclease

2.1. Zinc-Finger Nucleases (ZFNs)

ZFNs are a class of DNA-targeting components with two monomer subunits containing DNA-binding and cleavage domains. Each monomer is composed of three zinc fingers, which recognize nine base pairs and a *FokI* endonuclease domain. The DNA-binding zinc fingers can be engineered to bind to specific regions on the genome. *FokI* is enzymatically active as a dimer; therefore, two ZFN subunits are designed for each target sequence to facilitate the dimerization and cleavage [9]. The dimerization requirement of *FokI* and binding of fingers to the target sequence have increased ZFNs attractiveness as a tool for introducing DSB at desired locations on the genome, which is mostly repaired by NHEJ pathway, resulting in the disruption of the amino acid sequence and function of the gene [10,11]. ZFNs have been widely used to create mutations in a wide variety of organisms, including, drosophila, zebrafish, mouse, rats, sea urchins and frogs [11]. ZFNs have also been employed for therapeutic purposes, such as disrupting the *CCR5* gene to interrupt the expression of co-receptor and prevent HIV infection [12]. Moreover, homologous recombination with donor template DNA at the target site has also been achieved in mice and rat embryos [13,14]. However, gene targeting did not succeed in all the animals, such as zebrafish, despite a high rate of DNA cleavage and mutagenesis, potentially due to differences in DNA repair mechanisms [11]. ZFNs are smaller in size and are presumed to possess low immunogenic properties due to their similarity to mammalian transcription factors. Nevertheless, the complexity and cost of designing the domains are disadvantages of ZFNs.

2.2. Transcription Activator-Like Effector Nucleases (TALENs)

Similar to ZFNs, TALENs have a customizable DNA-binding domain and *FokI* nuclease domain. The TALE-DNA-binding domain is composed of conserved repeats domains derived from transcription activator-like effectors (TALEs) secreted by *Xanthomonas* bacteria to alter the transcription in host cells [15]. Each TALE repeat binds to a specific single base of DNA, and the number of repeats corresponds to the length of the target site. Two TALE repeats with target site binding domains fused with the catalytic domain of *FokI* endonuclease are used to create a DSB. TALENs exhibit higher specificity and efficiency than ZFNs. For this reason, TALENs have been widely used for genetic manipulation in different organisms [16]. Additionally, two pairs of TALENs have been used on the same chromosome to generate large deletions [17]. Moreover, TALENs have also been employed to introduce the donor sequences into the genome [18]. The single base pair recognition of TALE allows greater flexibility in designing the TALENs; however, the repeat arrays of TALE presents a technical challenge in cloning the identical sequences and also delivering in viral vectors. Additionally, the large size and immunogenicity of TALENs limit their clinical applications.

2.3. CRISPR-Cas System

The clustered regularly interspaced short palindromic repeats (CRISPR)/CRISPR-associated 9 (Cas9) nuclease is a recently identified system in prokaryotes with adaptive immunity against viruses and plasmids. Cas9 complexes with CRISPR RNA (crRNA) and trans-activating crRNA (tracrRNA) to form an endonuclease that can recognize and cleave foreign genetic sequences. The DNA binding occurs using a 20-base pair DNA sequence in the crRNA that complements the targeting region next to protospacer adjacent motif (PAM) that triggers Cas9 to create DSB. During the repair of DSB, primarily by NHEJ, small indels are created at the target site, which results in deletions, insertions or frameshift mutations leading to loss of function of the gene. The sequence of crRNA can be replaced with any synthetic target sequence without modifying the other components. The crRNA and tracrRNA were fused to form a single chimeric RNA (sgRNA) and complexed with Cas9 to induce site-specific DNA cleavage [19]. The applicability of CRISPR-Cas9 for genomic modifications was demonstrated in human cells [20–23]. The replacement of only the targeting sequence in the RNA component and higher targeting efficiency made the CRISPR-Cas9 an attractive genome editing tool. Moreover, the simplicity in design and cloning facilitated the adoption of the system to various labs around the globe. Notably, the size of the Cas9 nuclease also advantageously allowed the delivery of the system in vivo using adeno-associated viruses (AAVs) [24–29]. Recently, additional Cas9 orthologues that recognize different PAM sequences have been discovered [30]. The CRISPR-Cas9 has been widely used for genetic modification in several different organisms, including plants [31,32]. Importantly, the clinical potential of CRISPR-Cas9 to correct the genetic mutations that result in the manifestation of the diseases is demonstrated in several different animal models [31]. However, the presence of antibodies against certain types of Cas enzymes and a distinct cellular and molecular changes in the host raise concerns [33–36]. Thus, large-scale screening for antibodies in different populations and further studies in larger animals are required to reach a conclusion.

In an adult mammal, the majority of the cells in the body are post-mitotic, with a few exceptions like cells in the liver. The classical HDR mechanism is generally inefficient in non-dividing cells, which limits the possibility of performing a knock-in in these cells. We developed an NHEJ-based homology independent strategy using CRISPR-Cas9, named homology-independent target integration (HITI), for the integration of transgene in non-dividing cells [29,37]. Unlike the HDR-based CRISPR-Cas9 approach, the transgene that is integrated using the HITI method lacks homology regions but harbors Cas9 cleavage sites similar to the targeting sequence on the genome. The cleavage by Cas9 creates blunt ends on the transgene and at the targeting site, while the NHEJ pathway allows the integration of transgenes during the repair of genomic DSB. As the NHEJ pathway is active during all cell cycle phases, HITI opened the doors for targeted gene knock-in in non-dividing cells, including neurons and muscle [29]. However, HITI cannot repair existing mutations; therefore, it is limited in its ability to correct point or frameshift mutations. Recently, we developed another versatile knock-in method called intracellular linearized single homology arm donor mediated intron targeting integration (SATI) for gene knock-in in intronic regions using donor vector containing a single homology arm with a Cas9 cleavage site [38]. SATI has a bipotential capacity to use HDR and NHEJ DSB repair machinery, facilitating in targeting a broad range of mutations in different cell types. SATI was successfully used for gene knock-in in vivo to correct a dominant point mutation that causes premature aging in mice [38]. Similarly, several other gene-editing methods utilizing CRISPR-Cas9 and MMEJ were developed during the last couple of years for both in vitro and in vivo application [37].

In addition to the use of CRISPR-Cas9 for gene deletion and insertion, Cas9 nickase and catalytically deficient Cas9 (dCas9) are fused with deaminases for the conversion of single nucleotides. The cytosine base editor (CBE) is the first base editor developed that can convert C to T [39]. The commonly used third-generation CBE consists of a cytidine deaminase (APOBEC1), Cas nickase, and a uracil glycosylase inhibitor (UGI). In mammalian cells, an average of 37% permanent conversion at the target site is reported [39]. Nishida et al. also reported another cytosine base editing system using cytidine deaminase 1 (CDA1) [40]. Later, adenine base editor (ABE) was developed by replacing the cytidine deaminase with adenine deaminase (TadA) that can convert A to G [41]. The ABE comprises heterodimeric proteins (wild-type non-catalytic TadA monomer and evolved TadA* monomer) and Cas9 nickase in a single polypeptide chain. Base editors are successfully used in plants, zebrafish, mice and human embryos [30]. Additionally, RNA base editors (RBE) are created by fusing nucleobase deaminase with Cas13 protein to convert A to inosine (I) or C to uracil (U) in the targeted RNA [42].

Interestingly, three independent groups have recently reported the development of dual adenine and cytosine base editors by combining both the deaminases with Cas9 nickase [43–45]. Using the dual deaminase base editor, both A to G and C to T substitutions were achieved at the target site. The dual deaminase base editors will offer new possibilities that were not possible with single-deaminase base editors such as targeting multi-nucleotide variants and CA/TG-rich transcription factor binding sites [43]. Additionally, Zhao et al. developed glycosylase base editors that can cause C to A transversions in bacteria and C to G transversions in mammalian cells [46]. The glycosylase base editors contain Cas9 nickase, a cytidine deaminase and uracil-DNA glycosylase. In mammalian cells, editing efficiency of 5–53% was observed.

Base editors do not generate DSBs and the chances of undesired changes such as indels are low. However, the base editors sometimes show off-target specificity [47]. Moreover, the presence of multiple C and A nucleotides close to the target base called "bystander base" can result in multiple base conversions, which can affect the targeting efficiency of base editors. Notably, Arbab et al. reported the creation of a machine learning model called BE-Hive using experimental data from more than 38,000 target sites in human and mouse cells [48]. This tool facilitates in predicting the base editing efficiency at the target site, especially in the presence of bystander nucleotides.

Anzalone et al. reported a prime editing approach similar to base editors, where Cas9 nickase was fused to an engineered reverse transcriptase, which is guided by a two-part guide RNAs termed "search" and "replace". The "search" guide localizes the Cas9 to target loci, where it cuts the DNA and the "replace" guide sequence is used by reverse transcriptase to make complementary DNA to integrate at the cut site [49]. Since most of the genetic diseases occur due to point mutations, the therapeutic potential of base and prime editors for the treatment of human disorders is currently being explored [50–52].

Interestingly, the CRISPR-Cas complex was also found to be encoded in a class of bacterial Tn7-like transposons [53]. Due to the site-specific integration of Tn7 transposon downstream of the conserved genomic sequence in *Escherichia coli*, researchers have hypothesized that transposon encoded CRISPR-Cas promoted this process [53]. In a recent study, Klompe et al. demonstrated how transposons have used the RNA-guided DNA targeting mechanism for site-specific integration without the need of DSBs and homologous recombination [54]. The unique features of this system might help to overcome the issues that arise from potential DSBs at off-target sites and the requirement of a long-homology arm, which limits the size of the target sequence. However, the system has not been tested in human cells and the efficiency of integration of template DNA at the target site remains unknown [55].

In addition to the targeting of DNA, Cas9 is also directed to target the single-stranded RNA (ssRNA) matching the guide RNA sequence when PAM is presented in trans as a separate DNA oligonucleotide (PAMmers). The PAMmers were able to stimulate the Cas9 endonuclease activity on ssRNA, similar to DNA cleavage [56]. This approach was used to eliminate the toxic microsatellite repeat expansion RNA in myotonic dystrophy type 1 patient cells [57]. Later, a naturally existing CRISPR-Cas13 system with RNA-targeting endonuclease activity was discovered in bacteria. Cas13 has four family members (Cas13a-d) and each demonstrates specific base preferences; for example, Cas13a requires a protospacer flanking sequence consisting of a single A, U or C base pair [58]. Moreover, Cas13 subtypes differ in CRISPR RNA structure, direct repeat sequence and size. Although all exhibit promiscuous ribonuclease activity upon target recognition, Cas13d RNA cleavage is observed only in bacteria and not in the mammalian cells [59]. This unique characteristic of Cas13d allowed targeting RNAs in mammalian cells [59,60].

3. Specificity and Off-Target Effects of Customizable Nucleases

The specificity of nucleases used for genome editing is one of the essential criteria for success in both basic and translational research. The customizable nucleases are engineered to target the region of interest on the genome using sequence information; however, the shorter-targeting sequence length used for the identification and few mismatches might allow the binding of nucleases at off-target sites. The concern of off-target applies to all the customizable nucleases in general. For therapeutic use of nucleases, they need to demonstrate higher specificity, activity, and gene modification ability. They should also be easier to deliver. Along this line, re-engineering strategies have been implemented for Zinc finger proteins and TAL effectors to improve the targeting precision [61–63]. Since Zinc finger nucleases and TALENs have been actively used for a long time, they demonstrate a long track record in safety, including their use in patients for therapeutic purposes. Conversely, CRISPR is relatively new; due to the simplicity in its design and ease of use, it is widely used, but we are still understanding the specificity and repair outcomes [63]. In the initial studies using CRISPR-Cas9, depending on the number of mismatches in the guide RNA, the rate of off-target effects were observed [20,64,65]. Later, a Cas9 nickase mutant paired with two guide RNAs was used to create DSBs, which led to reduction of off-target effects by 50 to 1000-fold [66]. Similarly, base and prime editing approaches can be a good alternative way to correct the disease-causing mutations without introducing DSBs and thereby avoid unintended changes. Nevertheless, the development of advanced bioinformatics tools and high-throughput sequencing methods will help in screening and identification of guide RNAs that are specific and do not have any off-targets [67]. In addition, the use of cell- or tissue-specific promoters to restrict the expression of CRISPR in combination with the local delivery, short-term expression, and use of selective AAV serotype can also help to minimize the negative effects.

4. Applications of Customizable Nucleases

4.1. Modeling Genetic Diseases in Cells

The traditional approach of genetic modification in the cells is less efficient, especially in performing targeted gene knockout or knock-in of fluorescent reporters. The customizable nucleases allowed the generation of a variety of genetic modifications in mammalian cells to model diseases, including cancer, metabolic and neurodegenerative diseases [68]. Stem cells are routinely used in the laboratories as they can be differentiated to any cell type using a defined medium, but genome editing by homologous recombination is less efficient and possesses limited use in the modeling diseases. The generation of pluripotent stem cells from patient somatic cells by reprogramming opened the possibilities of generating personalized induced pluripotent stem cells (iPSCs) [69]. iPSCs are routinely used to generate disease causing mutations to mimic the disease phenotypes in cell culture, which aid in understanding the cellular and molecular changes that occur during the disease progression [70]. Also, the engineered iPSCs can be differentiated to other cell types and used them for large-scale drug screenings and CRISPR knockdown screenings to identify new gene networks that play a role in disease progression or prevention. Moreover, pluripotent stem cells are widely used to generate different types of organoids [71,72]. Interestingly, gene-editing tools are also used in the in vitro organoid system to model human diseases to understand the etiology of the disease as well as for drug screening [73]. Notably, the genetically engineered cells have been used to generate several different types of organoids, including the brain, intestine, liver, kidney and lung [70].

4.2. Correction of Disease-Causing Mutations

The correction of genetic mutations to treat human diseases has proven an exciting potential application for the genome editing tools. In this line, ZFNs, TALENs, and the CRISPR-Cas system have been used to correct mutations in cells in vitro and transplanting them back to the patients. ZFNs have been successfully employed in mammalian cells to deliver the vectors expressing the ZFN-coding sequences by transfection of DNA or infection with viruses [11]. The higher specificity and mutagenesis rate of ZFN provides an advantage for therapeutic applications. ZFNs have been used to knock out the *CCR5* gene in T-cell precursor cells isolated from HIV patients to avoid the infection of HIV-1 [12]. Currently, clinical trials are ongoing that use this approach with modifications in the delivery of ZFNs to T-cells and improvements in the engraftment of infused cells [74]., Moreover, the genetic mutation that causes β-thalassemia and sickle cell disease in hematopoietic stem cells has been corrected using ZFNs [75,76]. Similarly, TALENs are also used in chimeric antigen receptor (CAR) T-cell therapy, where the T-cells are genetically modified to produce artificial receptors that recognize a specific protein on the tumor cells. Many products based on TALEN-edited cells have begun clinical trials, especially those focused on immuno-oncology [74].

Similar to ZFN and TALEN, T-cells have been genetically edited using CRISPR to knockdown immune checkpoint inhibitor programmed cell death-1 (PD-1), which is upregulated during activation of T-cells to reduce the autoimmune reaction and aid cancer cells in evading the immune system [77]. Moreover, CRISPR is also used to induce exon skipping of defective exons in Duchenne muscular dystrophy (DMD), to inactivate faulty genes that lead to the manifestation of disease including amyotrophic lateral sclerosis and Huntington disease, correct a genetic mutation that causes premature aging and eliminate the entire chromosome in aneuploid stem cells [32,78,79]. Importantly, gene-editing tools have already been used to correct the mutation in *β-globin* gene in patient hematopoietic stem cells [31].

ZFNs and CRISPR-Cas9 have been used to edit the HIV-1 genome and block its expression in T-cells, microglia and promonocytes [80–82]. CRISPR-Cas9 has been used to directly target and disrupt the reverse-transcribed products of lentivirus RNA generated during their life cycle [83]. Although the use of nucleases to edit the HIV-1 genome from human cells may not be considered a correction of disease-causing mutations, the HIV-1 genome in the cells produces new viral particles that lead to the development of acquired immune deficiency syndrome (AIDS).

The recent development of the NHEJ based genome-editing approach in non-dividing cells now allows for correcting mutations that cover a wide range of diseases, including Parkinson's disease and amyotrophic lateral sclerosis. HITI was employed to correct a mutation that causes inherited degenerative eye disease, retinitis pigmentosa, in rats [29]. Likewise, SATI was used to knock-in a normal copy of *Lmna* and prevent the expression of mutated copy, which led to the extension of the lifespan of progeria mice [38]. Furthermore, other NHEJ and CRISPR-Cas9 based approaches were used to knock-in a normal copy of the gene to rescue diseases such as tyrosinemia type I in mice [37]. Notably, several clinical trials are ongoing using CRISPR for the treatment of genetic diseases, including a blood disorder, eye disease and muscular dystrophy [31]. Likewise, CRISPR single-base editors are now used for the correction of single-base mutations or to disable the expression of the mutant gene [52]. Although CRISPR-based gene editing was identified recently, it has been tested in almost all cell types.

4.3. Generation of Animal Models

The traditional approach for creating gene-edited animals requires a time-consuming method that involves the use of modified ES cells. The generation of modified ES cells is a time and labor-intensive process. Moreover, the low success rate of obtaining the founder mice with a higher contribution of injected ES cells to the germline also hindered the process. Furthermore, the lack of ES cells for certain animals, including rats, also limited the generation of genetically modified animals of different species. However, the development of customizable nucleases has helped to overcome the need for ES cells by performing the gene modifications directly in the zygotes. ZFNs were the first nucleases widely used for targeted mutagenesis and gene replacement, beginning with fruit fly and nematodes and progressing to other organisms such as silkworm and zebrafish, by injecting the ZFN pair at the early stages of zygote or embryo development. Notably, ZFNs opened the door to the possibility of creating genetically modified rats, which was not possible with other approaches [84]. In mice and rats, ZFNs have been able to induce both mono and biallelic gene disruption and homologous recombination with donor DNA at the target site. Furthermore, the germ cells carried the modifications. Similar to ZFNs, TALENs have been used to disrupt the expression of target genes in different animal models, including mice, rats, frog, zebrafish, pig and fruit fly [16]. In most of these studies, a single TALEN pair was used to create DSB to interrupt the function of the targeted gene. Moreover, to generate large deletions or chromosomal inversions, two pairs of TALENs were used to target the same chromosome [85,86]. The higher genome editing efficiency of TALEN is also used for generating animal models that mimic human diseases such as hypercholesterolemia.

Currently, the CRISPR-Cas system is the most favored customized nuclease and is widely used for performing in vivo genetic modification. Importantly, the CRISPR-Cas system allows the possibility of the simultaneous manipulation of several different genes, thereby dramatically reducing the amount of time required for the generation of double- or triple- knockout animals [87]. Moreover, in addition to mice, CRISPR has been successfully used in rats and other large animals, including dogs, pigs and monkeys [88]. In addition to performing gene knockout in vivo, the CRISPR-Cas system is also used to perform knock-in of reporters not only in dividing cells but also in non-dividing cells such as neurons [29,37]. Likewise, CRISPR-Cas9 along with NHEJ and MHMEJ-based methods have been used for transgene knock-in in mouse and monkey embryos [89]. Wang et al. reported the generation of non-human model of Hutchinson-Gilford progeria syndrome (HGPS) in monkey embryos using base editor to introduce C to T conversion in *LMNA* gene [90]. However, the microinjection of nucleases into zygotes requires special equipment and skill, which are not always available in all labs. To solve this problem, alternative methods are being developed, such as the injection of nucleases into the oviduct of pregnant females, followed by in vivo electroporation to deliver the components into zygotes [91].

4.4. Targeting Mitochondrial Genome

Among the different nucleases, so far, ZFNs and TALENs are the only ones so far that have been successfully used to target the mitochondrial genome. Unlike the nuclear genome, mitochondrial DNA (mtDNA) is mostly maternally inherited. The number of mitochondria and mtDNA can vary between different cell types and tissues. Moreover, multiple copies of mtDNA exist, ranging from a few hundred to thousands in each cell based on their energy demand. The mutations in the mtDNA lead to the degeneration of tissues and organs with high energy demand, including muscle and neurons, resulting in the manifestation of mitochondrial disease phenotypes [92]. Due to a lack of an efficient DNA repair mechanism in the mitochondria and the presence of multiple copies of both mutated and non-mutated mtDNA, the strategy of selective elimination of mutated mtDNA and re-population of normal mtDNA has been undertaken [93]. ZFNs and TALENs are localized into the mitochondria using a mitochondria localization signal and they selectively degrade the mtDNA with the disease-causing mutation in the cells obtained from mitochondrial disease patients [94–96]. Moreover, in a recent study, both ZFN and TALENs were delivered in vivo to reduce the mtDNA with a disease-causing mutation in muscle and heart and rescue the disease phenotypes in a mitochondrial disease mouse model [97,98]. Additionally, TALENs were also used in the mice embryos to target specific mitochondrial haplotypes and prevent their transmission to the next generation [99].

However, the CRISPR-Cas system has not been reported to be successfully used for targeting mtDNA. The major hurdle for the application of CRISPR-Cas system to mtDNA editing has been the successful import of gRNAs into the mitochondrial matrix, partially due to the inefficient RNA import mechanism present in the mitochondria of mammalian cells [100]. Although a few publications report the use of CRISPR-Cas9 to target mtDNA, the results presented in the studies lack proper experimental evidence and have not yet been independently validated by other groups [101,102]. Interestingly, a new study reports a CRISPR-free mitochondrial base editing approach, which is accomplished using an interbacterial cytidine deaminase toxin fused to TALE domains [103]. The cytidine deaminase was split into two halves to avoid the toxicity and is inactive until brought together at the target site. Using this new approach, the CG to TA base conversions in mtDNA are possible without the need of DSBs and five different genes on mtDNA were edited without any off-target effects [103]. Though this approach is promising to introduce base changes in the mtDNA, a strong preference for 5'-TC-3' is reported, which dramatically limits the number of target regions. In fact, only one mitochondrial mutation 8356T>C found in humans can fulfill this requirement. Nevertheless, the modification of current cytidine deaminase may allow us to overcome this requirement. Currently, we lack animal models for mitochondrial disease due to the inability to edit the mtDNA. However, a CRISPR-free mitochondrial base editing approach can be used to generate animal models by introducing pathogenic mutations in the mtDNA.

5. Applications Beyond Genome Editing

5.1. Epigenetic Modifications

Although initial applications of nucleases mostly focused on gene editing, they were quickly redirected for other purposes, such as gene regulation. Zinc-fingers and TALEs were fused to transcriptional activators, among the different activators, VP64 and p65 proved the strongest when targeted upstream of the transcription start site and in promoter regions [104]. Similarly, the catalytic inactive dCas9 was fused with different transcriptional activators, repressors, modifiers or fluorophores to modulate the expression of the target gene by modifying the epigenetic status at the promoter regions [30]. To repress the gene expression, dCas9 was fused with the transcription repressor domain Krüppel-associated box (KRAB), which induces heterochromatin formation and changes in chromatin structure. dCas9-KRAB has been shown to silence genes, non-coding RNA and proximal and distal enhancer elements [30]. For gene activation, multiple transcription activation domains were fused to dCas9 [105] or recruited using the dimerized MS2 bacteriophage coat proteins that bind to the minimal hairpin aptamer on the gRNA tetraloop and stem-loop 2 [106]. Using this approach, multiple genes were simultaneously activated at the same time for cellular reprogramming of somatic cells to pluripotent state or direct differentiation of fibroblasts to neurons [30]. Furthermore, other epigenetic modifications, such as the acetylation and methylation of DNA have also been performed by fusing histone acetyltransferase p300 or catalytic domain of methylcytosine dioxygenase TET1 to dCas9 [104]. Recently, a study achieved dose-dependent activation of genes was achieved using CRISPR and chemical epigenetic modifiers that recruit endogenous chromatin machinery [107].

We have shown, for the first time in vivo, that Cas9 and transcription activation complexes can be recruited to the target loci using modified guide RNAs to activate the expression of endogenous genes [108]. Using this approach, we treated acute kidney disease, diabetes and muscular dystrophy in mouse models [108]. Later, a transgenic mouse model expressing a modified dCas9 system was used in vivo to activate multiple neurogenic endogenous genes to directly convert astrocytes into functional neurons [109]. Recently, Matharu et al. delivered dCas9-VP64 using AAVs to rescue the obesity phenotypes in a haploinsufficient mouse model [110]. Moreover, CRISPR-Cas12a was fused to a transcriptional activation domain to enable multiplexed knockout and transcriptional activation in vivo [111]. Similarly, the CRISPR system was also used to repress the expression of genes in vivo. In the last few years, several studies have successfully delivered dCas9 fused with different transcriptional repressors to reduce the expression of genes that play a role in reducing brain function [112], lower circulating low-density lipoprotein (LDL) concentration [113], and to correct retinitis pigmentosa phenotypes [114]. All these studies demonstrate the therapeutic potential of CRISPR based epigenetic modifications in vivo in ameliorating disease phenotypes [115].

5.2. Live Cell Genome Imaging and Large-Scale Genetic Screenings

Among the different repurposes, nucleases were also used for labeling specific regions of chromatin using fluorescent proteins. Before the identification of CRISPR-Cas system, ZFN and TALE proteins were used to recruit the fluorescent protein to the regions such as telomeres and centromeres for live imaging in cells [116,117]. Higher targeting efficiencies of Cas9 and dCas9 have replaced the other nucleases. Moreover, in another study, the improvement to the gRNA scaffold containing multiple MS2 binding modules facilitated the increase of the fluorescent signal with as few as four gRNAs. This improvement facilitated better labeling of low-repetitive and non-repetitive regions and tracking of the transcriptionally active and inactive regions [118]. Among the different nucleases, CRISPR-Cas system is the popular choice for performing high-throughput screens. Additionally, the CRISPR-Cas system is also employed in large-scale functional screening using hundreds of gRNAs in the cells and is efficient compared to the traditional short hairpin RNA (shRNA) system [119]. This approach allows large-scale genetic screening in an unbiased way to understand the role of a gene on a specific phenotype [106,120,121]. CRISPR-Cas system is also used to perform large-scale knockout screens to identify causative drivers of cancer in a native tissue environment [122,123]. Notably, this type of screen can be performed in a regular laboratory with access to cell culture, and no automated robotics are required. However, it involves a significant amount of sequencing, data analysis, and validation of data [124].

5.3. Use of CRISPR to Detect Nucleic Acids for Diagnostic Purposes

The use of CRISPR for molecular diagnosis has provided another exciting development during the last couple of years. Initially, the promiscuous ribonuclease activity of Cas13a upon target recognition of the surrounding RNA molecules was used to develop a molecular detection platform termed specific high-sensitivity enzymatic reporter unlocking (SHERLOCK). This platform was used for the detection of the Zika and Dengue viruses [125]. Moreover, a new version of SHERLOCK (SHERLOCKv2) was developed that can simultaneously detect multiple targets in the same reaction using different Cas enzymes and fluorescent reporters [126]. The SHERLOCK system was also shown to identify single-nucleotide polymorphisms (SNPs) on the viral genome [127]. Similarly, Cas12a possesses a non-specific cleavage of ssDNA molecules upon recognition of targeted sequence; using this feature, a DNA detection platform termed DNA Endonuclease Targeted CRISPR Trans Reporter (DETECTR) was developed [128]. Interestingly, both SHERLOCK and DETECTR approaches have been used for the detection of SARS-CoV-2 from nasal swabs during the recent COVID19 pandemic [129]. Notably, in the case of both the approaches, the results can be obtained in less than one hour and can be observed on a lateral flow strip. Furthermore, SHERLOCK and DETECTR methods are specific and sensitive in detecting the nucleic acids at low concentrations. These features make them ideal as care diagnostic tools that can be deployed and used with minimal setup during pandemics such as COVID19.

Interestingly, the RNA targeting property of CRISPR was also tested to target the SARS-CoV-2 genome. A CRISPR-Cas13-based strategy, PAC-MAN (prophylactic antiviral CRISPR in human cells), was shown to target and degrade RNA from SARS-CoV-2 sequences and H1N1 IAV load in respiratory epithelial cells [130]. In this study, the PAC-MAN was tested in an in vitro setting; however, the successful translation of this approach in vivo requires a non-viral delivery vehicle. Nanoparticles can be used to deliver mRNAs encoding CasRx/gRNAs directly into the lungs in an aerosol format using a nebulizer, are an ideal choice. Nevertheless, directly targeting the virus RNA genome is a promising strategy to prevent viral replication without relying on the body's immune system, which is an important factor for patients with low immunity or older individuals that cannot fight the infection and develop antibodies efficiently [131,132].

6. Gene Editing in Human Embryos

Genetic mutations in the germline of parents are passed down to the next generation. Some of the mutations can be lethal and affect embryo development that may lead to the early termination of pregnancy. In some less severe cases, the mutation can lead to the development of disease later during life. With the advancements in diagnosis and availability of cutting-edge medical interventions, it is now possible to treat or prevent the progression of many diseases. However, we still lack effective methods for treating the majority of the diseases caused by the genetic mutations inherited from the parents, so the correction of these mutations in the early stage of embryo development has been considered. Nevertheless, genome editing in somatic cells and germline differs greatly, not only in terms of DNA repair mechanism, but also in long-term consequences. Genome editing in somatic cells involves the modification of patient cells to cure a disease, which can be performed by isolating the cells and transplanting them back after correcting the mutation. However, for germline editing, the correction needs to be performed during the early stages of embryo development, and all the cells from the embryo may carry the modification, including the germ cells, which will also impact the future generations. Alternatively, it is possible that only some cells in the embryo undergo correction, which can lead to the generation of a mosaic embryo.

In the last few years, several research groups have performed gene editing in human embryos. Until now, more than seven different studies have been carried out using human embryos to test the cleavage efficiency and off-targets using CRISPR-Cas system [133–136]. Interestingly, during the correction of a pathogenic mutation in human embryos, DSBs have been repaired using endogenous HDR mechanism and wild-type allele as a template, which differs from the HDR efficiency observed in pluripotent stem cells [135]. In addition to the correction of pathogenic mutations, gene editing has also been used performed in human embryos to understand the role of pluripotent transcription factor OCT4 during early embryogenesis [137]. Moreover, base editing technology has also been used in the human embryos to correct pathogenic mutations [138,139]. Interestingly, better correction efficiency and higher homozygotic nucleotide conversion with no overlapped mutations have been observed at two-cell and four-cell human embryos compared to zygote [139].

Interestingly, the development of a long-term in vitro culture system for human embryos (until 14 days) [140,141], opened up possibilities of culturing the gene-edited embryo to better understand the early developmental problems. Moreover, pluripotent stem cells are now cultured in vitro on different cellular matrices to allow them to self-organize and generate structures called synthetic embryos that are similar to normal embryos and mimic the early developmental program of natural embryos [142]. Recently, using a single stem cell type, extended pluripotent stem cells of mouse origin, and a 3D-differentiation system has been used to generate blastocyst-like structures [143]. A similar approach is currently being refined to create synthetic embryos using human pluripotent stem cells. We can foresee that in the near future, the synthetic embryos might help to replace the use of natural human embryos for basic research purposes, especially for gene editing, to generate various disease models. Notably, the successful generation of a synthetic human embryo can, to some extent, avoid the ethical issues surrounding the use of human embryos for basic research purposes [144,145].

Until recently, the goal of genome editing in human embryos was intended to better understand the efficacy of gene correction and early developmental problems without implanting the edited embryos. However, to prevent HIV infection, one researcher in China to prevent HIV infection attempted to modify the CCR5 gene in the human embryos that were later transferred to a human resulting in the birth of twin babies. This controversial experiment reignited an international debate on the necessity and ethical issues on genome editing in human embryos. Currently, in several different countries, a moratorium exists on genome editing in human embryos for clinical purposes. According to the guidelines developed by the National Academy of Science, clinical trials for heritable genome editing can be permitted when performed adhering to the regulatory framework and fulfilling a list of criteria that includes, among others things, the absence of reasonable alternatives, the prevention of the transmission of serious disease, the restriction of the conversion of genes to the versions already prevalent in the population, plans for long-term and multigenerational follow-up, and oversight to prevent the use for other purposes [146,147]. Reports from the World Health Organization and International Commission on the Clinical Use of Human Germline Genome editing organized by US National Academy are due later this year. In general, pre-implantation genetic diagnosis (PGD) can be used to select un-mutated embryos free of mutation for implantation and avoid genome editing. However, the selection-based approaches can be a challenge for families who produce a lower number of embryos or when one of the partners carries a homozygous autosomal dominant mutation [148].

7. Future Perspectives

Customizable nucleases have opened new possibilities in the treatment of genetic mutations. Promising results from in vitro experiments and animal models demonstrate the potential application of CRISPR-Cas system in both basic research and clinical settings. However, before these nucleases can be used in clinics, several improvements must be achieved, including more precise targeting efficiency, lower off-targets, fewer unintended changes and a good delivery vehicle that can target a wide range of tissues when delivered in vivo. Certainly, significant progress on these requirements has been made. Notably, the repair efficiency has been improved by delivering Cas protein, and the availability of different types of Cas nucleases isolated from other prokaryotes and nickases are used to avoid DSBs and reduce the off-target activity [31]. Moreover, to prevent the unintended changes at the targeting site during the correction, the intronic region upstream of the mutation site is targeted to perform gene knock-in; this approach will offer greater flexibility in designing the gRNAs, and any additional changes will potentially not affect the gene function [38]. Similarly, the use of delivery vehicles other than viruses, including nanoparticles, are being tested to deliver the CRISPR-Cas system efficiently and safely. Another factor that might affect the clinical use of CRISPR-Cas system is the pre-existing antibodies against Cas proteins due to their bacterial origin, which could lead to inflammation and lower stability of Cas proteins [31]. However, more evidence is needed to determine the minimal levels of Cas protein that can activate the immune system. Together, these improvements will aid in using the CRISPR-Cas system to correct the mutations in vivo and cure the genetic disease. Notably, people with some genetic variants are more susceptible to the development of neurological disorders and some cancers. Moreover, with age, the number of mutations in somatic cells increases dramatically, and some of these mutations can lead to the development of cancer [149]. The availability of an efficient CRISPR-Cas system might facilitate the modification of specific regions of the genome in the future to prevent the development of diseases, for example, a variant of the gene that encodes for less functional protein or familial mutation that can lead to the development of the neurodegenerative disease. Moreover, the development of efficient genome editing tools, including the base editors with high specificity and no off-target effects, will open the possibilities of using them in human embryos to avoid the transmission of the disease-causing mutation. Similarly, the newly developed CRISPR-free mitochondrial base editing approach promises tremendous potential in the future to correct the pathogenic mutations in the mtDNA present in the unfertilized oocytes or embryos and prevent the transmission of mitochondrial diseases to the next generation.

In addition to the application of customizable nucleases for gene editing, their use in modulating the expression of the genes by changing the epigenetic marks on the promoters offers great potential. Interestingly, genetic diseases are not only caused due to the mutations in a gene, but also due to the lower expression of said genes that can affect the function of tissues and organs. Notably, during aging, dysregulation of epigenetic marks leads to the decreased expression of several different genes that are important for the normal function of cells and tissue, which eventually leads to the manifestation of disease phenotypes [150–152]. Since customizable nucleases were shown to modulate the expression of target gene without modifying the genomic sequences, they can be an attractive method in clinical settings to treat various diseases. Notably, we have shown that the use of CRISPR-Cas system may allow the activation of endogenous genes in vivo and reverse disease phenotypes [108]. In vivo gene activation using a CRISPR-Cas system can also overcome several limitations posed by traditional gene therapy, including the size and number of transgenes that can be delivered. Age-associated disorders are not caused due to dysregulation of a single gene or pathway, and in such cases, multiple genes may need to be activated at the same time. For this reason, a multiplex system needs to be developed in which several gRNAs can be simultaneously delivered to every cell and activate multiple genes that will help to ameliorate the cellular hallmarks of aging and restore the function of the tissues. Furthermore, the use of tissue or cell-specific promoters will help to restrict the expression of Cas enzyme or gRNAs and prevent unintended gene activation in other tissues.

In conclusion, during the last couple of years, we have not only witnessed the discovery and development of new genome editing approaches, but also their implementation to treat various diseases. Currently, many clinical trials are underway that use the newly developed gene-editing tools, and in the next few years, some of them will be eventually used in clinics not just for the treatments of genetic diseases, but also to prevent or treat viral infections such as SARS-CoV-2.

Author Contributions: Writing-review and editing, P.R., F.V., J.C.I.B., and C.S. All authors have read and agreed to the published version of the manuscript.

Funding: This research was funded by the Moxie Foundation and Department of Defense (grant number W81XWH-17-1-0552) to J.C.I.B. Miguel Servet Program Type II of ISCIII [CPII18/00020], and a FIS project [PI18/00957] to F.V.

Conflicts of Interest: All the authors declare no conflict of interest.

References

1. Smithies, O.; Gregg, R.G.; Boggs, S.S.; Koralewski, M.A.; Kucherlapati, R.S. Insertion of DNA sequences into the human chromosomal β-globin locus by homologous recombination. *Nature* **1985**, *317*, 230–234. [CrossRef]
2. Capecchi, M.R. Altering the genome by homologous recombination. *Science* **1989**, *244*, 1288–1292. [CrossRef]
3. Capecchi, M.R. Gene targeting in mice: Functional analysis of the mammalian genome for the twenty-first century. *Nat. Rev. Genet.* **2005**, *6*, 507–512. [CrossRef]
4. Capecchi, M.R. Generating mice with targeted mutations. *Nat. Med.* **2001**, *7*, 1086–1090. [CrossRef]
5. Russell, D.W.; Hirata, R.K. Human gene targeting by viral vectors. *Nat. Genet.* **1998**, *18*, 325–330. [CrossRef]
6. Jasin, M. Genetic manipulation of genomes with rare-cutting endonucleases. *Trends Genet.* **1996**, *12*, 224–228. [CrossRef]
7. Segal, D.J.; Meckler, J.F. Genome Engineering at the Dawn of the Golden Age. *Annu. Rev. Genom. Hum. Genet.* **2013**, *14*, 135–158. [CrossRef]
8. Silva, G.; Poirot, L.; Galetto, R.; Smith, J.; Montoya, G.; Duchateau, P.; Paques, F. Meganucleases and Other Tools for Targeted Genome Engineering: Perspectives and Challenges for Gene Therapy. *Curr. Gene Ther.* **2011**, *11*, 11–27. [CrossRef] [PubMed]
9. Cathomen, T.; Keith Joung, J. Zinc-finger Nucleases: The Next Generation Emerges. *Mol. Ther.* **2008**, *16*, 1200–1207. [CrossRef] [PubMed]
10. Urnov, F.D.; Rebar, E.J.; Holmes, M.C.; Zhang, H.S.; Gregory, P.D. Genome editing with engineered zinc finger nucleases. *Nat. Rev. Genet.* **2010**, *11*, 636–646. [CrossRef] [PubMed]
11. Carroll, D. Genome Engineering with Zinc-Finger Nucleases. *Genetics* **2011**, *188*, 773–782. [CrossRef] [PubMed]
12. Perez, E.E.; Wang, J.; Miller, J.C.; Jouvenot, Y.; Kim, K.A.; Liu, O.; Wang, N.; Lee, G.; Bartsevich, V.V.; Lee, Y.-L.; et al. Establishment of HIV-1 resistance in CD4 + T cells by genome editing using zinc-finger nucleases. *Nat. Biotechnol.* **2008**, *26*, 808–816. [CrossRef] [PubMed]
13. Meyer, M.; de Angelis, M.H.; Wurst, W.; Kühn, R. Gene targeting by homologous recombination in mouse zygotes mediated by zinc-finger nucleases. *Proc. Natl. Acad. Sci. USA* **2010**, *107*, 15022–15026. [CrossRef] [PubMed]
14. Cui, X.; Ji, D.; Fisher, D.A.; Wu, Y.; Briner, D.M.; Weinstein, E.J. Targeted integration in rat and mouse embryos with zinc-finger nucleases. *Nat. Biotechnol.* **2011**, *29*, 64–67. [CrossRef]
15. Boch, J.; Bonas, U. XanthomonasAvrBs3 Family-Type III Effectors: Discovery and Function. *Annu. Rev. Phytopathol.* **2010**, *48*, 419–436. [CrossRef]

16. Joung, J.K.; Sander, J.D. TALENs: A widely applicable technology for targeted genome editing. *Nat. Rev. Mol. Cell. Biol.* **2012**, *14*, 49–55. [CrossRef]
17. Xiao, A.; Wang, Z.; Hu, Y.; Wu, Y.; Luo, Z.; Yang, Z.; Zu, Y.; Li, W.; Huang, P.; Tong, X.; et al. Chromosomal deletions and inversions mediated by TALENs and CRISPR/Cas in zebrafish. *Nucleic Acids Res.* **2013**, *41*, e141. [CrossRef]
18. Bedell, V.M.; Wang, Y.; Campbell, J.M.; Poshusta, T.L.; Starker, C.G.; Krug, R.G., II; Tan, W.; Penheiter, S.G.; Ma, A.C.; Leung, A.Y.H.; et al. In vivo genome editing using a high-efficiency TALEN system. *Nature* **2012**, *491*, 114–118. [CrossRef]
19. Jinek, M.; Chylinski, K.; Fonfara, I.; Hauer, M.; Doudna, J.A.; Charpentier, E. A Programmable Dual-RNA-Guided DNA Endonuclease in Adaptive Bacterial Immunity. *Science* **2012**, *337*, 816–821. [CrossRef]
20. Cong, L.; Ran, F.A.; Cox, D.; Lin, S.; Barretto, R.; Habib, N.; Hsu, P.D.; Wu, X.; Jiang, W.; Marraffini, L.A.; et al. Multiplex Genome Engineering Using CRISPR/Cas Systems. *Science* **2013**, *339*, 819–823. [CrossRef]
21. Mali, P.; Yang, L.; Esvelt, K.M.; Aach, J.; Guell, M.; DiCarlo, J.E.; Norville, J.E.; Church, G.M. RNA-Guided Human Genome Engineering via Cas. *Science* **2013**, *339*, 823–826. [CrossRef] [PubMed]
22. Cho, S.W.; Kim, S.; Kim, J.M.; Kim, J.-S. Targeted genome engineering in human cells with the Cas9 RNA-guided endonuclease. *Nat. Biotechnol.* **2013**, *31*, 230–232. [CrossRef] [PubMed]
23. Jinek, M.; East, A.; Cheng, A.; Lin, S.; Ma, E.; Doudna, J. RNA-programmed genome editing in human cells. *Elife Sci.* **2013**, *2*, 273. [CrossRef] [PubMed]
24. Tabebordbar, M.; Zhu, K.; Cheng, J.K.W.; Chew, W.L.; Widrick, J.J.; Yan, W.X.; Maesner, C.; Wu, E.Y.; Xiao, R.; Ran, F.A.; et al. In vivo gene editing in dystrophic mouse muscle and muscle stem cells. *Science* **2016**, *351*, 407–411. [CrossRef] [PubMed]
25. Nelson, C.E.; Hakim, C.H.; Ousterout, D.G.; Thakore, P.I.; Moreb, E.A.; Rivera, R.M.C.; Madhavan, S.; Pan, X.; Ran, F.A.; Yan, W.X.; et al. In vivo genome editing improves muscle function in a mouse model of Duchenne muscular dystrophy. *Science* **2016**, *351*, 403–407. [CrossRef]
26. Long, C.; Amoasii, L.; Mireault, A.A.; McAnally, J.R.; Li, H.; Sanchez-Ortiz, E.; Bhattacharyya, S.; Shelton, J.M.; Bassel-Duby, R.; Olson, E.N. Postnatal genome editing partially restores dystrophin expression in a mouse model of muscular dystrophy. *Science* **2016**, *351*, 400–403. [CrossRef]
27. Ran, F.A.; Cong, L.; Yan, W.X.; Scott, D.A.; Gootenberg, J.S.; Kriz, A.J.; Zetsche, B.; Shalem, O.; Wu, X.; Makarova, K.S.; et al. In vivo genome editing using Staphylococcus aureus Cas. *Nature* **2015**, *520*, 186–191. [CrossRef]
28. Yang, Y.; Wang, L.; Bell, P.; McMenamin, D.; He, Z.; White, J.; Yu, H.; Xu, C.; Morizono, H.; Musunuru, K.; et al. A dual AAV system enables the Cas9-mediated correction of a metabolic liver disease in newborn mice. *Nat. Biotechnol.* **2016**, *34*, 334–338. [CrossRef]
29. Suzuki, K.; Tsunekawa, Y.; Hernandez-Benitez, R.; Wu, J.; Zhu, J.; Kim, E.J.; Hatanaka, F.; Yamamoto, M.; Araoka, T.; Li, Z.; et al. In vivo genome editing via CRISPR/Cas9 mediated homology-independent targeted integration. *Nature* **2016**, *540*, 144–149. [CrossRef]
30. Pickar-Oliver, A.; Gersbach, C.A. The next generation of CRISPR–Cas technologies and applications. *Nat. Rev. Mol. Cell. Biol.* **2019**, *68*, 2913. [CrossRef]
31. Doudna, J.A. The promise and challenge of therapeutic genome editing. *Nature* **2020**, *578*, 229–236. [CrossRef] [PubMed]
32. Knott, G.J.; Doudna, J.A. CRISPR-Cas guides the future of genetic engineering. *Science* **2018**, *361*, 866–869. [CrossRef] [PubMed]
33. Charlesworth, C.T.; Deshpande, P.S.; Dever, D.P.; Camarena, J.; Lemgart, V.T.; Cromer, M.K.; Vakulskas, C.A.; Collingwood, M.A.; Zhang, L.; Bode, N.M.; et al. Identification of preexisting adaptive immunity to Cas9 proteins in humans. *Nat. Med.* **2019**, *25*, 249–254. [CrossRef] [PubMed]
34. Crudele, J.M.; Chamberlain, J.S. Cas9 immunity creates challenges for CRISPR gene editing therapies. *Nat. Commun.* **2018**, *9*, 1–3. [CrossRef] [PubMed]
35. Rath, D.; Amlinger, L.; Rath, A.; Lundgren, M. The CRISPR-Cas immune system: Biology, mechanisms and applications. *Biochimie* **2015**, *117*, 119–128. [CrossRef]
36. Chew, W.L.; Tabebordbar, M.; Cheng, J.K.W.; Mali, P.; Wu, E.Y.; Ng, A.H.M.; Zhu, K.; Wagers, A.J.; Church, G.M. A multifunctional AAV–CRISPR–Cas9 and its host response. *Nat. Meth.* **2016**, *13*, 868–874. [CrossRef]

37. Suzuki, K.; Belmonte, J.C.I. In vivo genome editing via the HITI method as a tool for gene therapy. *J. Hum. Genet.* **2018**, *63*, 157–164. [CrossRef]
38. Suzuki, K.; Yamamoto, M.; Hernandez-Benitez, R.; Li, Z.; Wei, C.; Soligalla, R.D.; Aizawa, E.; Hatanaka, F.; Kurita, M.; Reddy, P.; et al. Precise in vivo genome editing via single homology arm donor mediated intron-targeting gene integration for genetic disease correction. *Cell Res.* **2019**, *21*, 121. [CrossRef]
39. Komor, A.C.; Kim, Y.B.; Packer, M.S.; Zuris, J.A.; Liu, D.R. Programmable editing of a target base in genomic DNA without double-stranded DNA cleavage. *Nature* **2016**, *533*, 420–424. [CrossRef]
40. Nishida, K.; Arazoe, T.; Yachie, N.; Banno, S.; Kakimoto, M.; Tabata, M.; Mochizuki, M.; Miyabe, A.; Araki, M.; Hara, K.Y.; et al. Targeted nucleotide editing using hybrid prokaryotic and vertebrate adaptive immune systems. *Science* **2016**, *353*, aaf8729. [CrossRef]
41. Gaudelli, N.M.; Komor, A.C.; Rees, H.A.; Packer, M.S.; Badran, A.H.; Bryson, D.I.; Liu, D.R. Programmable base editing of A•T to G•C in genomic DNA without DNA cleavage. *Nature* **2017**, *551*, 464–471. [CrossRef] [PubMed]
42. Cox, D.B.T.; Gootenberg, J.S.; Abudayyeh, O.O.; Franklin, B.; Kellner, M.J.; Joung, J.; Zhang, F. RNA editing with CRISPR-Cas. *Science* **2017**, *358*, 1019–1027. [CrossRef] [PubMed]
43. Grünewald, J.; Zhou, R.; Lareau, C.A.; Garcia, S.P.; Iyer, S.; Miller, B.R.; Langner, L.M.; Hsu, J.Y.; Aryee, M.J.; Joung, J.K. A dual-deaminase CRISPR base editor enables concurrent adenine and cytosine editing. *Nat. Biotechnol.* **2020**, *38*, 861–864. [CrossRef] [PubMed]
44. Sakata, R.C.; Ishiguro, S.; Mori, H.; Tanaka, M.; Tatsuno, K.; Ueda, H.; Yamamoto, S.; Seki, M.; Masuyama, N.; Nishida, K.; et al. Base editors for simultaneous introduction of C-to-T and A-to-G mutations. *Nat. Biotechnol.* **2020**, *38*, 865–869. [CrossRef] [PubMed]
45. Zhang, X.; Zhu, B.; Chen, L.; Xie, L.; Yu, W.; Wang, Y.; Li, L.; Yin, S.; Yang, L.; Hu, H.; et al. Dual base editor catalyzes both cytosine and adenine base conversions in human cells. *Nat. Biotechnol.* **2020**, *38*, 856–860. [CrossRef] [PubMed]
46. Zhao, D.; Li, J.; Li, S.; Xin, X.; Hu, M.; Price, M.A.; Rosser, S.J.; Bi, C.; Zhang, X. Glycosylase base editors enable C-to-A and C-to-G base changes. *Nat. Biotechnol.* **2020**, *337*, 1–6. [CrossRef]
47. Rees, H.A.; Liu, D.R. Base editing: Precision chemistry on the genome and transcriptome of living cells. *Nat. Rev. Genet.* **2018**, *19*, 770–788. [CrossRef]
48. Arbab, M.; Shen, M.W.; Mok, B.; Wilson, C.; Matuszek, Ż.; Cassa, C.A.; Liu, D.R. Determinants of Base Editing Outcomes from Target Library Analysis and Machine Learning. *Cell* **2020**, *182*, 463–480.e30. [CrossRef]
49. Anzalone, A.V.; Randolph, P.B.; Davis, J.R.; Sousa, A.A.; Koblan, L.W.; Levy, J.M.; Chen, P.J.; Wilson, C.; Newby, G.A.; Raguram, A.; et al. Search-and-replace genome editing without double-strand breaks or donor DNA. *Nature* **2019**, *576*, 149–157. [CrossRef]
50. Yeh, W.-H.; Chiang, H.; Rees, H.A.; Edge, A.S.B.; Liu, D.R. In vivo base editing of post-mitotic sensory cells. *Nat. Commun.* **2018**, *9*, 1–10. [CrossRef]
51. Chadwick, A.C.; Wang, X.; Musunuru, K. In Vivo Base Editing of PCSK9 as a Therapeutic Alternative to Genome Editing. *Arterioscler. Thromb. Vasc. Biol.* **2017**, *37*, 1741–1747. [CrossRef] [PubMed]
52. Lim, C.K.W.; Gapinske, M.; Brooks, A.K.; Woods, W.S.; Powell, J.E.; Zeballos C., M.A.; Winter, J.; Perez-Pinera, P.; Gaj, T. Treatment of a Mouse Model of ALS by In Vivo Base Editing. *Mol. Ther.* **2020**, *28*, 1177–1189. [CrossRef] [PubMed]
53. Peters, J.E.; Makarova, K.S.; Shmakov, S.; Koonin, E.V. Recruitment of CRISPR-Cas systems by Tn7-like transposons. *Proc. Natl. Acad. Sci. USA* **2017**, *114*, E7358–E7366. [CrossRef] [PubMed]
54. Klompe, S.E.; Vo, P.L.H.; Halpin-Healy, T.S.; Sternberg, S.H. Transposon-encoded CRISPR–Cas systems direct RNA-guided DNA integration. *Nature* **2019**, *571*, 219–225. [CrossRef] [PubMed]
55. Urnov, F.D. Hijack of CRISPR defences by selfish genes holds clinical promise. *Nature* **2019**, *571*, 180–181. [CrossRef] [PubMed]
56. O'Connell, M.R.; Oakes, B.L.; Sternberg, S.H.; East-Seletsky, A.; Kaplan, M.; Doudna, J.A. Programmable RNA recognition and cleavage by CRISPR/Cas. *Nature* **2014**, *516*, 263–266. [CrossRef]
57. Batra, R.; Nelles, D.A.; Pirie, E.; Blue, S.M.; Marina, R.J.; Wang, H.; Chaim, I.A.; Thomas, J.D.; Zhang, N.; Nguyen, V.; et al. Elimination of Toxic Microsatellite Repeat Expansion RNA by RNA-Targeting Cas9.-PubMed-NCBI. *Cell* **2017**, *170*, 899–912.e10. [CrossRef]

58. Abudayyeh, O.O.; Gootenberg, J.S.; Konermann, S.; Joung, J.; Slaymaker, I.M.; Cox, D.B.T.; Shmakov, S.; Makarova, K.S.; Semenova, E.; Minakhin, L.; et al. C2c2 is a single-component programmable RNA-guided RNA-targeting CRISPR effector.-PubMed-NCBI. *Science* **2016**, *353*, aaf5573. [CrossRef]
59. Konermann, S.; Lotfy, P.; Brideau, N.J.; Oki, J.; Shokhirev, M.N.; Hsu, P.D. Transcriptome Engineering with RNA-Targeting Type VI-D CRISPR Effectors. *Cell* **2018**, *173*, 665–676.e14. [CrossRef]
60. Yan, W.X.; Chong, S.; Zhang, H.; Makarova, K.S.; Koonin, E.V.; Cheng, D.R.; Scott, D.A. Cas13d Is a Compact RNA-Targeting Type VI CRISPR Effector Positively Modulated by a WYL-Domain-Containing Accessory Protein. *Mol. Cell* **2018**, *70*, 327–339.e5. [CrossRef]
61. Perez-Pinera, P.; Ousterout, D.G.; Gersbach, C.A. Advances in targeted genome editing. *Curr. Opin. Chem. Biol.* **2012**, *16*, 268–277. [CrossRef] [PubMed]
62. Paschon, D.E.; Lussier, S.; Wangzor, T.; Xia, D.F.; Li, P.W.; Hinkley, S.J.; Scarlott, N.A.; Lam, S.C.; Waite, A.J.; Truong, L.N.; et al. Diversifying the structure of zinc finger nucleases for high-precision genome editing. *Nat. Commun.* **2019**, *10*, 1–12. [CrossRef] [PubMed]
63. Bogdanove, A.J.; Bohm, A.; Miller, J.C.; Morgan, R.D.; Stoddard, B.L. Engineering altered protein–DNA recognition specificity. *Nucleic Acids Res.* **2018**, *46*, 4845–4871. [CrossRef] [PubMed]
64. Fu, Y.; Foden, J.A.; Khayter, C.; Maeder, M.L.; Reyon, D.; Joung, J.K.; Sander, J.D. High-frequency off-target mutagenesis induced by CRISPR-Cas nucleases in human cells. *Nat. Biotechnol.* **2013**, *31*, 822–826. [CrossRef] [PubMed]
65. Hsu, P.D.; Scott, D.A.; Weinstein, J.A.; Ran, F.A.; Konermann, S.; Agarwala, V.; Li, Y.; Fine, E.J.; Wu, X.; Shalem, O.; et al. DNA targeting specificity of RNA-guided Cas9 nucleases. *Nat. Biotechnol.* **2013**, *31*, 827–832. [CrossRef]
66. Ran, F.A.; Hsu, P.D.; Lin, C.-Y.; Gootenberg, J.S.; Konermann, S.; Trevino, A.E.; Scott, D.A.; Inoue, A.; Matoba, S.; Zhang, Y.; et al. Double Nicking by RNA-Guided CRISPR Cas9 for Enhanced Genome Editing Specificity. *Cell* **2013**, *154*, 1380–1389. [CrossRef]
67. Hsu, P.D.; Lander, E.S.; Zhang, F. Development and Applications of CRISPR-Cas9 for Genome Engineering. *Cell* **2014**, *157*, 1262–1278. [CrossRef]
68. Li, H.; Yang, Y.; Hong, W.; Huang, M.; Wu, M.; Zhao, X. Applications of genome editing technology in the targeted therapy of human diseases: Mechanisms, advances and prospects. *Sig. Transduct. Target* **2020**, *5*, 1–23. [CrossRef]
69. Takahashi, K.; Tanabe, K.; Ohnuki, M.; Narita, M.; Ichisaka, T.; Tomoda, K.; Yamanaka, S. Induction of Pluripotent Stem Cells from Adult Human Fibroblasts by Defined Factors. *Cell* **2007**, *131*, 861–872. [CrossRef]
70. Gopal, S.; Rodrigues, A.L.; Dordick, J.S. Exploiting CRISPR Cas9 in Three-Dimensional Stem Cell Cultures to Model Disease. *Front. Bioeng. Biotechnol.* **2020**, *8*, 64. [CrossRef]
71. Takebe, T.; Wells, J.M. Organoids by design. *Science* **2019**, *364*, 956–959. [CrossRef] [PubMed]
72. Xia, Y.; Belmonte, J.C.I. Design Approaches for Generating Organ Constructs. *Cell Stem Cell* **2019**, *24*, 877–894. [CrossRef] [PubMed]
73. Artegiani, B.; Hendriks, D.; Beumer, J.; Kok, R.; Zheng, X.; Joore, I.; de Sousa Lopes, S.C.; van Zon, J.; Tans, S.; Clevers, H. Fast and efficient generation of knock-in human organoids using homology-independent CRISPR–Cas9 precision genome editing. *Nat. Cell. Biol.* **2020**, *22*, 321–331. [CrossRef] [PubMed]
74. Ashmore-Harris, C.; Fruhwirth, G.O. The clinical potential of gene editing as a tool to engineer cell-based therapeutics. *Clin. Trans. Med.* **2020**, *9*, 1445. [CrossRef]
75. Hoban, M.D.; Cost, G.J.; Mendel, M.C.; Romero, Z.; Kaufman, M.L.; Joglekar, A.V.; Ho, M.; Lumaquin, D.; Gray, D.; Lill, G.R.; et al. Correction of the sickle cell disease mutation in human hematopoietic stem/progenitor cells. *Blood* **2015**, *125*, 2597–2604. [CrossRef]
76. Sebastiano, V.; Maeder, M.L.; Angstman, J.F.; Haddad, B.; Khayter, C.; Yeo, D.T.; Goodwin, M.J.; Hawkins, J.S.; Ramirez, C.L.; Batista, L.F.Z.; et al. In Situ Genetic Correction of the Sickle Cell Anemia Mutation in Human Induced Pluripotent Stem Cells Using Engineered Zinc Finger Nucleases. *Stem Cells* **2011**, *29*, 1717–1726. [CrossRef]
77. Rupp, L.J.; Schumann, K.; Roybal, K.T.; Gate, R.E.; Ye, C.J.; Lim, W.A.; Marson, A. CRISPR/Cas9-mediated PD-1 disruption enhances anti-tumor efficacy of human chimeric antigen receptor T cells. -PubMed-NCBI. *Sci. Rep.* **2017**, *7*, 189. [CrossRef]

78. Santiago-Fernández, O.; Osorio, F.G.; Quesada, V.; Rodríguez, F.; Basso, S.; Maeso, D.; Rolas, L.; Barkaway, A.; Nourshargh, S.; Folgueras, A.R.; et al. Development of a CRISPR/Cas9-based therapy for Hutchinson–Gilford progeria syndrome. *Nat. Med.* **2019**, *25*, 423–426. [CrossRef]
79. Beyret, E.; Liao, H.-K.; Yamamoto, M.; Hernandez-Benitez, R.; Fu, Y.; Erikson, G.; Reddy, P.; Izpisua Belmonte, J.C. Single-dose CRISPR–Cas9 therapy extends lifespan of mice with Hutchinson–Gilford progeria syndrome. *Nat. Med.* **2019**, *119*, 1825. [CrossRef]
80. Qu, X.; Wang, P.; Ding, D.; Li, L.; Wang, H.; Ma, L.; Zhou, X.; Liu, S.; Lin, S.; Wang, X.; et al. Zinc-finger-nucleases mediate specific and efficient excision of HIV-1 proviral DNA from infected and latently infected human T cells. *Nucleic Acids Res.* **2013**, *41*, 7771–7782. [CrossRef]
81. Ebina, H.; Misawa, N.; Kanemura, Y.; Koyanagi, Y. Harnessing the CRISPR/Cas9 system to disrupt latent HIV-1 provirus. *Sci. Rep.* **2013**, *3*, a006890. [CrossRef] [PubMed]
82. Hu, W.; Kaminski, R.; Yang, F.; Zhang, Y.; Cosentino, L.; Li, F.; Luo, B.; Alvarez-Carbonell, D.; Garcia-Mesa, Y.; Karn, J.; et al. RNA-directed gene editing specifically eradicates latent and prevents new HIV-1 infection. *Proc. Natl. Acad. Sci. USA* **2014**, *111*, 11461–11466. [CrossRef] [PubMed]
83. Liao, H.-K.; Gu, Y.; Diaz, A.; Marlett, J.; Takahashi, Y.; Li, M.; Suzuki, K.; Xu, R.; Hishida, T.; Chang, C.-J.; et al. Use of the CRISPR/Cas9 system as an intracellular defense against HIV-1 infection in human cells. *Nat. Commun.* **2015**, *6*, 1011. [CrossRef] [PubMed]
84. Geurts, A.M.; Cost, G.J.; Freyvert, Y.; Zeitler, B.; Miller, J.C.; Choi, V.M.; Jenkins, S.S.; Wood, A.; Cui, X.; Meng, X.; et al. Knockout Rats via Embryo Microinjection of Zinc-Finger Nucleases. *Science* **2009**, *325*, 433. [CrossRef]
85. Carlson, D.F.; Tan, W.; Lillico, S.G.; Stverakova, D.; Proudfoot, C.; Christian, M.; Voytas, D.F.; Long, C.R.; Whitelaw, C.B.A.; Fahrenkrug, S.C. Efficient TALEN-mediated gene knockout in livestock. *Proc. Natl. Acad. Sci. USA* **2012**, *109*, 17382–17387. [CrossRef]
86. Ma, S.; Zhang, S.; Wang, F.; Liu, Y.; Liu, Y.; Xu, H.; Liu, C.; Lin, Y.; Zhao, P.; Xia, Q. Highly Efficient and Specific Genome Editing in Silkworm Using Custom TALENs. *PLoS ONE* **2012**, *7*, e45035. [CrossRef]
87. Wang, H.; Yang, H.; Shivalila, C.S.; Dawlaty, M.M.; Cheng, A.W.; Zhang, F.; Jaenisch, R. One-Step Generation of Mice Carrying Mutations in Multiple Genes by CRISPR/Cas-Mediated Genome Engineering. *Cell* **2013**, *153*, 910–918. [CrossRef]
88. Jacinto, F.V.; Link, W.; Ferreira, B.I. CRISPR/Cas9-mediated genome editing: From basic research to translational medicine. *J. Cell. Mol. Med.* **2020**, *24*, 3766–3778. [CrossRef]
89. Yao, X.; Wang, X.; Hu, X.; Liu, Z.; Liu, J.; Zhou, H.; Shen, X.; Wei, Y.; Huang, Z.; Ying, W.; et al. Homology-mediated end joining-based targeted integration using CRISPR/Cas. *Cell Res.* **2017**, *27*, 801–814. [CrossRef]
90. Wang, F.; Zhang, W.; Yang, Q.; Kang, Y.; Fan, Y.; Wei, J.; Liu, Z.; Dai, S.; Li, H.; Li, Z.; et al. Generation of a Hutchinson–Gilford progeria syndrome monkey model by base editing. *Protein Cell* **2020**, *4*, 1–16. [CrossRef]
91. Gurumurthy, C.B.; Sato, M.; Nakamura, A.; Inui, M.; Kawano, N.; Islam, M.A.; Ogiwara, S.; Takabayashi, S.; Matsuyama, M.; Nakagawa, S.; et al. Creation of CRISPR-based germline-genome-engineered mice without ex vivo handling of zygotes by i-GONAD. *Nat. Protoc.* **2019**, *14*, 2452–2482. [CrossRef] [PubMed]
92. Taylor, R.W.; Turnbull, D.M. Mitochondrial DNA mutations in human disease. *Nat. Rev. Genet.* **2005**, *6*, 389–402. [CrossRef] [PubMed]
93. Nissanka, N.; Moraes, C.T. Mitochondrial DNA heteroplasmy in disease and targeted nuclease-based therapeutic approaches. *EMBO Rep.* **2020**, *46*, e49612. [CrossRef] [PubMed]
94. Minczuk, M.; Papworth, M.A.; Miller, J.C.; Murphy, M.P.; Klug, A. Development of a single-chain, quasi-dimeric zinc-finger nuclease for the selective degradation of mutated human mitochondrial DNA. *Nucleic Acids Res.* **2008**, *36*, 3926–3938. [CrossRef] [PubMed]
95. Bacman, S.R.; Williams, S.L.; Pinto, M.; Peralta, S.; Moraes, C.T. Specific elimination of mutant mitochondrial genomes in patient-derived cells by mitoTALENs. *Nat. Med.* **2013**, *19*, 1111–1113. [CrossRef] [PubMed]
96. Gammage, P.A.; Rorbach, J.; Vincent, A.I.; Rebar, E.J.; Minczuk, M. Mitochondrially targeted ZFNs for selective degradation of pathogenic mitochondrial genomes bearing large-scale deletions or point mutations. *EMBO Mol. Med.* **2014**, *6*, 458–466. [CrossRef]
97. Gammage, P.A.; Viscomi, C.; Simard, M.-L.; Costa, A.S.H.; Gaude, E.; Powell, C.A.; Van Haute, L.; McCann, B.J.; Rebelo-Guiomar, P.; Cerutti, R.; et al. Genome editing in mitochondria corrects a pathogenic mtDNA mutation in vivo. *Nat. Med.* **2018**, *24*, 1691–1695. [CrossRef]

98. Bacman, S.R.; Kauppila, J.H.K.; Pereira, C.V.; Nissanka, N.; Miranda, M.; Pinto, M.; Williams, S.L.; Larsson, N.-G.; Stewart, J.B.; Moraes, C.T. MitoTALEN reduces mutant mtDNA load and restores tRNA Ala levels in a mouse model of heteroplasmic mtDNA mutation. *Nat. Med.* **2018**, *24*, 1696–1700. [CrossRef]
99. Reddy, P.; Ocampo, A.; Suzuki, K.; Luo, J.; Bacman, S.R.; Williams, S.L.; Sugawara, A.; Okamura, D.; Tsunekawa, Y.; Wu, J.; et al. Selective elimination of mitochondrial mutations in the germline by genome editing. *Cell* **2015**, *161*, 459–469. [CrossRef]
100. Gammage, P.A.; Moraes, C.T.; Minczuk, M. Mitochondrial Genome Engineering: The Revolution May Not Be CRISPR-Ized. *Trends Genet.* **2017**, *34*, 101–110. [CrossRef]
101. Jo, A.; Ham, S.; Lee, G.H.; Lee, Y.-I.; Kim, S.; Lee, Y.-S.; Shin, J.-H.; Lee, Y. Efficient Mitochondrial Genome Editing by CRISPR/Cas. *BioMed Res. Int.* **2015**, *2015*, 1–10. [CrossRef] [PubMed]
102. Hussain, S.-R.A.; Yalvac, M.E.; Khoo, B.; Eckardt, S.; McLaughlin, K.J. Adapting CRISPR/Cas9 System for Targeting Mitochondrial Genome. *bioRxiv* **2020**, 759. [CrossRef]
103. Mok, B.Y.; de Moraes, M.H.; Zeng, J.; Bosch, D.E.; Kotrys, A.V.; Raguram, A.; Hsu, F.; Radey, M.C.; Peterson, S.B.; Mootha, V.K.; et al. A bacterial cytidine deaminase toxin enables CRISPR-free mitochondrial base editing. *Nature* **2020**, *19*, 1–7.
104. Thakore, P.I.; Black, J.B.; Hilton, I.B.; Gersbach, C.A. Editing the epigenome: Technologies for programmable transcription and epigenetic modulation. *Nat. Meth.* **2016**, *13*, 127–137. [CrossRef]
105. Chavez, A.; Scheiman, J.; Vora, S.; Pruitt, B.W.; Tuttle, M.; Iyer, E.P.R.; Lin, S.; Kiani, S.; Guzman, C.D.; Wiegand, D.J.; et al. Highly efficient Cas9-mediated transcriptional programming. *Nat. Meth.* **2015**, *12*, 326–328. [CrossRef]
106. Konermann, S.; Brigham, M.D.; Trevino, A.E.; Joung, J.; Abudayyeh, O.O.; Barcena, C.; Hsu, P.D.; Habib, N.; Gootenberg, J.S.; Nishimasu, H.; et al. Genome-scale transcriptional activation by an engineered CRISPR-Cas9 complex. *Nature* **2015**, *517*, 583–588. [CrossRef]
107. Chiarella, A.M.; Butler, K.V.; Gryder, B.E.; Lu, D.; Wang, T.A.; Yu, X.; Pomella, S.; Khan, J.; Jin, J.; Hathaway, N.A. Dose-dependent activation of gene expression is achieved using CRISPR and small molecules that recruit endogenous chromatin machinery. *Nat. Biotechnol.* **2020**, *38*, 50–55. [CrossRef]
108. Liao, H.-K.; Hatanaka, F.; Araoka, T.; Reddy, P.; Wu, M.-Z.; Sui, Y.; Yamauchi, T.; Sakurai, M.; O'Keefe, D.D.; Nuñez Delicado, E.; et al. In Vivo Target Gene Activation via CRISPR/Cas9-Mediated Trans-epigenetic Modulation. *Cell* **2017**, *171*, 1495–1507.e15. [CrossRef]
109. Zhou, H.; Liu, J.; Zhou, C.; Gao, N.; Rao, Z.; Li, H.; Hu, X.; Li, C.; Yao, X.; Shen, X.; et al. In vivo simultaneous transcriptional activation of multiple genes in the brain using CRISPR–dCas9-activator transgenic mice. *Nat. Neurosci.* **2018**, *21*, 440–446. [CrossRef]
110. Matharu, N.; Rattanasopha, S.; Tamura, S.; Maliskova, L.; Wang, Y.; Bernard, A.; Hardin, A.; Eckalbar, W.L.; Vaisse, C.; Ahituv, N. CRISPR-mediated activation of a promoter or enhancer rescues obesity caused by haploinsufficiency. *Science* **2018**, *39*, eaau0629. [CrossRef]
111. Breinig, M.; Schweitzer, A.Y.; Herianto, A.M.; Revia, S.; Schaefer, L.; Wendler, L.; Galvez, A.C.; Tschaharganeh, D.F. Multiplexed orthogonal genome editing and transcriptional activation by Cas12a. *Nat. Meth.* **2019**, *16*, 51–54. [CrossRef] [PubMed]
112. Zheng, Y.; Shen, W.; Zhang, J.; Yang, B.; Liu, Y.-N.; Qi, H.; Yu, X.; Lu, S.-Y.; Chen, Y.; Xu, Y.-Z.; et al. CRISPR interference-based specific and efficient gene inactivation in the brain. *Nat. Neurosci.* **2018**, *21*, 447–454. [CrossRef] [PubMed]
113. Thakore, P.I.; Kwon, J.B.; Nelson, C.E.; Rouse, D.C.; Gemberling, M.P.; Oliver, M.L.; Gersbach, C.A. RNA-guided transcriptional silencing in vivo with S. aureus CRISPR-Cas9 repressors. *Nat. Commun.* **2018**, *9*, 1–9. [CrossRef] [PubMed]
114. Moreno, A.M.; Fu, X.; Zhu, J.; Katrekar, D.; Shih, Y.-R.V.; Marlett, J.; Cabotaje, J.; Tat, J.; Naughton, J.; Lisowski, L.; et al. In Situ Gene Therapy via AAV-CRISPR-Cas9-Mediated Targeted Gene Regulation. *Mol. Ther.* **2018**, *26*, 1818–1827. [CrossRef]
115. Pandelakis, M.; Delgado, E.; Ebrahimkhani, M.R. CRISPR-Based Synthetic Transcription Factors In Vivo: The Future of Therapeutic Cellular Programming. *Cell Syst.* **2020**, *10*, 1–14. [CrossRef]
116. Lindhout, B.I.; Fransz, P.; Tessadori, F.; Meckel, T.; Hooykaas, P.J.J.; van der Zaal, B.J. Live cell imaging of repetitive DNA sequences via GFP-tagged polydactyl zinc finger proteins. *Nucleic Acids Res.* **2007**, *35*, e107. [CrossRef]

117. Miyanari, Y.; Ziegler-Birling, C.; Torres-Padilla, M.-E. Live visualization of chromatin dynamics with fluorescent TALEs. *Nat. Struct. Mol. Biol.* **2013**, *20*, 1321–1324. [CrossRef]
118. Adli, M. The CRISPR tool kit for genome editing and beyond. *Nat. Commun.* **2018**, *9*, 1–13. [CrossRef]
119. Evers, B.; Jastrzebski, K.; Heijmans, J.P.M.; Grernrum, W.; Beijersbergen, R.L.; Bernards, R. CRISPR knockout screening outperforms shRNA and CRISPRi in identifying essential genes. *Nat. Biotechnol.* **2016**, *34*, 631–633. [CrossRef]
120. Wang, T.; Wei, J.J.; Sabatini, D.M.; Lander, E.S. Genetic Screens in Human Cells Using the CRISPR-Cas9 System. *Science* **2014**, *343*, 80–84. [CrossRef]
121. Shalem, O.; Sanjana, N.E.; Hartenian, E.; Shi, X.; Scott, D.A.; Mikkelsen, T.S.; Heckl, D.; Ebert, B.L.; Root, D.E.; Doench, J.G.; et al. Genome-Scale CRISPR-Cas9 Knockout Screening in Human Cells. *Science* **2014**, *343*, 84–87. [CrossRef] [PubMed]
122. Chow, R.D.; Chen, S. Cancer CRISPR Screens In Vivo. *Trends Cancer* **2018**, *4*, 349–358. [CrossRef] [PubMed]
123. Sánchez-Rivera, F.J.; Jacks, T. Applications of the CRISPR–Cas9 system in cancer biology. *Nat. Rev. Cancer* **2015**, *15*, 387–393. [CrossRef] [PubMed]
124. Doench, J.G. Am I ready for CRISPR? A user's guide to genetic screens. *Nat. Publ. Group* **2018**, *19*, 67–80. [CrossRef] [PubMed]
125. Gootenberg, J.S.; Abudayyeh, O.O.; Lee, J.W.; Essletzbichler, P.; Dy, A.J.; Joung, J.; Verdine, V.; Donghia, N.; Daringer, N.M.; Freije, C.A.; et al. Nucleic acid detection with CRISPR-Cas13a/C2c. *Science* **2017**, *356*, 438–442. [CrossRef]
126. Gootenberg, J.S.; Abudayyeh, O.O.; Kellner, M.J.; Joung, J.; Collins, J.J.; Zhang, F. Multiplexed and portable nucleic acid detection platform with Cas13, Cas12a, and Csm. *Science* **2018**, *360*, 439–444. [CrossRef]
127. Myhrvold, C.; Freije, C.A.; Gootenberg, J.S.; Abudayyeh, O.O.; Metsky, H.C.; Durbin, A.F.; Kellner, M.J.; Tan, A.L.; Paul, L.M.; Parham, L.A.; et al. Field-deployable viral diagnostics using CRISPR-Cas. *Science* **2018**, *360*, 444–448. [CrossRef]
128. Chen, J.S.; Ma, E.; Harrington, L.B.; Da Costa, M.; Tian, X.; Palefsky, J.M.; Doudna, J.A. CRISPR-Cas12a target binding unleashes indiscriminate single-stranded DNase activity. *Science* **2018**, *360*, 436–439. [CrossRef]
129. Broughton, J.P.; Deng, X.; Yu, G.; Fasching, C.L.; Servellita, V.; Singh, J.; Miao, X.; Streithorst, J.A.; Granados, A.; Sotomayor-Gonzalez, A.; et al. CRISPR–Cas12-based detection of SARS-CoV. *Nat. Biotechnol.* **2020**, *395*, 1–5. [CrossRef]
130. Abbott, T.R.; Dhamdhere, G.; Liu, Y.; Lin, X.; Goudy, L.; Zeng, L.; Chemparathy, A.; Chmura, S.; Heaton, N.S.; Debs, R.; et al. Development of CRISPR as an Antiviral Strategy to Combat SARS-CoV-2 and Influenza. *Cell* **2020**, *181*, 1–12. [CrossRef]
131. Cancro, M.P. Age-Associated B Cells. *Annu. Rev. Immunol.* **2020**, *38*, 315–340. [CrossRef] [PubMed]
132. Wagner, A.; Garner-Spitzer, E.; Jasinska, J.; Kollaritsch, H.; Stiasny, K.; Kundi, M.; Wiedermann, U. Age-related differences in humoral and cellular immune responses after primary immunisation: Indications for stratified vaccination schedules. *Sci. Rep.* **2018**, *8*, 1–12. [CrossRef] [PubMed]
133. Liang, P.; Xu, Y.; Zhang, X.; Ding, C.; Huang, R.; Zhang, Z.; Lv, J.; Xie, X.; Chen, Y.; Li, Y.; et al. CRISPR/Cas9-mediated gene editing in human tripronuclear zygotes. *Protein Cell* **2015**, *6*, 363–372. [CrossRef] [PubMed]
134. Tang, L.; Zeng, Y.; Du, H.; Gong, M.; Peng, J.; Zhang, B.; Lei, M.; Zhao, F.; Wang, W.; Li, X.; et al. CRISPR/Cas9-mediated gene editing in human zygotes using Cas9 protein. *Mol. Genet. Genom.* **2017**, *292*, 525–533. [CrossRef]
135. Ma, H.; Marti-Gutierrez, N.; Park, S.-W.; Wu, J.; Lee, Y.; Suzuki, K.; Koski, A.; Ji, D.; Hayama, T.; Ahmed, R.; et al. Correction of a pathogenic gene mutation in human embryos. *Nature* **2017**, *548*, 413–419. [CrossRef]
136. Kang, X.; He, W.; Huang, Y.; Yu, Q.; Chen, Y.; Gao, X.; Sun, X.; Fan, Y. Introducing precise genetic modifications into human 3PN embryos by CRISPR/Cas-mediated genome editing. *J. Assist. Reprod. Genet.* **2016**, *33*, 581–588. [CrossRef]
137. Fogarty, N.M.E.; McCarthy, A.; Snijders, K.E.; Powell, B.E.; Kubikova, N.; Blakeley, P.; Lea, R.; Elder, K.; Wamaitha, S.E.; Kim, D.; et al. Genome editing reveals a role for OCT4 in human embryogenesis. *Nature* **2017**, *550*, 67–73. [CrossRef]
138. Zeng, Y.; Li, J.; Li, G.; Huang, S.; Yu, W.; Zhang, Y.; Chen, D.; Chen, J.; Liu, J.; Huang, X. Correction of the Marfan Syndrome Pathogenic FBN1 Mutation by Base Editing in Human Cells and Heterozygous Embryos. *Mol. Ther.* **2018**, *26*, 2631–2637. [CrossRef]

139. Zhang, M.; Zhou, C.; Wei, Y.; Xu, C.; Pan, H.; Ying, W.; Sun, Y.; Sun, Y.; Xiao, Q.; Yao, N.; et al. Human cleaving embryos enable robust homozygotic nucleotide substitutions by base editors. *Genome Biol.* **2019**, *20*, 772. [CrossRef]
140. Shahbazi, M.N.; Jedrusik, A.; Vuoristo, S.; Recher, G.; Hupalowska, A.; Bolton, V.; Fogarty, N.M.E.; Campbell, A.; Devito, L.G.; Ilic, D.; et al. Self-organization of the human embryo in the absence of maternal tissues. *Nat. Cell. Biol.* **2016**, *18*, 700–708. [CrossRef]
141. Deglincerti, A.; Croft, G.F.; Pietila, L.N.; Zernicka-Goetz, M.; Siggia, E.D.; Brivanlou, A.H. Self-organization of the in vitro attached human embryo. *Nature* **2016**, *533*, 251–254. [CrossRef] [PubMed]
142. Harrison, S.E.; Sozen, B.; Christodoulou, N.; Kyprianou, C.; Zernicka-Goetz, M. Assembly of embryonic and extraembryonic stem cells to mimic embryogenesis in vitro. *Science* **2017**, *356*, eaal1810. [CrossRef] [PubMed]
143. Li, R.; Zhong, C.; Yu, Y.; Liu, H.; Sakurai, M.; Yu, L.; Min, Z.; Shi, L.; Wei, Y.; Takahashi, Y.; et al. Generation of Blastocyst-like Structures from Mouse Embryonic and Adult Cell Cultures. *Cell* **2019**, *179*, 687–702.e18. [CrossRef] [PubMed]
144. Rivron, N.; Pera, M.; Rossant, J.; Martinez Arias, A.; Zernicka-Goetz, M.; Fu, J.; van den Brink, S.; Bredenoord, A.; Dondorp, W.; de Wert, G.; et al. Debate ethics of embryo models from stem cells. *Nature* **2018**, *564*, 183–185. [CrossRef]
145. Hyun, I.; Munsie, M.; Pera, M.F.; Rivron, N.C.; Rossant, J. Toward Guidelines for Research on Human Embryo Models Formed from Stem Cells. *Stem Cell Rep.* **2020**, *14*, 169–174. [CrossRef]
146. Pei, D.; Beier, D.W.; Levy-Lahad, E.; Marchant, G.; Rossant, J.; Izpisua Belmonte, J.C.; Lovell-Badge, R.; Jaenisch, R.; Charo, A.; Baltimore, D. Human Embryo Editing: Opportunities and Importance of Transnational Cooperation. *Cell Stem Cell* **2017**, *21*, 423–426. [CrossRef]
147. National Academies of Sciences, Engineering, and Medicine. *Human Genome Editing: Science, Ethics, and Governance*; National Academies Press: Washington, DC, USA, 2017.
148. Wolf, D.P.; Mitalipov, P.A.; Mitalipov, S.M. Principles of and strategies for germline gene therapy. *Nat. Med.* **2019**, *25*, 890–897. [CrossRef]
149. Risques, R.-A.; Kennedy, S.R. Aging and the rise of somatic cancer-associated mutations in normal tissues. *PLoS Genet* **2018**, *14*, e1007108. [CrossRef]
150. Zhang, W.; Qu, J.; Liu, G.-H.; Belmonte, J.C.I. The ageing epigenome and its rejuvenation. *Nat. Rev. Mol. Cell. Biol.* **2020**, *21*, 137–150. [CrossRef]
151. Ocampo, A.; Reddy, P.; Belmonte, J.C.I. Anti-Aging Strategies Based on Cellular Reprogramming. *Trends Mol. Med.* **2016**, *22*, 725–738. [CrossRef]
152. López-Otín, C.; Blasco, M.A.; Partridge, L.; Serrano, M.; Kroemer, G. The Hallmarks of Aging. *Cell* **2013**, *153*, 1194–1217. [CrossRef] [PubMed]

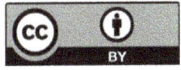

© 2020 by the authors. Licensee MDPI, Basel, Switzerland. This article is an open access article distributed under the terms and conditions of the Creative Commons Attribution (CC BY) license (http://creativecommons.org/licenses/by/4.0/).

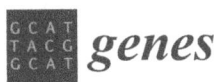

Article

Characteristics of the IVF Cycle that Contribute to the Incidence of Mosaicism

Lorena Rodrigo [1,*], Mónica Clemente-Císcar [2], Inmaculada Campos-Galindo [1], Vanessa Peinado [1], Carlos Simón [3,4,5,6] and Carmen Rubio [7]

1. Preimplantation Genetic Testing Department, Igenomix, 46980 Valencia, Spain; inmaculada.campos@igenomix.com (I.C.-G.); vanessa.peinado@igenomix.com (V.P.)
2. Functional Genomix & Bioinformatics Lab, Igenomix, 46980 Valencia, Spain; monica.clemente@igenomix.com
3. Department of Obstetrics and Gynecology, University of Valencia/Instituto de Investigación Sanitaria (INCLIVA), 46016 Valencia, Spain; carlos.simon@igenomix.com
4. Department of Obstetrics and Gynecology, School of Medicine, Stanford University, Stanford, CA 94305, USA
5. Department of Obstetrics and Gynecology, Baylor College of Medicine, Houston, TX 77030, USA
6. Head of Scientific Advisory Board, Igenomix and Igenomix Foundation, 46980 Valencia, Spain
7. Research & Development Department, Igenomix and Igenomix Foundation, 46980 Valencia, Spain; carmen.rubio@igenomix.com
* Correspondence: lorena.rodrigo@igenomix.com; Tel.: +34-96-390-53-10

Received: 18 August 2020; Accepted: 26 September 2020; Published: 30 September 2020

Abstract: Highly sensitive next-generation sequencing (NGS) platforms applied to preimplantation genetic testing for aneuploidy (PGT-A) allow the classification of mosaicism in trophectoderm biopsies. However, the incidence of mosaicism reported by these tests can be affected by a wide number of analytical, biological, and clinical factors. With the use of a proprietary algorithm for automated diagnosis of aneuploidy and mosaicism, we retrospectively analyzed a large series of 115,368 trophectoderm biopsies from 27,436 PGT-A cycles to determine whether certain biological factors and *in vitro* fertilization (IVF) practices influence the incidence of overall aneuploidy, whole uniform aneuploidy, mosaicism, and TE biopsies with only segmental aneuploidy. Older female and male patients showed higher rates of high-mosaic degree and whole uniform aneuploidies and severe oligozoospermic patients had higher rates of mosaicism and only segmental aneuploidies. Logistic regression analysis identified a positive effect of female age but a negative effect of embryo vitrification on the incidence of overall aneuploid embryos. Female age increased whole uniform aneuploidy rates but decreased only segmental aneuploidy and mosaicism, mainly low-mosaics. Conversely, higher ovarian response decreased whole uniform aneuploidy rates but increased only segmental aneuploidies. Finally, embryo vitrification decreased whole uniform aneuploidy rates but increased mosaicism, mainly low-mosaics, compared to PGT-A cycles with fresh oocytes. These results could be useful for clinician's management of the IVF cycles.

Keywords: PGT-A; NGS; aneuploidy; mosaicism; segmental; vitrification; ovarian response; female age

1. Introduction

Current genetic analysis platforms used in preimplantation genetic testing for aneuploidy (PGT-A) are highly sensitive and, when applied to trophectoderm embryo biopsies (TE), identify mosaicism when not only euploid or aneuploid cells, but a combination of both are present in the TE biopsy. Embryonic mosaicism is mitotic in origin and is caused by improper separation and segregation of chromosomes during cell division [1]. Next-generation sequencing (NGS)-based platforms are most commonly used in PGT-A programs; however, differences in platform sensitivity and specificity, the threshold established for data interpretation and the cut-offs applied for low-level mosaicism classification affect the percentage of mosaicism reported among genetic laboratories and the number of euploid embryos deemed suitable for transfer [2]. Other factors related to biopsy technique, the number of cells biopsied, and the conditions surrounding the cell loading can also affect the results [3]. Studies by Popovic et al. [4,5] on the inner cell mass (ICM) and TE analysis from aneuploid and mosaic embryos suggest limitations in the accuracy of diagnosing mosaicism in PGT-A due to difficulty distinguishing technical bias from biological mosaicism. As a result, the use of validated NGS platforms and the development of algorithms to improve mosaicism diagnosis have become priorities for many genetic laboratories [6–8].

Ovarian stimulation protocols during the IVF cycle can influence the incidence of euploid embryos [9]. Additionally, the fertilization method [10] and conditions in the clinical IVF laboratory, such as the embryo culture media, pH, oxygen, osmolality, temperature or plastics, are linked to increased aneuploidy and mosaicism [3]. Accurate mosaicism determination describes incidences of euploid/aneuploid mosaicism from 31% at the cleavage stage to 4–5% at the blastocyst stage [11,12]. Maternal age is a major influence on aneuploidy, but primarily related to incidence of uniform aneuploidies. Isolated mosaicism may be independent of maternal age, but Rubio et al. [13] described a slight decrease in mosaicism in women over 37 compared to younger patients. The same study, however, did not observe an effect of the ovarian response and vitrification of oocytes on mosaicism rate. Finally, the use of PGT-A in couples with compromised semen quality shows higher rates of mosaic embryos with low sperm concentrations [14,15].

Since the first pregnancies reported by Greco in 2015 [16] transferring mosaic embryos after PGT-A analysis, more clinicians are considering transfer in the absence of euploid embryos. Clinical outcomes are poorest for high-mosaic compared to low-mosaic embryo transfers [17]; therefore, mosaic degree classification is critical to the decision-making process for clinicians and patients. We evaluated the distribution of euploid and aneuploid cells in a large series of 115,368 TE biopsies to assess whether the distribution was affected by characteristics of the IVF cycle, including the indication to perform a PGT-A cycle, the use of fresh or vitrified oocyte/embryos, the ovarian response, sperm concentration, and maternal and paternal ages. Aneuploidies were analyzed considering uniform aneuploidies, low- and high-degree mosaicism, and segmental aneuploidy. Logistic regression analysis identified maternal age, ovarian response, and PGT-A cycles with vitrified embryos as the factors with the most influence on aneuploidy.

2. Materials and Methods

2.1. Study Design

This was a retrospective observational study carried out between October 2018 and December 2019 that included TE embryo biopsies from PGT-A cycles analyzed in our laboratory subsidiaries (Igenomix, Valencia, Spain). Every TE biopsy was classified as euploid or aneuploid. The aneuploidies observed in the TE biopsies were distributed among four categories: (i) only segmental aneuploidy, when only partial deletion/duplications were observed; (ii) low-mosaic, when one or two low-mosaic degree aneuploidies without additional uniform or segmental aneuploidies were observed; (iii) high-mosaic, when one or two high-mosaic degree aneuploidies or one low- and one high-mosaic degree aneuploidies without additional uniform or segmental aneuploidies were observed; or (iv) whole uniform aneuploidy, when at least one aneuploidy for a whole chromosome was observed in the TE biopsy, combined or not combined with additional segmental or mosaic aneuploidies.

The distribution of euploid and aneuploid results within the four categories of aneuploidies (whole uniform aneuploidy, low-mosaic, high-mosaic, and only segmental) were evaluated according to the following characteristics of the IVF cycle: the indication to perform the PGT-A cycle, the origin of the embryos, ovarian response, sperm count, and maternal and paternal age. Patients with altered karyotype, cycles with females aged ≥ 45 years at embryo biopsy, as well as ovum donation cycles where excluded from analysis.

2.2. Study Population

The study included 115,368 day 5, 6, or 7 TE biopsies from 27,436 PGT-A cycles. Clinical indications for PGT-A were: (1) advanced maternal age, ≥37 years old (AMA; $n = 48,174$ TE biopsies); (2) repetitive implantation failure with ≥2 failures (RIF; $n = 6742$ TE biopsies); (3) recurrent pregnancy loss with ≥2 miscarriages (RPL; $n = 5244$ TE biopsies); (4) male factor infertility with impaired sperm parameters and/or increase in the incidence of aneuploid sperm (MF; $n = 6562$ TE biopsies); (5) previous aneuploid conception (PAC; $n = 512$ TE); (6) mixed causes (MIX; $n = 2199$ TE biopsies); or (7) aneuploidy screening (AS; $n = 45,935$ TE biopsies). Female age in RIF, RPL, MF, PAC, MIX, and AS indications was <37 years old.

Information on embryo origin was available in 34,346 (29.8%) of the embryos analyzed, distributed as fresh oocyte origin (FO; $n = 30,312$ TE biopsies), vitrified oocyte origin (VO; $n = 1649$ TE biopsies), and vitrified embryo origin (VE; $n = 2385$ TE biopsies). A total of 14,092 (12.2%) TE biopsies had information regarding the ovarian response, considered as the total number of MII oocytes retrieved in the IVF cycle. These were distributed as: (i) ≤5 MII oocytes ($n = 1677$); (ii) 6–10 MII oocytes ($n = 3302$); (iii) 11–15 MII oocytes ($n = 2646$); (iv) 16–20 MII oocytes ($n = 2373$); and (v) >20 MII oocytes ($n = 4094$). The sperm count of the samples used in IVF cycles was available for 8360 (7.3%) of the TE biopsies analyzed, classified as: (i) normozoospermia with $\geq 15 \times 10^6$ sperm/mL (N; $n = 6428$); (ii) moderate oligozoospermia between $>5 \times 10^6$ and $<15 \times 10^6$ sperm/mL (MO; $n = 911$); and (iii) severe oligozoospermia with $\leq 5 \times 10^6$ sperm/mL (SO; $n = 1021$).

2.3. Next-Generation Sequencing of TE Biopsies

TE biopsies were performed on day 5, 6, or 7 of blastocyst growth. NGS analysis was conducted using an Ion ReproSeq™PGS kit for 24 chromosome aneuploidy screening (Thermo Fisher Scientific, Waltham, MA, USA) and was performed on the Ion Chef™ and Ion S5 System instruments (Thermo Fisher Scientific). Data were analyzed with Ion Reporter Software using the human genome build (hg19) (Thermo Fisher Scientific). An internally validated algorithm was applied for automatic mosaicism calling. Low mosaic degree was determined when the TE biopsy had 30% to <50% of aneuploidy cells while a high mosaic degree was determined by 50% to <70% aneuploid cells. TE biopsies with <30% aneuploid cells were classified as euploid and those with ≥70% were classified as uniform aneuploid [13]. TE biopsies showing another uniform aneuploidy were not reported as mosaic but as uniform aneuploid. Partial deletions/duplications were determined by >10 Mb.

2.4. Statistical Analyses

Univariant analysis using pairwise comparisons between pairs of proportions with correction for multiple testing (based on Pearson's Chi-squared test) was applied to evaluate the distribution of embryo ploidy (euploid and aneuploid) and the category of aneuploidy (whole uniform aneuploidy, only segmental aneuploidy, low-mosaic degree, or high-mosaic degree) according to the indication to perform PGT-A (AMA, RIF, RPL, MF, PAC, MIX, or AS), the ovarian response (≤5 MII oocytes; 6–10 MII oocytes; 11–15 MII oocytes; 16–20 MII oocytes; >20 MII oocytes), the classification of sperm count (N, MO, or SO) and the embryo origin (FO, VO, or VE). To evaluate the distribution of the four categories of aneuploidies according to maternal and paternal age, a pairwise comparison between means (± standard deviation, SD) with corrections for multiple testing (based on t-test) was used.

Multivariant analysis was performed in 4885 TE biopsies for which all variables were present (4.4% of the informative embryos). A binary logistic regression model was applied to evaluate the variables affecting embryo ploidy and the four categories of aneuploidies. Maternal and paternal age, sperm concentration, and ovarian response defined as the number of mature oocytes retrieved (MII) were considered as quantitative variables and the embryo origin and the indication for the PGT-A were considered qualitative variables in the model, considering FO for the embryo origin and AS for the indication for the PGT-A as references. The odds ratio for each coefficient and the confidence interval at 95% were computed in the case of a significant variable to analyze the effect of each parameter.

Statistical analysis was performed using R Free software (R Foundation for Statistical Computing, Vienna, Austria) and GraphPad InStat v3.10 for Windows (GraphPad Software, Inc., San Diego, CA, USA). Differences were considered statistically significant when $p < 0.05$, highly significant when $p < 0.01$, and extremely significant when $p < 0.001$.

3. Results

We retrospectively analyzed 115,368 TE biopsies and 111,860 were informative. From the informative TE biopsies, 46.1% were euploid and 53.9% were aneuploid, mainly due to whole uniform aneuploidies (42.6%) followed by mosaicism (6.2%) and TE biopsies with only segmental aneuploidies (5.1%) (Table 1). When analyzing the data per day of biopsy from day-5 to day-7, the percentage of euploid TE biopsies decreased significantly (49.4% in day 5; 42.1% in day 6; 35.7% in day 7; $p < 0.0001$) and the percentage of aneuploid embryos increased significantly (50.6% in day 5; 57.9% in day 6; 64.3% in day 7; $p < 0.0001$). The incidence of TE biopsies with whole uniform aneuploidy increased significantly from day-5 to day-7 (39.5%, 46.5% and 52.8 in day-5, day-6 and day-7, respectively; $p < 0.0001$). No significant differences in the percentage of TE biopsies with mosaicism or only segmental aneuploidies were observed in different biopsy day.

Table 1. NGS results of 27,436 PGT-A cycles performed in TE biopsies.

	TE Embryo Biopsy			TOTAL
	Day 5	Day 6	Day 7	
No. embryos analyzed	64,578	50,054	736	115,368
Mean female age (SD)	35.7 (4.6) [j]	36.3 (4.3) [k]	36.9 (4.1) [l]	36.0 (4.5)
Mean male age (SD)	38.5 (6.3) [m]	38.4 (6.1) [n]	39.2 (6.6) [o]	38.6 (6.2)
Informative embryos (%)	62,435 (96.7)	48,703 (97.3)	722 (98.1)	111,860 (97.0)
Euploid embryos (%)	30,819 (49.4) [a]	20,509 (42.1) [b]	258 (35.7) [c]	51,586 (46.1)
Aneuploid embryos (%)	31,616 (50.6) [d]	28,194 (57.9) [e]	464 (64.3) [f]	60,274 (53.9)
Whole uniform aneuploidy (%)	24,672 (39.5) [g]	22,638 (46.5) [h]	381 (52.8) [i]	47,691 (42.6)
Only segmental aneuploidy (%)	3187 (5.1)	2474 (5.1)	38 (5.3)	5699 (5.1)
Mosaic aneuploidy (%)	3757 (6.0)	3082 (6.3)	45 (6.2)	6884 (6.2)
Low-mosaic aneuploidy (%)	2439 (3.9)	1951 (4.0)	25 (3.5)	4415 (4.0)
High-mosaic aneuploidy (%)	1318 (2.1)	1131 (2.3)	20 (2.7)	2469 (2.2)

Note: [a-b, a-c, d-e, d-f, g-h, g-i, j-k, j-l, k-l] $p < 0.0001$; [b-c, e-f, h-i] $p < 0.001$; [n-o] $p < 0.01$; [m-o] $p < 0.05$; Fisher's Exact test and Welch's t test.

3.1. Univariant Analysis

3.1.1. Maternal and Paternal Age

Euploid TE biopsies showed significantly lower mean female and male age compared to aneuploid TE biopsies (34.8 ± 4.2 vs. 37.0 ± 4.4 for female, and 37.6 ± 6.0 vs. 39.4 ± 6.2 for male, respectively; $p < 0.0001$). When considering the categories of aneuploidies, mean female age was similar in the groups of euploid (34.8 ± 4.2) and low-mosaic degree (34.9 ± 4.2) TE biopsies and both were slightly but significantly higher compared to only segmental aneuploidy TE biopsies (34.6 ± 2.2; $p < 0.001$) and significantly lower compared to the high-mosaic degree (36.5 ± 4.3) and whole uniform aneuploidy TE biopsies (37.5 ± 4.2) ($p < 0.0001$) (Figure 1a). Mean paternal age was similar in the euploid (37.6 ± 6.0), low-mosaic degree (37.8 ± 6.0), and only segmental aneuploidy (37.5 ± 6.0) TE biopsies and these were significantly lower compared to the groups of high-mosaic degree (39.0 ± 6.1) and whole uniform aneuploid (39.8 ± 6.1) TE biopsies ($p < 0.0001$) (Figure 1b). In summary, whole uniform aneuploidy had the highest mean maternal and paternal age, significantly increased compared to the other categories of aneuploid TE biopsies ($p < 0.0001$).

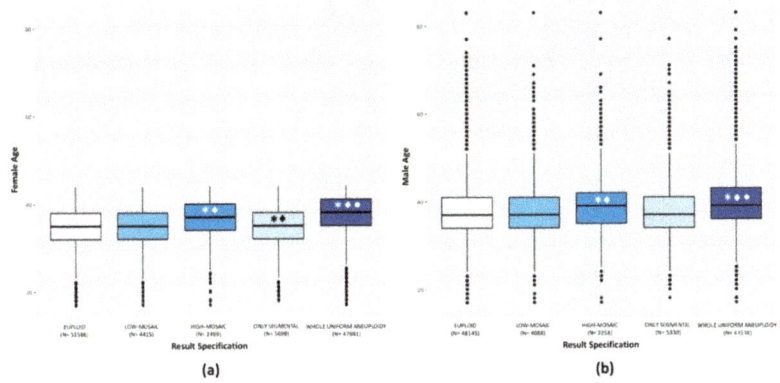

Figure 1. Box plot distribution of mean maternal age (**a**) and mean paternal age (**b**) expressed in years in the results categories of euploid, low-mosaic, high-mosaic, only segmental, and whole uniform aneuploid TE biopsies.

3.1.2. Ovarian Response

Figure 2 shows the distribution of aneuploidies in TE biopsies according to the number of mature oocytes (MII) retrieved. The percentage of aneuploid TE biopsies decreased progressively as the number of MII oocytes increased. The percentage of whole uniform aneuploidies was significantly higher in patients with less than 11 MII oocytes compared to patients with more than 11 MII oocytes ($p < 0.01$). No significant differences in the percentage of TE biopsies with mosaicism or only segmental aneuploidies were observed within the ovarian response.

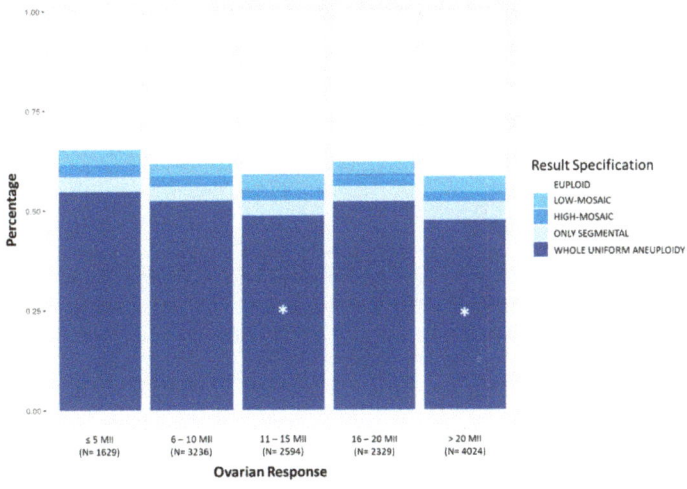

Figure 2. Distribution of chromosomal abnormalities in TE biopsies (euploid, low-mosaic, high-mosaic, only segmental, and whole uniform aneuploidy) according to categories of ovarian response considering the number of mature oocytes retrieved (≤5 MII oocytes; 6–10 MII oocytes; 11–15 MII oocytes; 16–20 MII oocytes; >20 MII oocytes). The mean number of embryos biopsied (SD) per case was 2.6 (1.9) for ≤5 MII oocytes category, 3.4 (2.1) for 6–10 MII, 4.5 (2.9) for 11–15 MII, 4.8 (2.7) for 16–20 MII and 6.5 (3.9) for >20 MII oocytes category.

Mean maternal age was significantly higher in the group with ≤5 MII (38.9 ± 2.7) compared to the other groups (38.1 ± 3.3 in 6–10 MII, 37.6 ± 3.5 in 11–15 MII, 38.0 ± 3.4 in 16–20 MII, 37.4 ± 3.8 in >20 MII; $p < 0.0001$). The group with 6–10 MII compared to the group with 16–20 MI, and the group with 11–15 MII compared to the group with >20 MII showed similar mean maternal ages.

3.1.3. Classification of Sperm Count

Analysis of TE biopsies considering patient sperm count showed significantly higher incidence of aneuploid embryos in patients with N (63.8%) compared to patients with MO (57.6%, $p < 0.001$) and SO (54.2%, $p < 0.0001$) (Figure 3). Mean maternal age was also significantly higher in the N group (38.8 ± 3.1) compared to MO (37.4 ± 3.5) and SO (35.9 ± 3.8) ($p < 0.001$, among groups). The N group showed significantly higher incidence of embryos with whole uniform aneuploidy (53.8%) compared to MO (47.5%) and SO (41.5%) groups, $p < 0.001$. Although the percentage of embryos with mosaicism (6.1% in N; 6.4% in MO; 7.9% in SO) and only segmental aneuploidy (3.9% in N; 3.7% in MO; 4.9% in SO) was slightly increased in patients with SO, no statistical differences were observed among groups. However, the incidence of embryos with aneuploidies due to mosaicism or only segmental instead of uniform aneuploidy was significantly higher in the SO compared to the N group (12.7% vs. 10.0%, respectively; $p < 0.05$).

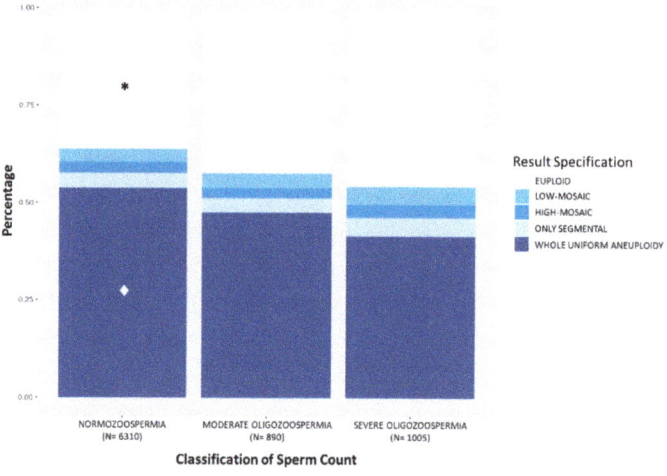

Figure 3. Distribution of the percentages of chromosomal abnormalities in TE biopsies (euploid, low-mosaic, high-mosaic, only segmental, and whole uniform aneuploidy) according to the classification of sperm count (normozoospermia, with ≥15 × 10^6 sperm/mL; moderate oligozoospermia, between >5 × 10^6 and <15 × 10^6 sperm/mL; severe oligozoospermia, with ≤5 × 10^6 sperm/mL). The mean number of embryos biopsied (SD) per case was 4.6 (3.2) for N category, 5.2 (4.1) for MO and 5.1 (3.7) for SO category.

3.1.4. Embryo Origin

Figure 4 shows the distribution of aneuploidies in TE biopsies according to embryo origin. The percentage of euploid embryos was significantly higher in the VE group (46.5%) compared to FO (41.3%) and VO (39.2%) groups, $p < 0.0001$. Comparing the four categories of aneuploidies, the VE group showed significantly lower percentage of embryos with whole uniform aneuploidy (40.6%) compared to FO (47.5%) and VO (48.7%) groups, $p < 0.0001$. The percentage of embryos with only segmental aneuploidy was significantly higher in the VE groups (6.5%) compared to the FO group (5.2%), $p < 0.05$. No differences were observed in the incidence of mosaic embryos among the three groups (6.0%, 6.9% and 6.3% in FO, VO, and VE groups respectively, NS). The VO group had the highest mean maternal age (38.7 ± 3.7), followed by the group of FO (36.6 ± 4.5), and the VE group showed the lowest maternal age (35.7 ± 4.6) ($p < 0.0001$ among groups).

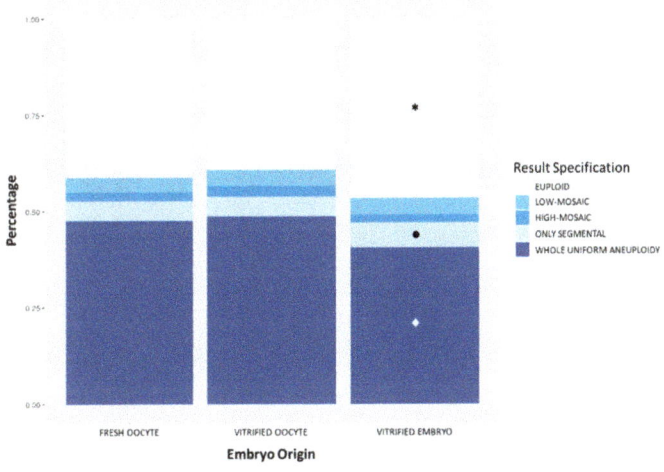

Figure 4. Distribution of the percentages of chromosomal abnormalities in TE biopsies (euploid, low-mosaic, high-mosaic, only segmental, and whole uniform aneuploidy) according to the embryo origin (fresh oocyte, vitrified oocyte, and vitrified embryo). The mean number of embryos biopsied (SD) per case was 4.8 (3.3) for fresh oocyte category, 4.7 (3.4) for vitrified oocyte and 4.5 (3.5) for vitrified embryo category.

3.1.5. Indication for PGT-A

PGT-A cycles with indication of AMA showed significantly lower percentage of euploid embryos (32.1%) compared to cycles with indication of RIF (54.2%), RPL (53.9%), MF (56.7%), PAC (54.9%), MIX (55.5%), and AS (56.8%), $p < 0.0001$ (Figure 5). Considering the four categories of aneuploidies evaluated, AMA showed significantly higher percentage of embryos with whole uniform aneuploidy (59.1%) compared to RIF (32.9%), RPL (32.5%), MF (29.6%), PAC (31.4%), MIX (31.5%), and AS (30.4%), $p < 0.0001$. Moreover, the percentage of whole uniform aneuploidy in MF and AS cycles was significantly lower than that observed in RIF and RPL cycles.

The percentage of embryos with only segmental aneuploidy was significantly lower in AMA cycles (3.5%) compared to RIF (6.4%), RPL (6.4%), MF (7.0%), PAC (8.1%), MIX (6.3%), and AS (6.1%), $p < 0.0001$, and significantly higher in MF compared to AS ($p < 0.05$). A similar trend was observed for the overall incidence of mosaicism, which was significantly lower in AMA (5.4%) compared to RIF (6.4%, $p < 0.01$), RPL (7.3%, $p < 0.0001$), MF (6.7%, $p < 0.001$), MIX (6.7%, <0.05%) and AS (6.7%, $p < 0.0001$). The percentage of embryos with low-mosaic degree was significantly lower in AMA (2.9%) compared to RIF (4.4%), RPL (5.1%), MF (4.7%), MIX (4.4%), and AS (5.7%) ($p < 0.0001$). However, TE biopsies with high-mosaic degree were significantly increased in AMA compared to AS (2.4% vs. 2.0%, respectively; $p < 0.001$). Mean maternal age was 40.1 ± 1.7 in AMA, 33.0 ± 3.1 in RIF, 32.8 ± 3.4 in RPL, 32.6 ± 3.6 in MF, 33.5 ± 2.9 in PAC, 33.1 ± 3.2 in MIX, and 33.1 ± 3.3 in AS.

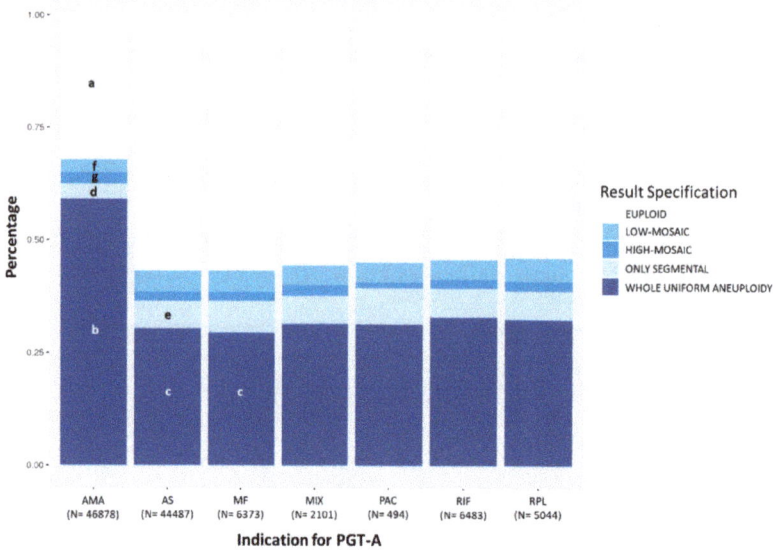

Figure 5. Distribution of the percentages of chromosomal abnormalities in TE biopsies (euploid, low-mosaic, high-mosaic, only segmental, and whole uniform aneuploidy) according to the indication for PGT-A (AMA: advanced maternal age ≥ 37 years; AS: aneuploidy screening; MF: male factor infertility; MIX: mixed causes; PAC: previous aneuploid conception; RIF: repetitive implantation failure; RPL: recurrent pregnancy loss). Female age was <37 years in AS, MF, MIX, PAC, RIF, and RPL groups. The mean number of embryos biopsied (SD) per case was 4.4 (3.4) for AMA indication, 6.1 (6.6) for AS, 6.0 (3.7) for MF, 5.2 (3.6) for MIX, 5.1 (2.7) for PAC, 4.8 (3.5) for RIF and 5.4 (3.8) for RPL indication.

3.2. Multivariant Analysis

Female and male age, ovarian response, sperm count, embryo origin, and indication for PGT-A were assessed to identify which could be an independent variable affecting the overall incidence of aneuploidy and the different sub-categories (whole uniform aneuploidy, only segmental aneuploidy, low-mosaic, and high-mosaic). Logistic regression analysis showed that the percentage of aneuploid TE biopsies increased with female age (OR: 1.168, 95% CI 1.130–1.208, $p < 0.0001$), and decreased in PGT_A cycles with vitrified embryos (OR: 0.488, 95% CI 0.315–0.754, $p < 0.01$). Among the different types of aneuploidy, the percentage of whole uniform aneuploidy increased with female age (OR: 1.178, 95% CI 1.117–1.242, $p < 0.0001$). However, it decreased with higher ovarian response (OR: 0.991, 95% CI 0.985–0.998, $p < 0.05$) and in PGT-A cycles with vitrified embryos (OR: 0.416, 95% CI 0.213–0.862, $p < 0.05$). The percentage of TE biopsies with only segmental aneuploidy decreased when the female age increased (OR: 0.816, 95% CI 0.851–0.965, $p < 0.0001$) and increased when the ovarian response increased (OR: 1.011, 95% CI 0.995–1.012, $p < 0.05$). The percentage of mosaic TE biopsies decreased when female age increased (OR: 0.906, 95% CI 0.851–0.965, $p < 0.01$) and increased in PGT-A cycles with vitrified embryos (OR: 2.344, 95% CI 0.990–4.930, $p < 0.05$). Finally, analysis of the two grades of mosaicism revealed that the percentage of embryos with low-mosaic degree decreased with higher female age (OR: 0.884, 95% CI 0.817–0.958, $p < 0.01$) and increased in PGT-A cycles with vitrified embryos (OR: 3.456, 95% CI 1.279–7.879, $p < 0.01$). The percentage of TE biopsies with high-mosaic degree was not affected by any of the variables evaluated.

4. Discussion

PGT-A results are influenced by many analytical and biological factors. Our laboratory uses a proprietary algorithm for the automated diagnosis of aneuploidy and mosaicism in TE biopsies, resulting in an objective and robust system to minimize variability in the diagnosis [8]. We have mainly observed whole uniform aneuploidies, followed by mosaic aneuploidies and only segmental aneuploidies. Interestingly, the incidence of aneuploid embryos significantly increased from day-5 to day-7 TE biopsies, due to the increase of whole uniform aneuploidy, whereas the incidence of mosaic aneuploidy and only segmental aneuploidy remained constant regardless the day of biopsy. The increased incidence of aneuploidies in day-7 TE biopsies can be related to the lower embryo quality and significantly higher female age compared to day-5 and day-6 TE biopsies. However, other factors may contribute to differences in the overall incidence of aneuploidy and the different subtypes. To assess the influence of these other factors, we retrospectively analyzed our PGT-A results to determine if certain biological factors and IVF practices have an effect on the incidence of overall aneuploidy, whole uniform aneuploidy, mosaicism, and TE biopsies with only segmental aneuploidy. Logistic regression analysis identified maternal age, ovarian response, and PGT-A cycles with vitrified embryos as the factors with the most impact on aneuploidy determination.

Female age is one of the primary biological factors that influences infertility. The presence of meiotic errors in oocytes increases with female age [18], which hinders successful pregnancies and makes advanced maternal age the most common indication for PGT-A. We observed a significant increase in aneuploidy with higher female age, mainly due to the increase of whole uniform aneuploidies. Girardi et al. [19] recently described a predominant meiotic origin for whole-chromosome errors, which justifies the increase in the percentage of this category of aneuploidy observed in our study. However, for other types of chromosomal abnormalities, such as segmental aneuploidies and low-mosaic degree, female age showed a negative correlation. Both could be considered as mitotic in origin [1,20]. In fact, Girardi et al. [19] showed that 67.9% of the segmental aneuploidies from preimplantation embryos had a mitotic origin, confirming previous publications [21,22]. Interestingly, mean maternal and paternal age were higher in the group of TE biopsies with whole uniform aneuploidy and high-mosaic degree compared to the group of TE biopsies with low-mosaic degree and only segmental aneuploidy. Moreover, logistic regression analysis showed a significant decrease in low-mosaic degree with female age, suggesting that this decrease is the main contributor to the overall decrease in mosaicism as female age increases.

Regarding ovarian response, we observed a significant increase in the percentage of aneuploid embryos with the decrease in the number of MII oocytes: 58.4% in PGT-A cycles with >20 MII oocytes retrieved and 65.3% with ≤5 MII oocytes. This confirms a trend described in our previous publication [13] where there was a decrease in aneuploidies in PGT-A cycles with >20 MII oocytes (41.7%) compared to ≤5 MII oocytes (47.5%) without statistical significance. In contrast, a recent publication in cycles with oocyte donation did not find an association between the proportion of aneuploid embryos and the number of MII oocytes retrieved, although the absolute number of euploid blastocysts was higher with higher oocyte number [9]. The nature of our population could explain these differences when female age is a factor. Logistic regression analysis showed that the percentage of aneuploid embryos increases with female age, but decreases with higher ovarian response, with a stronger effect of maternal age than the ovarian response. In our population, there was a correlation between female age and the ovarian response in which patients with ovarian response below 11 MII oocytes were older than those with 11 or more MII oocytes. Female age is a risk factor for decreased ovarian reserve [23], which explains the inverse effect that both variables exerted on the overall aneuploidy rates of our population. In fact, we observed that the percentage of aneuploid embryos in the group of 16–20 MII oocytes (62.1%) was similar to the group of low responders (65.3%). This finding could be explained by the fact that female age in the group of 16–20 MII was similar to the female age in the group of low responders and significantly higher than the group with more than 22 MII oocytes.

Contrary to the effect of maternal age, ovarian response was positively correlated with the incidence of TE biopsies with only segmental aneuploidies.

Vitrification of oocytes and embryos is a widespread practice in IVF laboratories, which allows multiple possibilities in managing fertility treatment. The incidence of aneuploid embryos derived from fresh or vitrified oocytes was similar in our study, confirming previous results from our group and others [13,24]. Interestingly, we observed lower incidence of aneuploid embryos when TE biopsies derived from vitrified embryos with a decrease in whole uniform aneuploidies and an increase in TE biopsies with only segmental aneuploidies. Maternal age was lower in our group of patients using vitrified embryos compared to fresh and vitrified oocytes. Lower maternal age could explain the lower incidence of aneuploid embryos, but logistic regression analysis identified embryo vitrification as an independent factor reducing the incidence of embryo aneuploidy and increasing the probability of mosaicism mainly of low-mosaic degree.

The contribution of sperm to embryo aneuploidy is controversial. The incidence of mosaic and chaotic patterns in cleavage stage embryos from oligozoospermic and azoospermic patients ranges from 35% to 68% [25–32]. Although the incidence is lower at the blastocyst stage, two recent studies described a higher rate of mosaic blastocysts in PGT-A cycles with male factor indication compared to couples with normal sperm parameters, with the highest rate of mosaicism correlated with the severity of male infertility [14,15]. We also observed an increase in mosaicism with a decrease in sperm count, with the highest mosaicism rate in patients with severe oligozoospermia (7.9%) similar to the 7.7% described by Tarozzi's group and 10.9–15.6% described by Kharaman's group [14,15]. Our group of severe oligozoospermia had the highest incidence of TE biopsies with only segmental aneuploidy. Interestingly, whereas whole chromosomal aneuploidies in TE biopsies are predominantly maternally derived aneuploidies, segmental aneuploidies are mostly paternally derived [33]. Moreover, SNP data in the same study showed 76.7% of mosaic segmental aneuploidies affecting paternally derived aneuploidies. Our group previously described sperm count as the parameter primarily associated with increased risk of sperm aneuploidies [34]. We also described a clear effect of specific sperm aneuploidies on the chromosomal constitution of preimplantation embryos [32]. Moreover, the incidence of TE biopsies with only segmental aneuploidy in male factor indication to perform PGT-A was significantly increased compared to patients performing PGT-A without a specific clinical indication (aneuploidy screening—AS). These results highlight male infertility as a factor influencing the risk of mosaicism and segmental aneuploidies in preimplantation embryos. Nevertheless, neither the sperm count nor the male factor as an indication for PGT-A were identified in the logistic regression analysis as factors affecting aneuploidy rates. The low number of samples included in the logistic regression analysis for sperm parameters (only 4.4% of the informative TE biopsies) could explain the differences observed in the univariant analysis.

5. Conclusions

Female age is the most influential on the overall incidence of aneuploid embryos and mosaicism, showing an inverse effect on both. While the incidence of aneuploid embryos increases, mainly due to whole uniform aneuploidies, the incidence of mosaic embryos and only segmental aneuploidies decrease with age. Other biological and IVF factors, such as the ovarian response and PGT-A cycles with vitrified embryos also affect aneuploidy incidence, with an effect contrary to female age. While the incidence of whole uniform aneuploid embryos decreases with the ovarian response and the use of vitrified embryos, the incidence of only segmental aneuploidies increases with the ovarian response, and the incidence of mosaicism increases with the use of vitrified embryos compared to fresh oocytes. Considering the two grades of mosaicism, high mosaic degree is not affected by any of the variables evaluated. However, the incidence of low-mosaic degree decreases with female age but increases in PGT-A cycles with vitrified embryos.

Author Contributions: C.S., C.R., and L.R. participated in conceptualizing the study; I.C.-G., V.P. and L.R. curated the data; M.C.-C. and L.R. analyzed the data; the manuscript was written by L.R. and reviewed by C.S. and C.R. All authors have read and agreed to the published version of the manuscript.

Funding: This research received no external funding.

Acknowledgments: The authors would like to thank all the Igenomix laboratories for sharing the PGT-A data analyzed in this study.

Conflicts of Interest: L.R., M.C.-C., I.C.-G., V.P., C.S. and C.R. are employees of Igenomix. Authors declare no conflict of interest.

References

1. Taylor, T.H.; Gitlin, S.A.; Patrick, J.L.; Crain, J.L.; Wilson, J.M.; Griffin, D.K. The origin, mechanisms, incidence and clinical consequences of chromosomal mosaicism in humans. *Hum. Reprod. Update* **2014**, *20*, 571–581. [CrossRef] [PubMed]
2. Monahan, D.; Harton, G.; Griffin, D.; Angle, M.; Smikle, C. Clinical comparison of two PGT-A platforms utilizing different thresholds to determine ploidy status. *Reprod. Biomed. Online* **2019**, *39*, e27–e28.2. [CrossRef]
3. Swain, J.E. Controversies in ART: Can the IVF laboratory influence preimplantation embryo aneuploidy? *Reprod. Biomed. Online* **2019**, *39*, 599–607. [CrossRef] [PubMed]
4. Popovic, M.; Dheedene, A.; Christodoulou, C.; Taelman, J.; Dhaenens, L.; Van Nieuwerburgh, F.; Deforce, D.; Van den Abbeel, E.; De Sutter, P.; Menten, B.; et al. Chromosomal mosaicism in human blastocysts: The ultimate challenge of preimplantation genetic testing? *Hum. Reprod.* **2018**, *33*, 1342–1354. [CrossRef] [PubMed]
5. Popovic, M.; Dhaenens, L.; Taelman, J.; Dheedene, A.; Bialecka, M.; De Sutter, P.; Chuva de Sousa Lopes, S.M.; Menten, B.; Heindryckx, B. Extended in vitro culture of human embryos demonstrates the complex nature of diagnosing chromosomal mosaicism for a single trophectoderm biopsy. *Hum. Reprod.* **2019**, *34*, 758–769. [CrossRef]
6. Goodrich, D.; Tao, X.; Bohrer, C.; Lonczak, A.; Xing, T.; Zimmerman, R.; Zhan, Y.; Scott, R.T., Jr.; Treff, N.R. A randomized and blinded comparison of qPCR and NGS-based detection of aneuploidy in a cell line mixture model of blastocyst biopsy mosaicism. *J. Assist. Reprod. Genet.* **2016**, *33*, 1473–1480. [CrossRef] [PubMed]
7. Goodrich, D.; Xing, T.; Tao, X.; Lonczak, A.; Zhan, Y.; Landis, J.; Zimmerman, R.; Scott, R.T., Jr.; Treff, N.R. Evaluation of comprehensive chromosome screening platforms for the detection of mosaic segmental aneuploidy. *J. Assist. Reprod. Genet.* **2017**, *34*, 975–981. [CrossRef]
8. García-Pascual, C.M.; Navarro-Sánchez, L.; Navarro, R.; Martínez, L.; Jiménez, J.; Rodrigo, L.; Simón, C.; Rubio, C. Optimized NGS approach for detection of aneuploidies and mosaicism in PGT-A and imbalances in PGT-SR. *Genes* **2020**, *11*, 724. [CrossRef]
9. McCulloh, D.H.; Alikani, M.; Norian, J.; Kolb, B.; Arbones, J.M.; Munné, S. Controlled ovarian hyperstimulation (COH) parameters associated with euploid rates in donor oocytes. *Eur. J. Med. Genet.* **2019**, *62*, 103707. [CrossRef]
10. Palmerola, K.L.; Vitez, S.F.; Amrane, S.; Fishcer, C.P.; Forman, E.J. Minimizing mosaicism: Assessing the impact of fertilization method on rate of mosaicism after next-generation sequencing (NGS) preimplantation genetic testing for aneuploidy (PGT-A). *J. Assist. Reprod. Genet.* **2019**, *36*, 153–157. [CrossRef]
11. Treff, N.R.; Levy, B.; Su, J.; Northrop, L.E.; Tao, X.; Scott, R.T., Jr. SNP microarray-based 24 chromosome aneuploidy screening is significantly more consistent than FISH. *Mol. Hum. Reprod.* **2010**, *16*, 583–589. [CrossRef] [PubMed]
12. Capalbo, A.; Ubaldi, F.M.; Rienzi, L.; Scott, R.; Treff, N. Detecting mosaicism in trophectoderm biopsies: Current challenges and future possibilities. *Hum. Reprod.* **2017**, *32*, 492–498. [CrossRef] [PubMed]
13. Rubio, C.; Rodrigo, L.; Garcia-Pascual, C.; Peinado, V.; Campos-Galindo, I.; Garcia-Herrero, S.; Simón, C. Clinical application of embryo aneuploidy testing by next-generation sequencing. *Biol. Reprod.* **2019**, *101*, 1083–1090. [CrossRef] [PubMed]

14. Tarozzi, N.; Nadalini, M.; Lagalla, C.; Coticchio, G.; Zacà, C.; Borini, A. Male factor infertility impacts the rate of mosaic blastocysts in cycles of preimplantation genetic testing for aneuploidy. *J. Assist. Reprod. Genet.* **2019**, *36*, 2047–2055. [CrossRef] [PubMed]
15. Kahraman, S.; Sahin, Y.; Yelke, H.; Kumtepe, Y.; Tufekci, M.A.; Yapan, C.C.; Yesil, M.; Cetinkaya, M. High rates of aneuploidy, mosaicism and abnormal morphokitetic development in cases with low sperm concentration. *J. Assist. Reprod. Genet.* **2020**, *37*, 629–640. [CrossRef] [PubMed]
16. Greco, E.; Minasi, M.G.; Fiorentino, F. Healthy babies after intrauterine transfer of mosaic aneuploid blastocysts. *N. Engl. J. Med.* **2015**, *373*, 2089–2090. [CrossRef]
17. Munné, S.; Spinella, F.; Grifo, J.; Zhang, J.; Beltran, M.P.; Fragouli, E.; Fiorentino, F. Clinical outcomes after the transfer of blastocysts characterized as mosaic by high resolution Next Generation Sequencing-futher insights. *Eur. J. Med. Genet.* **2020**, *63*, 103741. [CrossRef]
18. Hassold, T.; Hunt, P. To err (meiotically) is human: The genesis of human aneuploidy. *Nat. Rev. Genet.* **2001**, *2*, 280–291. [CrossRef]
19. Girardi, L.; Serdarogullari, M.; Patassini, C.; Poli, M.; Fabiani, M.; Caroselli, S.; Coban, O.; Findikli, N.; Kubra Boynukalin, F.; Bahceci, M.; et al. Incidence, origin, and predictive model for the detection and clinical management of segmental aneuploidies in human embryos. *Am. J. Hum. Genet.* **2020**, *106*, 525–534. [CrossRef]
20. Vera-Rodriguez, M.; Rubio, C. Assessing the true incidence of mosaicism in preimplantation embryos. *Fertil. Steril.* **2017**, *107*, 1107–1112. [CrossRef]
21. Vera-Rodríguez, M.; Claude-Edouard, M.; Mercader, A.; Bladon, A.J.; Rodrigo, L.; Kokocinski, F.; Mateu, E.; Al-Asmar, N.; Blesa, D.; Simón, C.; et al. Distribution patterns of segmental aneuploidies in human blastocysts identified by next-generation sequencing. *Fertil. Steril.* **2016**, *105*, 1047–1055. [CrossRef] [PubMed]
22. Babariya, D.; Fragouli, E.; Alfarawati, S.; Spath, K.; Wells, D. The incidence and origin of segmental aneuploidy in human oocytes and preimplantation embryos. *Hum. Reprod.* **2017**, *32*, 2549–2560. [CrossRef] [PubMed]
23. Ferraretti, A.P.; La Marca, A.; Fauser, B.C.J.M.; Tarlatzis, B.; Nargund, G.; Gianaroli, L. ESHRE working group on Poor Ovarian Response Definition. ESHRE consensus on the definition of "poor response" to ovarian stimulation for in vitro fertilization: The Bologna criteria. *Hum. Reprod.* **2011**, *26*, 1616–1624. [CrossRef]
24. Forman, E.J.; Li, X.; Ferry, K.M.; Scott, K.; Treff, N.R.; Scott, R.T., Jr. Oocyte vitrification does not increase the risk of embryonic aneuploidy or diminish the implantation potential of blastocysts created after intracytoplasmic sperm injection: A novel, paired randomized controlled trial using DNA fingerprinting. *Fertil. Steril.* **2012**, *98*, 644–649. [CrossRef]
25. Silber, S.; Escudero, T.; Lenahan, K.; Abdelhadi, I.; Kilani, Z.; Munné, S. Chromosomal abnormalities in embryos derived from testicular sperm extraction. *Fertil. Steril.* **2003**, *79*, 30–38. [CrossRef]
26. Aran, B.; Veiga, A.; Vidal, F.; Parriego, M.; Vendrell, J.M.; Santaló, J.; Egozcue, J.; Barri, N. Preimplantation genetic diagnosis in patients with male meiotic abnormalities. *Reprod. Biomed. Online* **2004**, *8*, 470–476. [CrossRef]
27. Platteau, P.; Staessen, C.; Michiels, A.; Tournaye, H.; Van Steirteghem, A.; Liebaers, I.; Devroey, P. Comparison of the aneuploidy frequency in embryos derived from testicular sperm extraction in obstructive and non-obstructive azoospermic men. *Hum. Reprod.* **2004**, *19*, 1570–1574. [CrossRef]
28. Gianaroli, L.; Magli, M.C.; Ferraretti, A.P. Sperm and blastomere aneuploidy detection in reproductive genetics and medicine. *J. Histochem. Cytochem.* **2005**, *53*, 261–267. [CrossRef]
29. Rubio, C.; Rodrigo, L.; Pérez-Cano, I.; Mercader, A.; Mateu, E.; Buendía, P.; Remohí, J.; Simón, C.; Pellicer, A. FISH screening of aneuploidies in preimplantation embryos to improve IVF outcome. *Reprod. Biomed. Online* **2005**, *11*, 497–506. [CrossRef]
30. Sánchez-Castro, M.; Jiménez-Macedo, A.R.; Sandalinas, M.; Blanco, J. Prognostic value of sperm fluorescence in situ hybridization analysis over PGD. *Hum. Reprod.* **2009**, *24*, 1516–1521. [CrossRef]
31. Magli, C.; Gianaroli, L.; Ferraretti, A.P.; Gordts, S.; Fredericks, V.; Crippa, A. Paternal contribution to aneuploidy in preimplantation embryos. *Reprod. Biomed. Online* **2009**, *18*, 536–542. [CrossRef]
32. Rodrigo, L.; Peinado, V.; Mateu, E.; Remohí, J.; Pellicer, A.; Simón, C.; Gil-Salom, M.; Rubio, C. Impact of different patterns of sperm chromosomal abnormalities on the chromosomal constitution of preimplantation embryos. *Fertil. Steril.* **2010**, *94*, 1380–1386. [CrossRef] [PubMed]

33. Kubicek, D.; Hornak, M.; Horak, J.; Navratil, R.; Tauwinklova, G.; Rubes, J.; Vesela, K. Incidence and origin of meiotic whole and segmental chromosomal aneuploidies detected by karyomapping. *Reprod. Biomed. Online* **2019**, *38*, 330–339. [CrossRef] [PubMed]
34. Rodrigo, L.; Meseguer, M.; Mateu, E.; Mercader, A.; Peinado, V.; Bori, L.; Campos-Galindo, I.; Milán, M.; García-Herrero, S.; Simón, C.; et al. Sperm chromosomal abnormalities and their contribution to human embryo aneuploidy. *Biol. Reprod.* **2019**, *101*, 1091–1101. [CrossRef]

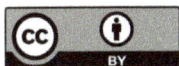

© 2020 by the authors. Licensee MDPI, Basel, Switzerland. This article is an open access article distributed under the terms and conditions of the Creative Commons Attribution (CC BY) license (http://creativecommons.org/licenses/by/4.0/).

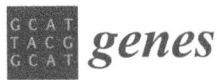 *genes*

Review

The Reproductive Journey in the Genomic Era: From Preconception to Childhood

Sandra Garcia-Herrero, Blanca Simon and Javier Garcia-Planells *

IGENOMIX, Valencia, 46980 Paterna, Spain; sandra.garcia@igenomix.com (S.G.-H.); blanca.simon@igenomix.com (B.S.)
* Correspondence: javier.garcia@igenomix.com

Received: 7 October 2020; Accepted: 14 December 2020; Published: 19 December 2020

Abstract: It is estimated that around 10–15% of the population have problems achieving a pregnancy. Assisted reproduction techniques implemented and enforced by personalized genomic medicine have paved the way for millions of infertile patients to become parents. Nevertheless, having a baby is just the first challenge to overcome in the reproductive journey, the most important is to obtain a healthy baby free of any genetic condition that can be prevented. Prevention of congenital anomalies throughout the lifespan of the patient must be a global health priority. Congenital disorders can be defined as structural or functional anomalies that occur during intrauterine life and can be identified prenatally, at birth, or sometimes may only be detected later during childhood. It is considered a frequent group of disorders, affecting 3–6% of the population, and one of the leading causes of morbidity and mortality. Congenital anomalies can represent up to 30–50% of infant mortality in developed countries. Genetics plays a substantial role in the pathogenesis of congenital anomalies. This becomes especially important in some ethnic communities or populations where the incidence and levels of consanguinity are higher. The impact of genetic disorders during childhood is high, representing 20–30% of all infant deaths and 11.1% of pediatric hospital admissions. With these data, obtaining a precise genetic diagnosis is one of the main aspects of a preventive medicine approach in developed countries. The field of reproductive health has changed dramatically from traditional non-molecular visual microscope-based techniques (i.e., fluorescence in situ hybridization (FISH) or G-banding karyotype), to the latest molecular high-throughput techniques such as next-generation sequencing (NGS). Genome-wide technologies are applied along the different stages of the reproductive health lifecycle from preconception carrier screening and pre-implantation genetic testing, to prenatal and postnatal testing. The aim of this paper is to assess the new horizon opened by technologies such as next-generation sequencing (NGS), in new strategies, as a genomic precision diagnostic tool to understand the mechanisms underlying genetic conditions during the "reproductive journey".

Keywords: genetic testing; reproductive health; next-generation sequencing; whole exome sequencing; perinatal care

---

1. Introduction

The odyssey of an infertile couple to become parents can be compared to the odyssey of those parents who realize that their child has some type of problem or illness but there are no answers or name for that "condition". It can also be compared to adults that suffer from a genetic condition and want to know what it is, how to deal with it and their reproductive options, embarking on a long, emotionally draining and financially costly journey.

There is an indisputable advancement that the emergence of molecular genetic techniques, such as next-generation sequencing (NGS), has allowed, which is to standardize pathways to achieve an accurate diagnosis. Genomic high-resolution and high-throughput technologies have opened new diagnostic pathways, allowing a more personalized clinical management paired with new challenges, such as the use, management and interpretation of generated databases needing great bioinformatic support.

2. The Reproductive Journey

2.1. First Stage: Pre-Conceptional Care

Increasingly often, more couples assess their reproductive potential without acknowledging the reproductive roulette of the risk for an associated genetic disease (Figure 1). The growing knowledge on the impact of genetic diseases in soon to become newborns, as well as the development of new technologies, has led to an increase of the pre-conceptional care field. Nevertheless, genetics is not the only area covered by pre-conceptional assessment. Genetic analysis can be implemented at any stage of the reproductive journey, starting from preconception to detect genetic carriers of frequent diseases like cystic fibrosis, hemophilia or fragile X syndrome, pre-implantation to ensure a chromosomal and genetically normal embryo is transferred, decreasing the risk of monogenetic disease like Duchenne muscular dystrophy, aneuploidies such as Down's syndrome or structural diseases like DiGeorge's syndrome or Prader Willi syndrome. Genetic analysis is also useful for prenatal diagnosis of these kinds of diseases, high-risk pregnancies and in case of spontaneous abortions, the analysis of the products of conception. Lastly, it can be utilized to perform newborn screening of common and actionable diseases, personalized genetic analyses such as single gene analysis for monogenic diseases and genetic panels or whole exome sequencing for complex or clinically unspecific diseases (Figure 1).

The WHO (World Health Organization) defines preconception care as the provision of biomedical, behavioral and social health interventions for women and couples before conception occurs. Its main aim is to improve maternal and child health, in both the short and long term [1]. Preconception counseling must cover all known barriers that may have a detrimental effect on fertility or pregnancy which include:

- An evaluation of the overall well-being
- Medical history
- Surgical history
- Social and behavioral history
- Medication
- Occupational and education risks

There are many areas addressed by preconception care assessment including nutrition, environmental conditions, toxic habits (i.e., tobacco and alcohol consumption), mental health and genetic conditions. We are going to focus on the last one, genetic conditions.

Most genetic disorders that result in sterility or childhood death are caused by recessive mutations. Nonetheless, these variants can cause devastating diseases like cystic fibrosis when the patient carries both copies of the mutation. It is estimated that humans carry an average of one to two mutations per person that can cause severe genetic disorders or prenatal death when two copies of the same mutation are inherited [2]. This means that if two carriers of the same mutation have a child, it could be affected by a genetic disease.

Currently, there are many genetic tests that assess the "mutational state" of a patient or a couple to reduce the probability of having a baby with a genetic disorder. Genetic carriers screening based on NGS test the existence of mutations causing a vast number of recessive genetic conditions in an individual, that can be passed on to their offspring if the couple carries the mutation. Even though the standard of practice is to offer carrier testing only to those individuals who have a strong family history of a genetic disorder, or a history of genetic disorder in the partner and/or relatives of identified carriers, only a minority of carrier couples are identified. These reduced indications for testing can lead to children affected by recessive disorders with no known family or medical history [3].

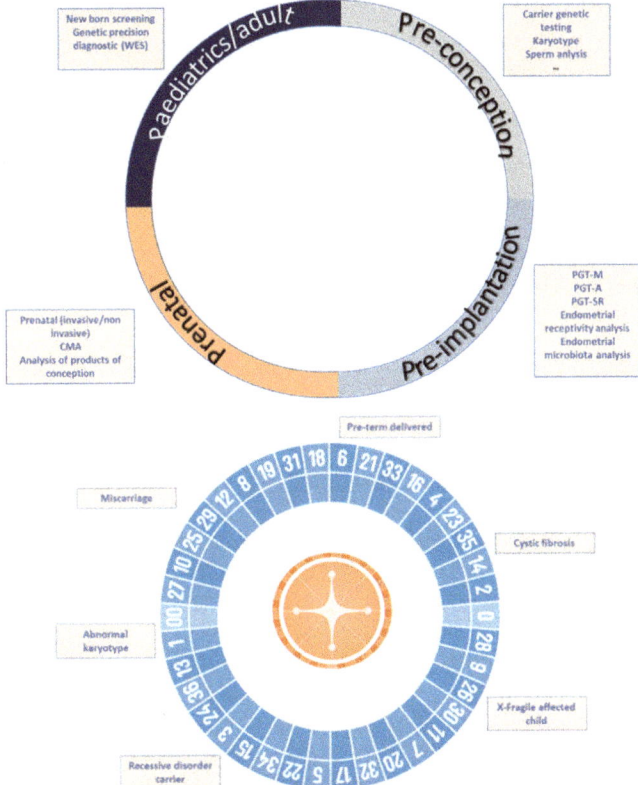

Figure 1. Reproductive journey vs. reproductive roulette: Genetic analysis can be implemented at any stage of the reproductive journey, starting from preconception to detect genetic carriers of frequent diseases, pre-implantation to ensure chromosomal and genetically normal embryos, prenatal diagnosis and lastly, for newborn screening of common and actionable diseases. The reproductive roulette is a term that aims to explain the unknown risk of having any form of genetic disease given the risk factors of the parents or purely by chance. The possibility of reducing this probability can be done by an adequate and directed genetic analysis or screening approaches.

Autosomal/X-linked recessive disorders are more frequent than autosomal/X-linked dominant because the latter present a higher deleterious effect. The reproductive approach is different in these cases because patients are not only carriers, but they also suffer the illness, and so are aware that they can transmit the genetic condition to 50% of their offspring.

When it is known that an autosomal and/or dominant disease is present in a couple, preconception counselling is crucial. During this process, we must evaluate the medical and family history to obtain an accurate clinical diagnosis. From here, the next step will be to carry out the most appropriate genetic analyses to identify the molecular cause of the disease, an essential requirement for any subsequent family study, including prenatal and pre-implantation analyses.

2.2. Second Stage: Pre-Implantation Diagnosis

At this stage of the reproductive journey, it is useful to group together couples with known reproductive problems (infertility, miscarriages, previously affected child ...) as well as those couples that have never tried but know there is a genetic condition running in the family. Therefore, all of them could benefit from assisted reproduction techniques such as pre-implantation genetic testing for monogenic diseases (PGT-M) and pre-implantation genetic testing for aneuploidies (PGT-A).

PGT-M allows us to detect embryos affected by a known monogenic that has been previously detected in their parents. Molecular technologies used to perform the PGT-M test were several, for example:

- Multiplex PCR (Polymerase Chain Reaction): Multiplex PCR uses targeted primers designed specifically for the mutation of interest combined with other markers for linked short tandem repeat (STR) markers.
- Whole-genome amplification (WGA).
- Karyomapping: High-density SNP (Single Nucleotide Polymorphism) array that allows evaluation of DNA haplotypes).
- Sanger sequencing.
- Multiplex Ligation-dependent Probe Amplification (MLPA) [4].

Besides genetic disorders caused by gene mutations/variations, other genetic conditions can have an impact on fertility, pregnancy, parents and newborns: the so-called chromosomal disorders.

As women age, their fertility declines and there is an increased risk of numerical and structural chromosomal abnormalities, which can lead to implantation failure, early pregnancy loss, greater risk of congenital birth defects or severe chromosomal congenital diseases such as Down's and Patau syndromes. Aneuploidy ranks as the most common genetic abnormality accounting for approximately 50% of miscarriages. More than half of the embryos produced by in vitro fertilization (IVF) are aneuploid [5].

The process of detecting numeric or structural chromosomal abnormalities for the purpose of embryo selection is generally referred to as pre-implantation genetic testing for aneuploidies (PGT-A), introduced in the 2000s to increase implantation and pregnancy rates, decrease miscarriage rates and the risk of aneuploid offspring, as well as decrease the time to conceive [4,6,7]. Early PGT-A utilized fluorescence in situ hybridization (FISH) screening. However, data from several studies questioned the efficiency of FISH screening [8–11], which is restricted due to the limited panel of chromosomes that it is able to analyze. In recent years, PGT-A using FISH screening has been initially replaced by comprehensive approaches, including comparative genomic hybridization arrays (CGH) or single nucleotide polymorphism microarrays, and more recently, by next-generation sequencing (NGS)-based techniques.

Currently, embryo biopsy is required for PGT-A testing. In the event of a poor blastocyst quality at biopsy, new effective approaches involving the sequencing of cfDNA (cell free DNA) secreted into the culture medium from the human blastocyst have been developed. In addition, PGT-A could mitigate the potential adverse effects associated with embryo biopsy [12,13].

Aside from the assessment of the embryo's mutational/chromosomal status, additional genetic tests assessing fertility, based on high-throughput techniques such as NGS, are beyond the scope of an ordinary clinical practice to increase the reproductive chances of a couple, i.e., endometrial receptivity analysis and more recently, endometrial microbiome test [14,15].

2.3. Third Stage: Prenatal Diagnostis

Prenatal screening is the risk estimation of fetal aneuploidies based on high-resolution ultrasound scans, in order to assess ultrasonographic markers including nuchal translucency, combined with biochemical determinations in maternal blood samples of free beta-subunit of human chorionic gonadotropin (fβ-hCG) and pregnancy-associated plasma protein-A (PAPP-A) in the first trimester, and the alpha-fetoprotein (AFP) and beta-human chorionic gonadotropin (βhCG) in the second trimester [15]. If this risk of congenital defect is high, invasive procedures such as chorionic villus sampling (CVS) or amniocentesis are recommended [16]. Fetal chromosomal assessment traditionally performed using Giemsa banding (G-banding) on cultured cells in metaphase is considered as the gold standard detection method [17,18]. Although the accuracy and reliability of this technique is very high, 99.4–99.8% and 97.5–99.6% for amniocentesis and CV respectively [19], there are considerable disadvantages that must be highlighted: prenatal tissue must be cultured for several days to obtain metaphase nuclei prior to analysis, increasing maternal anxiety and the risk of fetal loss up to 0.5–2% due to an invasive technique used for fetal tissue extraction (i.e., amniocentesis to obtain amniotic fluid).

Currently, a rapid noninvasive prenatal test for the most common aneuploidies in the live newborn (i.e., Down or Turner syndrome) can be performed by sequencing fetal DNA present in maternal blood. The genomics-based non-invasive prenatal test (NIPT) could be considered as a candidate to replace the conventional karyotype as a first-tier test in unselected populations of pregnant women undergoing aneuploidy screening or as a second-tier test in pregnant women considered to be high risk after first-tier screening for common fetal aneuploidies [20].

Despite that cytogenetic conventional karyotype has been considered the gold standard for chromosomal assessment, new molecular microarray-based genomic copy-number techniques like chromosomal microarray (CMA) present some advantages.

The resolution of chromosomal analysis by karyotyping is limited to 5–10 Mb in size [21]. Most chromosomal anomalies identified in early pregnancy are aneuploidies, which are detected using conventional karyotyping. CMA resolution is higher than karyotype, therefore offering additional diagnostic benefits by revealing sub-microscopic imbalances or copy-number variations (CNV) that are too small to be detected using a standard G-banded chromosome preparation. Clinically significant copy-number variations not identifiable by standard karyotyping occur in 1–1.7% of routine pregnancies [22]. Most of these CNVs are responsible for:

- A variety of phenotypes.
- Multiple malformations.
- Congenital anomalies.
- Intellectual disabilities.
- Developmental delay.
- Epilepsy.
- Cerebral palsy.
- Neuropsychiatric disorders [23].

Alternatively, there are trade-offs, however, DNA extraction needed for prenatal purposes in order to perform a CMA still requires invasive techniques such as amniocentesis or chorionic villus sampling. Furthermore, a high resolution increases the probability of incidental findings of unknown clinical significance that, in turn, add a level of complexity to the genetic counselling as well as parent anxiety. We must take into consideration that CMA does not detect polyploidies or balanced rearrangements. In the vast majority of cases, the presence of a balanced rearrangement does not imply major clinical significance for the ongoing pregnancies, but there are still reproductive ramifications for future pregnancies if one of the parents is a carrier [24].

Although aneuploidies are the most frequent genetic alteration during the prenatal stage, as well as one of the main genetic causes of congenital defects (10–15%), monogenic alterations are of considerable importance throughout this stage, reaching up to 10% of the congenital defects.

Some of the clinical features of these monogenic disorders, especially those associated with syndromic forms, can be identified throughout pregnancy by ultrasonography analyses. In these cases, and depending on the clinical impression, specific tests can be used to analyze certain genes or variants, as well as more complex and nonspecific technologies, such as CMA, NGS gene panels or whole exome sequencing (WES), when a precise clinical guidance is not possible. In any case, when an ultrasound finding is detected during pregnancy, that pregnancy is labelled as high risk for a genetic disease, therefore an invasive test will be indicated to obtain a fetal sample to analyze using the most suitable technique depending on the type of ultrasound finding.

Another significant and relatively frequent issue is when the couple first finds out about the presence of a genetic disease or knows that they are at high risk of being a carrier during an advanced stage of their pregnancy. As we have described previously, it is strongly recommended to face this situation in the pre-conceptional stage in order to approach the diagnostic process with sufficient guarantees and time. Once the pregnancy has started, the gestational age and prenatal diagnosis can be time-limiting, being critical in some complex cases. In any case, and whenever possible, it is recommended to identify the molecular cause of the familial disease prior to taking the fetal sample using an invasive approach.

Unfortunately, miscarriages are the most common complication during early pregnancy. Clinically recognized pregnancy losses occur in approximately 15–25% of pregnancies, most of them occurring during the first trimester [25]. Although there are many known causes and risk factors for early pregnancy loss, about 60% of those cases are caused by sporadic chromosomal abnormalities which are usually numerical (86%) [26–29]. These cytogenetic anomalies include autosomal trisomies (27%), polyploidies (10%), chromosome X monosomy (9%) and structural rearrangements (2%) [30]; double trisomies, as well as multiple trisomies, which are infrequent, have an incidence of about 0.7% [31,32].

Until now, products of conception (POC) studies have been carried out using cell culture followed by conventional karyotyping. However, when using these techniques, the incidence of chromosomal abnormalities in miscarriages in the general population ranges between 40% and 80%, depending on the culture methods adopted [33,34]. Proper chromosomal analysis of POC samples is not always feasible, for several reasons:

- Cell culture growth failure (the failure rate in POC samples cultured after curettage ranges between 5% and 42% [35]).
- Suboptimal chromosome preparations.
- Maternal cell contamination (MCC).
- Low-resolution limit that does not allow the detection of submicroscopic deletions and duplications that can cause miscarriages.

Molecular biology techniques such as NGS or CMA that are culture-independent can avoid such limitations, increasing the karyotype resolution [36,37]. Given this, new genomic technologies are positioning themselves as the first-choice technologies for the analysis of miscarriages and POC.

Whole exome sequencing (WES) is very useful for the detection of alterations in the sequence of any gene that may be related to the potential genetic condition that may have caused the spontaneous termination of the pregnancy in progress. This is especially important in the second trimester of gestation when monogenic disorders acquire a higher frequency. In these cases, identification of the molecular causes of the miscarriage can be very useful to prevent new similar situations in the couple.

When miscarriage occurs in an advanced pregnancy, the clinical and anatomopathological evaluation of the fetus can be very useful to guide the genomic analysis. When clinical assessment is not possible, WES provides a high capability to identify sequence variants in genes associated to complex syndromes, but also, the optimization of bioinformatic analyses, making possible the identification of copy-number variations in these cases.

2.4. Fourth Step: Newborn Screening and Neonatal Care

Currently, 3% of live newborns will have a congenital alteration despite great efforts made in the different stages of the reproductive process, growing capacities of available technologies and the implementation of prevention programs. This is because, on one hand, technologies, although increasingly precise, are not infallible, and on the other, the use of prevention techniques and programs are not universal.

In this stage, as in other previous stages, we will be able to apply screening measures in order to reduce the impact of congenital diseases. An example would be extended neonatal screening aimed for early identification of apparently healthy newborns that are at immediate risk of a congenital disease if an early and accurate diagnosis is not established and therapeutic measures are not taken as soon as possible.

The neonatal screening allows us to detect a wide number of genetic disorders, causing health problems starting in infancy or early childhood, mainly metabolic disorders like phenylketonuria. Newborn screening programs are well-established as the standard of care in most developed countries, but the number of diseases and approaches differ between countries and health systems. Early detection and treatment can help prevent inborn errors of metabolism, intellectual and physical disabilities and life-threatening illnesses during the first hours of life. The advent of next-generation sequencing has resulted in attempts to expand the use of DNA sequencing in newborn screening to improve diagnostic and prognostic utility. Currently, in the market, we can find different commercial options for newborn screening panels that can detect, not only the most common metabolic disorders, but a great number of genetic disorders, or even gene susceptibility. Still, unexpected and medically irrelevant incidental findings must be carefully considered [38].

On the other hand, we can also apply diagnostic methods in those neonates who have developed symptoms, especially for newborns admitted to the intensive care unit when disease progression is extremely rapid and a quick molecular diagnostic is relevant for clinical decision making, establishing a prognosis, defining specific therapeutic measures and providing genetic counselling and access to family studies aiming to reduce the risks of recurrence in the family. Monogenic diseases have a high impact in the neonatal morbimortality, accounting for ~20% of infant deaths and ~18% of pediatric hospitalizations. Genomic testing of these patients aims to provide a comprehensive molecular diagnosis that allows for early intervention of the patient and proper genetic counseling of the family in order to reduce the time spent in the diagnostic odyssey [39,40]. These tests provide a high clinical utility and are cost-effective, especially in patients involved in neonatal intensive care units.

Both genetic assessment and diagnosis have a special impact during this stage of the reproductive journey, especially in young adults that may be developing a career, forming partnerships and potentially becoming parents. Pre-symptomatic testing may affect many facets of their future lives as well as the future of their upcoming families [41], but also raises profound ethical challenges.

NGS technologies, especially introduction of the WES, has become a turning point, especially in the rare genetic diseases research. It has allowed development and implementation of strategies to uncover the mechanisms behind all rare diseases to sketch a "molecular atlas" showing links between molecular genetic profiles and states of health or disease. Rare genetic conditions affect around 2–3% of the worldwide population, usually causing diseases that drastically reduce life expectancy and quality of life as well as reproductive consequences in their offspring.

3. Genomic Precision Diagnostic

Recent advent of genomic technologies and its clinical applications has allowed the scientific community, especially those involved in patient care and clinical management, to evolve from a diagnosis-based approach of fragmented or isolated data to a diagnostic-based approach of the "overall picture" point of view. This can be done as a result of huge datasets, using their unique genetic and physiologic characteristics to tailor the diagnosis and treatment of individual patients.

To reach an accurate and reliable genetic diagnosis, or in other words, to interpret these data in a meaningful and useful manner for the patient's clinical management, it is mandatory to develop bioinformatic tools, including novel data pipelines or computational tools, and also, acquire knowledge to manage and to interpret combined analysis of multi-dimensional data produced by these technological and scientific innovations. This is where clinical bioinformatics comes into play as an essential element to integrate laboratory and clinical data as well as the use of database-computational methods, algorithms, customized pipelines and other resources and methods, including machine learning or even artificial intelligence [42].

Whole exome sequencing (WES) and whole genome sequencing (WGS) are the most recent technologies based on NGS that are developed for genomic diagnostic purposes when a genetic disorder for which single-gene or limited gene testing fails to provide a genetic explanation. WGS and WES—wherein the genome or the protein-coding parts of the genome are sequenced in its entirety—would be an option to replace panel tests in the near future. There is no doubt that genomic tools, especially WES and WGS, give us a global view of the disease, increasing the knowledge on the underlying mechanism causing this rare genetic condition, but also increases the probability to find variants associated with other health conditions which may or may not be medically actionable and are unexpectedly so named secondary or incidental findings. How to report and manage this secondary finding as well as how to assess patients are some of the main genomic diagnostic challenges [43].

4. Conclusions

It is estimated that 350 million people globally suffer from a genetic disorder causing a rare condition. Genetic disorders can be assessed in several stages of our life, generating a different impact in our lifestyle and personal decision-making, in particular those involved with our reproductive options.

Frequently, searching for an answer and an accurate diagnosis in those patients suffering from a genetic disorder can turn into an odyssey, especially in those cases where children or pregnant women are involved.

Sometimes, patients and their families bounce back and forth from physician to specialist and back again only to receive multiple misdiagnoses. Genetic diagnosis serves to provide a linear or step-by-step flowchart with plenty of medical tests, reports and documentation of clinical manifestations. These lead to the concatenation of several visits, usually to different specialists, only to end up with the final step, which was a genetic analysis, usually by Sanger sequencing or NGS of a limited/selected gene panel when there was a suspicion of a genetic disorder. The emergence of a massive gene analysis tool like NGS has changed this diagnostic workflow in genetic diseases by providing a higher diagnostic yield, rapid, powerful and cost-effectiveness alternative for genetic analysis in the early stages of the process (Figure 2). This new workflow has drastically reduced waiting times and anxiety that many patients have to undergo to know their prognosis [44].

Currently, NGS-based tools can point to the implication of a single gene (or a small number of genes) and help establish a rapid diagnosis in just a few weeks or even less in a large percentage of cases.

Lately, we have experienced a noticeable increase in the demand of NGS technologies in the clinical setting. Increasing the diagnostic precision of these technologies has been one of the main levers for change, alongside the optimization of processes, reduction of costs and development of new applications. These adjustments contribute to an improvement in the diagnostic capacity, improving the life of patients with monogenic and widely known diseases, patients with heterogeneous conditions, gene-associated phenotypes or even complex differential diagnoses.

Genomics provides the tools and knowledge necessary to achieve an accurate diagnosis, making a difference in the lives of a growing number of patients suffering from genetic diseases. Relying on an accurate diagnosis enables a greater availability to different reproductive options, allowing the "reproductive journey" to be a comfortable and safe experience for the patient (Figure 3).

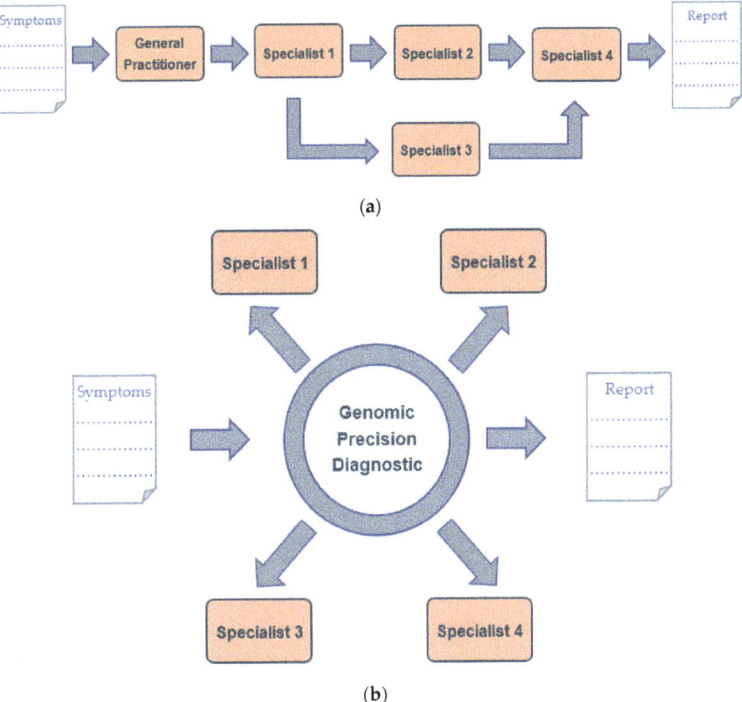

Figure 2. Classic genetic diagnostic (**a**) vs. Genomic diagnostic (**b**) flow-charts: Genomic Precision Diagnostic is an innovative approach that ultimately not only provides a precise diagnosis of a genetic alteration at every stage of the reproductive journey, it also alleviates the healthcare burden of a patient that has to go from specialist to specialist, increasing the degree of uncertainty and preoccupation. This can decrease the economic cost, psychological deterioration of the patient and the healthcare provider, and all in all, simplify the diagnosis for a more directed treatment and patient care, allowing the patient to be the center of the diagnostic axis.

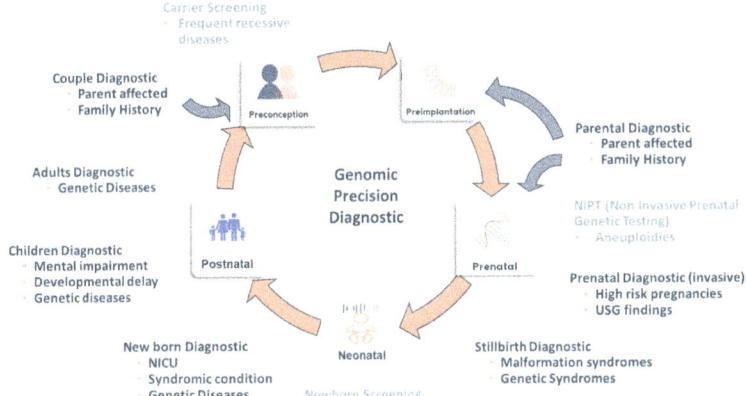

Figure 3. Closing the circle of the Reproductive Journey: Impact of the genomic diagnostic (dark blue) and screening (light blue) application along the different stages of the reproductive journey. Blue-gray arrows show new "access ways" to the reproductive journey driven by a precise diagnostic.

Author Contributions: All authors have contributed equally to the discussion and redaction of the manuscript. All authors have read and agreed to the published version of the manuscript.

Funding: This research received no external funding.

Conflicts of Interest: Authors are employees of Igenomix. Authors declare no conflict of interest.

References

1. Fowler, J.R.; Mahdy, H.; Jack, B.W. *Preconception Counseling*; StatPearls Publishing: Treasure Island, FL, USA, 2020.
2. Gao, Z.; Waggoner, D.; Stephens, M.; Ober, C.; Przeworski, M. An estimate of the average number of recessive lethal mutations carried by humans. *Genetics* **2015**, *199*, 1243–1254. [CrossRef] [PubMed]
3. Henneman, L.; Borry, P.; Chokoshvili, D.; Cornel, M.C.; van El, C.G.; Forzano, F.; Hall, A.; Howard, H.C.; Janssens, S.; Kayserili, H.; et al. Responsible implementation of expanded carrier screening. *Eur. J. Hum. Genet.* **2017**, *25*, 1291. [CrossRef] [PubMed]
4. Overcoming Challenges in Reproductive Health Applications by Deploying More Sensitive and Accurate Molecular Technologies. *EMJ Repro Health* **2019**, *5* (Suppl. 1), 2–12.
5. Rubio, C.; Bellver, J.; Rodrigo, L.; Castillón, G.; Guillén, A.; Vidal, C.; Giles, J.; Ferrando, M.; Cabanillas, S.; Remohí, J.; et al. In vitro fertilization with preimplantation genetic diagnosis for aneuploidies in advanced maternal age: A randomized, controlled study. *Fertil. Steril.* **2017**, *107*, 1122–1129. [CrossRef] [PubMed]
6. Garcia-Herrero, S.; Cervero, A.; Mateu, E.; Mir, P.; Póo, M.E.; Rodrigo, L.; Vera, M.; Rubio, C. Genetic Analysis of Human Preimplantation Embryos. *Curr. Top. Dev. Biol.* **2016**, *120*, 421–447. [PubMed]
7. Vera-Rodriguez, M.; Rubio, C. Assessing the true incidence of mosaicism in preimplantation embryos. *Fertil. Steril.* **2017**, *107*, 1107–1112.
8. Hardarson, T.; Hanson, C.; Lundin, K.; Hillensjö, T.; Nilsson, L.; Stevic, J.; Reismer, E.; Borg, K.; Wikland, M.; Bergh, C. Preimplantation genetic screening in women of advanced maternal age caused a decrease in clinical pregnancy rate: A randomized controlled trial. *Hum. Reprod.* **2008**, *23*, 2806–2812. [CrossRef]
9. Staessen, C.; Verpoest, W.; Donoso, P.; Haentjens, P.; Van der Elst, J.; Liebaers, I.; Devroey, P. Preimplantation genetic screening does not improve delivery rate in women under the age of 36 following single-embryo transfer. *Hum. Reprod.* **2008**, *23*, 2818–2825. [CrossRef]
10. Northrop, L.E.; Treff, N.R.; Levy, B.; Scott, R.T. SNP microarray-based 24 chromosome aneuploidy screening demonstrates that cleavage-stage FISH poorly predicts aneuploidy in embryos that develop to morphologically normal blastocysts. *Mol. Hum. Reprod.* **2010**, *16*, 590–600.
11. Treff, N.R.; Levy, B.; Su, J.; Northrop, L.E.; Tao, X.; Scott, R.T. SNP microarray-based 24 chromosome aneuploidy screening is significantly more consistent than FISH. *Mol. Hum. Reprod.* **2010**, *16*, 583–589. [CrossRef]
12. Rubio, C.; Navarro-Sánchez, L.; García-Pascual, C.M.; Ocali, O.; Cimadomo, D.; Venier, W.; Barroso, G.; Kopcow, L.; Bahçeci, M.; Iuri Roos Kulmann, M.; et al. Multicenter prospective study of concordance between embryonic cell-free DNA and trophectoderm biopsies from 1301 human blastocysts. *Am. J. Obstet. Gynecol.* **2020**, *223*, 751.e1–751.e13. [CrossRef] [PubMed]
13. Ho, J.R.; Arrach, N.; Rhodes-Long, K.; Ahmady, A.; Ingles, S.; Chung, K.; Bendikson, K.A.; Paulson, R.J.; McGinnis, L.K. Pushing the limits of detection: Investigation of cell-free DNA for aneuploidy screening in embryos. *Fertil. Steril.* **2018**, *110*, 467–475.e2. [CrossRef] [PubMed]
14. Simón, C.; Gómez, C.; Cabanillas, S.; Vladimirov, I.; Castillón, G.; Giles, J.; Boynukalin, K.; Findikli, N.; Bahçeci, M.; Ortega, I.; et al. A 5-year multicentre randomized controlled trial comparing personalized, frozen and fresh blastocyst transfer in IVF. *Reprod. Biomed. Online* **2020**, *41*, 402–415. [CrossRef] [PubMed]
15. Garcia-Grau, I.; Perez-Villaroya, D.; Bau, D.; Gonzalez-Monfort, M.; Vilella, F.; Moreno, I.; Simón, C. Taxonomical and Functional Assessment of the Endometrial Microbiota in A Context of Recurrent Reproductive Failure: A Case Report. *Pathogens* **2019**, *8*, 205. [CrossRef]
16. Generalitat de Catalunya Departamento de Salud. Protocolo de diagnóstico prenatal de anomalías congénitas fetales. *Maternidad* **2009**, *24*, 1–43.
17. Nicolini, U.; Lalatta, F.; Natacci, F.; Curcio, C.; Bui, T.-H. The introduction of QF-PCR in prenatal diagnosis of fetal aneuploidies: Time for reconsideration. *Hum. Reprod. Update* **2004**, *10*, 541–548. [CrossRef]

18. Bayani, J.; Squire, J.A. Traditional banding of chromosomes for cytogenetic analysis. *Curr. Protoc. Cell. Biol.* **2004**, *23*, 22–23. [CrossRef]
19. Midtrimester amniocentesis for prenatal diagnosis. Safety and accuracy. *JAMA* **1976**, *236*, 1471–1476. [CrossRef]
20. Badeau, M.; Lindsay, C.; Blais, J.; Nshimyumukiza, L.; Takwoingi, Y.; Langlois, S.; Légaré, F.; Giguère, Y.; Turgeon, A.F.; Witteman, W.; et al. Genomics-based non-invasive prenatal testing for detection of fetal chromosomal aneuploidy in pregnant women. *Cochrane Database Syst. Rev.* **2017**, *11*, CD011767. [CrossRef]
21. Rosenfeld, J.A.; Patel, A. Chromosomal Microarrays: Understanding Genetics of Neurodevelopmental Disorders and Congenital Anomalies. *J. Pediatr. Genet.* **2017**, *6*, 42–50.
22. Stosic, M.; Levy, B.; Wapner, R. The Use of Chromosomal Microarray Analysis in Prenatal Diagnosis. *Obstet. Gynecol. Clin.* **2017**, *45*, 55–68. [CrossRef] [PubMed]
23. Miller, D.T.; Adam, M.P.; Aradhya, S.; Biesecker, L.G.; Brothman, A.R.; Carter, N.P.; Church, D.M.; Crolla, J.A.; Eichler, E.E.; Epstein, C.J.; et al. Consensus statement: Chromosomal microarray is a first-tier clinical diagnostic test for individuals with developmental disabilities or congenital anomalies. *Am. J. Hum. Genet.* **2010**, *86*, 749–764. [CrossRef] [PubMed]
24. Levy, B.; Wapner, R. Prenatal diagnosis by chromosomal microarray analysis. *Fertil. Steril.* **2018**, *109*, 201–212. [CrossRef] [PubMed]
25. Jacobs, P.A.; Hassold, T.J. 4 The origin of numerical chromosome abnormalities. In *Advances in Genetics*; Elsevier: Amsterdam, The Netherlands, 1995; Volume 33, pp. 101–133.
26. Hassold, T.; Chen, N.; Funkhouser, J.; Jooss, T.; Manuel, B.; Matsuura, J.; Matsuyama, A.; Wilson, C.; Yamane, J.A.; Jacobs, P.A. A cytogenetic study of 1000 spontaneous abortions. *Ann. Hum. Genet.* **1980**, *44*, 151–178. [CrossRef] [PubMed]
27. Simpson, J.L. Incidence and timing of pregnancy losses: Relevance to evaluating safety of early prenatal diagnosis. *Am. J. Med. Genet.* **1990**, *35*, 165–173. [CrossRef] [PubMed]
28. Boué, J.; Bou, A.; Lazar, P. Retrospective and prospective epidemiological studies of 1500 karyotyped spontaneous human abortions. *Teratology* **1975**, *12*, 11–26. [CrossRef]
29. Kajii, T.; Ferrier, A.; Niikawa, N.; Takahara, H.; Ohama, K.; Avirachan, S. Anatomic and chromosomal anomalies in 639 spontaneous abortuses. *Hum. Genet.* **1980**, *55*, 87–98. [CrossRef]
30. Dimmick, J.E.; Kalousek, D.K. Developmental pathology of the embryo and fetus. *Am. J. Clin. Pathol.* **1992**, *98*. [CrossRef]
31. Reddy, K.S. Double trisomy in spontaneous abortions. *Hum. Genet.* **1997**, *101*, 339–345. [CrossRef]
32. Nagaishi, M.; Yamamoto, T.; Iinuma, K.; Shimomura, K.; Berend, S.A.; Knops, J. Chromosome abnormalities identified in 347 spontaneous abortions collected in Japan. *J. Obstet. Gynaecol. Res.* **2004**, *30*, 237–241. [CrossRef]
33. Yusuf, R.Z.; Naeem, R. Cytogenetic Abnormalities in Products of Conception: A Relationship Revisited. *Am. J. Reprod. Immunol.* **2004**, *52*, 88–96. [CrossRef] [PubMed]
34. Morales, C.; Sánchez, A.; Bruguera, J.; Margarit, E.; Borrell, A.; Borobio, V.; Soler, A. Cytogenetic study of spontaneous abortions using semi-direct analysis of chorionic villi samples detects the broadest spectrum of chromosome abnormalities. *Am. J. Med. Genet. Part A* **2008**, *146A*, 66–70. [CrossRef] [PubMed]
35. Robberecht, C.; Pexsters, A.; Deprest, J.; Fryns, J.P.; D'Hooghe, T.; Vermeesch, J.R. Cytogenetic and morphological analysis of early products of conception following hystero-embryoscopy from couples with recurrent pregnancy loss. *Prenat. Diagn.* **2012**, *32*, 933–942. [CrossRef] [PubMed]
36. Xu, J.; Chen, M.; Liu, Q.Y.; Hu, S.Q.; Li, L.R.; Li, J.; Ma, R.M. Detecting trisomy in products of conception from first-trimester spontaneous miscarriages by next-generation sequencing (NGS). *Medicine* **2020**, *99*, e18731. [CrossRef]
37. Campos-Galindo, I.; García-Herrero, S.; Martínez-Conejero, J.A.; Ferro, J.; Simón, C.; Rubio, C. Molecular analysis of products of conception obtained by hysteroembryoscopy from infertile couples. *J. Assist. Reprod. Genet.* **2015**, *32*, 839–848. [CrossRef]
38. Kingsmore, S. Comprehensive carrier screening and molecular diagnostic testing for recessive childhood diseases. *PLoS Curr.* **2012**, *4*, e4f9877ab8ffa9. [CrossRef]
39. Ceyhan-Birsoy, O.; Machini, K.; Lebo, M.S.; Yu, T.W.; Agrawal, P.B.; Parad, R.B.; Holm, I.A.; McGuire, A.; Green, R.C.; Beggs, A.H.; et al. A curated gene list for reporting results of newborn genomic sequencing. *Genet. Med.* **2017**, *19*, 809–818.

40. Godino, L.; Turchetti, D.; Jackson, L.; Hennessy, C.; Skirton, H. Impact of presymptomatic genetic testing on young adults: A systematic review. *Eur. J. Hum. Genet.* **2016**, *24*, 496–503. [CrossRef]
41. Van Campen, J.C.; Sollars, E.S.A.; Thomas, R.C.; Bartlett, C.M.; Milano, A.; Parker, M.D.; Dawe, J.; Winship, P.R.; Peck, G.; Grafham, D.; et al. Next Generation Sequencing in Newborn Screening in the United Kingdom National Health Service. *Int. J. Neonatal Screen.* **2019**, *5*, 40. [CrossRef]
42. Beckmann, J.S.; Lew, D. Reconciling evidence-based medicine and precision medicine in the era of big data: Challenges and opportunities. *Genome Med.* **2016**, *8*, 134. [CrossRef]
43. Mackley, M.P.; Fletcher, B.; Parker, M.; Watkins, H.; Ormondroyd, E. Stakeholder views on secondary findings in whole-genome and whole-exome sequencing: A systematic review of quantitative and qualitative studies. *Genet. Med.* **2017**, *19*, 283–293. [CrossRef] [PubMed]
44. Fernandez-Marmiesse, A.; Gouveia, S.; Couce, M.L. NGS Technologies as a Turning Point in Rare Disease Research, Diagnosis and Treatment. *Curr. Med. Chem.* **2018**, *25*, 404–432. [CrossRef] [PubMed]

Publisher's Note: MDPI stays neutral with regard to jurisdictional claims in published maps and institutional affiliations.

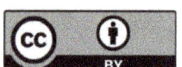

© 2020 by the authors. Licensee MDPI, Basel, Switzerland. This article is an open access article distributed under the terms and conditions of the Creative Commons Attribution (CC BY) license (http://creativecommons.org/licenses/by/4.0/).

MDPI
St. Alban-Anlage 66
4052 Basel
Switzerland
Tel. +41 61 683 77 34
Fax +41 61 302 89 18
www.mdpi.com

Genes Editorial Office
E-mail: genes@mdpi.com
www.mdpi.com/journal/genes